3/11

# VIRAL TAKEOVER

# 3/11 VIRAL TAKEOVER

**On March 11, 2020, a Pandemic was Declared and Our World Changed Forever**

SONIA ELIJAH

ELIJAH
LIGHT PRESS

*3/11 Viral Takeover*
*On March 11, 2020, a Pandemic was Declared*
*and Our World Changed Forever*



This book is a work of investigative journalism based on publicly available records, Freedom of Information responses, leaked documents, scientific and academic literature, and interviews. All statements, opinions, interpretations, conclusions, and allegations are those of the author, attributed sources, or matters of public interest and legitimate debate. Where facts remain disputed or unproven in a court of law, no assertion is made of proven misconduct, criminal activity, or established fact.

The author and publisher have made every effort to ensure the accuracy of the information presented as of the date of publication. However, they assume no responsibility for errors, omissions, or any consequences arising from the use of this book.

This book is for informational purposes only and does not constitute legal, medical, or financial advice. Readers are encouraged to conduct their own independent research and seek professional advice where appropriate. The author and publisher disclaim any liability for actions taken based on the contents of this book.

Published by Elijah Light Press

First edition

ISBN (paperback): 978-1-9195265-1-5
ISBN (hardcover): 978-1-9195265-2-2
ISBN (eBook): 978-1-9195265-0-8

For permissions requests, bulk orders, or inquiries, contact:

Elijah Light Press

soniaelijah@protonmail.com

www.soniaelijah.com

*"My people are destroyed for lack of knowledge."*

HOSEA 4:6 (King James Version)

*This book is dedicated*

*to all who have perished from*

*Covid countermeasures.*

# CONTENTS

# FOREWORD

The Covid period was a turning point in our lives. We saw how the system that rules us truly operates and that of which it is capable. We experienced the apotheosis of the corporatist planning state, as close to dystopian-level totalitarianism as we ever knew. We observed how the media, tech, elected and unelected government, and the medical industry all work together when the stakes are high. And we observed and experienced just how completely controlling this cartel can be once it is unleashed on the entire population.

All the sloganeering – buy some time, slow the spread, flatten the curve, we are all in this together, socially distance, be careful, mask up, get the jab, ban disinformation and malinformation, it's a pandemic of the unvaccinated, and a thousand other cliches – turned over time into a tissue of lies. They all point to the same nefarious scheme, to weaponize public trust in a way that results in the consumption of a mislabeled product based on a gene-invading technology that had never before been deployed.

Even now, typing those words and trying to mentally grasp all that we went through still shocks me, even if I have written probably thousands of articles and two books on the topic. In so many ways, the Covid period feels like a war complete with the legendary fog and long period of recovery. The response to the pathogen left large parts of the world in shambles: illiteracy, substance abuse, tech addiction, health crisis, broken supply chains, bankrupted businesses, discredited medical elites, indebted governments running the presses full time, flat wages despite stimulus payments once corrected for the inevitable inflation, and the building of a surveillance state that began with disease tracking and mutated into the ambition of a digital system of vaccine passports.

In each nation, there were malfactors. But what's more remarkable is how similar the policies were in nearly every country on earth, thanks to the World Health Organization's messaging. I have attended post-apocalyptic briefings in several counties and I'm struck by how nearly every country adopted the same cockamamie protocols, from sanitizer dousing to forced masking to business closures to vaccine mandates. The outlying nations can be named on one hand and include unpredictables such as Tanzania, Nicaragua, and Sweden.

The topic absolutely requires a book-length treatment. Even then, there is no way to cover the entire calamity. What's more, such a book bears a huge burden of documentation in several areas of policy, science, and history. This is because the deck still remains stacked against anyone who would dare question that not all that transpired was the best they could do with the information they had. How many times have we heard that? How many commissions have concluded with this same claim and even promise to do more earlier the next time? Even as of this writing, there have been precious few admissions of wrong doing much less apologies. The medical journals and major media have just moved on as if none of this matters.

Which brings us to this masterful treatise by science journalist Sonia Elijah. She has been, from the very beginning, an essential source of reporting and truth telling on the Covid calamity, writing from the point of view of a British journalist who followed every detail, day by day and hour by hour. She is the master of her topic. The book is five years in the writing and includes a level of documentation that will amaze you. This piety toward facts is backed by a fiery passion that is entirely appropriate to her subject.

The result is a book for the ages, one that will end the whitewashing that is taking place right now. Indeed, the appearance of *3/11: Viral Takeover* becomes on its publication date the most exhaustive and authoritative account of the UK experience to appear in print. It will likely be years before it is surpassed if it ever will be.

Every lover of freedom and civilization owes Elijah a deep debt of gratitude from the scrupulous attention to detail she has provided and the personal discipline it took to complete this book. Her book makes it impossible for the history books to reflect the official view that is being preached daily in the papers and journals. The reality is gritty and often terrifying but the truth needs to be told.

Congratulations to all readers and all those who recommend this work to others for your discernment in choosing literature, and to all those who will be inspired by this research to right the wrong and seek reforms that make it impossible to repeat this experience.

**Jeffrey Tucker**
Brownstone Institute
*February 2026*

# PREFACE

One late afternoon in early 2020, I vividly remember walking through a supermarket where every human face was masked, and every shopper shuffled obediently along one-way arrows taped to the floor. A small child froze mid-step, terrified he had broken the rules; already learning to fear his own footsteps.

In that moment, it became crystal clear to me: it was never about a virus. It was about control. Overcome by a deep yearning to dig out the truth, for the next several years, I sought to do just that.

This book is a forensic investigation of a "once-in-a-century pandemic" and of what was done in its name.

# INTRODUCTION

It is still hard to comprehend. A respiratory virus with an infection fatality rate (IFR) of roughly 0.1% for those under 70 (comparable to a severe flu season) was used to justify one of the greatest peacetime curtailments of civil liberties in history. The images from Wuhan, China, did the convincing: a city of eleven million sealed overnight, citizens welded into apartments, and viral videos of bodies collapsing in the street. Fear became the true contagion, spreading faster than any pathogen.

On 11 March 2020, which I mark as 3/11, the World Health Organization (WHO) declared COVID-19 a global pandemic. That single announcement marked the dawn of a new era. What began that day appeared to be more than a health response; it resembled a global reset executed with a speed and coordination no previous crisis had ever achieved.

History shows us that societal resets are precipitated by crises or disruptive events. 9/11 and the 2001 anthrax attacks birthed the PATRIOT Act, amplifying U.S. surveillance and igniting the global war on terror, complete with invasions of Afghanistan and Iraq. Similarly, post-3/11, we have seen an extraordinary surge in state biosecurity measures, enacted through laws like the UK's Coronavirus Act 2020 and its global counterparts. These granted governments sweeping new powers under the guise of public health to confine the healthy, close borders, suspend parliaments, and coerce medical interventions, often enforced through digital vaccine certificates. While 9/11 led to state surveillance of citizens, 3/11 led to citizen compliance with the state.

These policies did not merely "combat COVID-19," they laid groundwork for permanent biosecurity governance. This can be epitomized by the World Health Organization's proposed "Pandemic Treaty," International Health Regulations amendments, and its Global Digital Health Certification Network, aimed at bolstering readiness and response to pandemics.

In his book, *The Symbolic Life*, the Swiss psychiatrist Carl Jung notably wrote: "Indeed, it is becoming ever more obvious that it is not famine, not earthquakes, not microbes, not cancer, but man himself who is man's greatest danger to man, for the simple reason that there is no adequate protection against psychic epidemics, which are infinitely more devastating than the worst of natural catastrophes."

The fallout from 3/11 proved Jung right. Western democracies abandoned their own pre-2020 pandemic plans and imported authoritarian containment concepts pioneered by the Chinese Communist Party.

Hundreds of millions were spent on behavioral-science units and messaging campaigns that, in my view, weaponized fear. Dissent was often rebranded as public health endangerment and, in some cases, equated to terrorism. Behind the scenes, decisions were shaped by unelected committees and lavishly funded non-governmental organizations (NGOs): the WHO, World Economic Forum, Gates Foundation, Wellcome Trust, and their satellites.

Several years on, the dust may have settled, yet the architecture remains: the laws and the censorship machinery now entrenched in frameworks like the UK's Online Safety Act and the European Union's Digital Services Act, alongside the continued attempt to expand digital ID systems.

This book is based on evidence that powerful interests fought fiercely to suppress: thousands of pages of documents obtained through Freedom of Information Act (FOIA) requests, leaked internal records and emails. Drawing on exclusive interviews with leading experts and courageous whistleblowers, it is grounded in rigorous, in-depth research.

3/11: Viral Takeover is not a post-mortem. It is a live indictment of a turning point that is still unfolding.

# APPENDIX A

The following timeline consists exclusively of documented facts, statements, decisions, and actions recorded in government filings, scientific papers, FOIA releases, and contemporaneous news reports. It has been compiled to offer essential context for the reader.

**2019**

---

**January-August** U.S. Department of Health and Human Services (HHS) runs a pandemic simulation event code-named "Crimson Contagion[1]." A series of joint exercises involving a scenario in which a group of tourists returning from China spread a novel influenza virus in the United States.
**June 26** U.S. Government Accountability Office (GAO) issues report[2]: "The Nation Faces Long-Standing Challenges Related to Defending Against Biological Threats"
**July 11** Two people die and 18 others are hospitalized after a "respiratory outbreak[3]" at a Virginia retirement community in the United States.
**July 11** Biodefence Commission holds a panel discussion entitled "A Manhattan Project for Biodefense: Taking Biological Threats Off the Table[4]" to assess and recommend improvements to U.S. biodefense policies against biological threats (natural, accidental, or intentional).
**August 5** New York Times reports[5] on a germ lab creating vaccines for deadly microbes at the United States Army Medical Research Institute of Infectious Diseases, (USAMRIID), in Fort Detrick, Maryland, being shut down after failing CDC inspections.
**September 12** The Wuhan Institute of Virology's (WIV) essential database, Batvirus.whiov.ac.cn[6], goes offline. It is the most important bat coronavirus database in China, holding the samples and sequences from the WIV.
**October 18** Bill and Melinda Gates Foundation and The John Hopkins Center for Health Security in partnership with the World Economic Forum conduct Event 201[7]. A training tabletop exercise "aimed to educate senior leaders at the highest level of U.S. and international governments and leaders in global industries" practice the steps that would be taken during a fictional coronavirus pandemic.
**October 18-27** The City of Wuhan hosts the Military World Games[8]. Numerous foreign athletes later report severe COVID-like illness after returning home.

**October 25** USAID-run PREDICT program is quietly shut down [9]by the U.S. government.
**November 17** *South China Morning Post* [10]cites government data suggesting "patient zero" could be traced back to this date.
**November (exact date unknown)** According to U.S. intelligence report, three researchers at Wuhan Institute of Virology (WIV) seek hospital care for illness. This information was not made public until May 23, 2021[11].
**Late November** According to an April 9, 2020 *ABC News* [12]investigation, the National Center for Medical Intelligence (NCMI) warned the military and White House about a contagion in Wuhan posing a serious threat (potentially cataclysmic) to the population and U.S. forces in Asia, as early as late November 2019.
**December 12** Cluster of cases[13] in China's Hubei Province, in the city of Wuhan begin to experience symptoms of an atypical pneumonia-like illness that does not respond well to standard treatments.
**December 16** U.S. Congress moves forward with a spending package providing increases for several key U.S. biological defense programs, including an increase of $95 million[14] for the Strategic National Stockpile (SNS).
**December 30** Urgent notice[15] goes online from Wuhan municipal health commission describing a cluster of pneumonia cases of unknown origins: states first patient came from Hunan Seafood Market in Wuhan.
**December 31** First official report[16] of a cluster of cases of a respiratory virus of an unknown cause with symptoms including shortness of breath and fever, occurring in Wuhan, China, is reported to WHO.

**2020**

---

**January 1** Huanan Seafood Market in Wuhan is shut down[17] by order of the Chinese authorities with no (reported) effort to sample the most suspect forms of wildlife.
**January 2** Central Hospital of Wuhan bans its staff [18]from discussing the disease publicly.
**January 3** Wuhan doctor Li Wenliang is arrested[19] for "making false comments on the internet." after attempting to warn others about the new SARS-like virus.
**January 7** WHO officials announce[20] they have identified a new virus named SARS-CoV-2- belongs to the coronavirus family which includes SARS, MERS and the common cold.
**January 8** CDC issues an official health advisory[21] on its website.

**January 10** GISAID reports[22] it received SARS-CoV-2 genome sequence from the Chinese CDC on that date.
**January 10** Virologist Edward Holmes submits the viral genome sequence of SARS-CoV-2 on virological.org[23] on behalf of a Chinese-led consortium headed by Professor Yong-Zhen Zhang (Fudan University, Shanghai).
**January 11** China announces the first death[24] linked to the novel coronavirus.
**January 13** National Institute of Health's Vaccine Research Center (VRC) and Moderna decide on mRNA-1273 vaccine sequence[25].
**January 13** Prof Christian Drosten's RT (Reverse Transcription)-PCR test protocol to detect SARS-CoV-2 is accepted[26] by the WHO.
**January 14** Moderna initiates [27]current Good Manufacturing Practice (cGMP) production of mRNA-1273, its investigational mRNA vaccine candidate against SARS-CoV-2.
**January 14** Reporters from Hong Kong taken to a police station[28] after trying to film the situation within Wuhan hospital.
**January 16** COVID-19, first classified as a High Consequence Infectious Disease[29] (HCID) in the UK.
**January 20-24** World Economic Forum's annual meeting in Davos, Switzerland takes place.
**January 20** Chinese authorities first acknowledge human-to-human transmission[30] of SARS-CoV-2.
**January 23** Coronavirus specialist, Shi Zheng-Li and her team from Wuhan Institute of Virology (WIV) release a report on the preprint server[31] bioRxiv that the novel virus is 96.2% similar to bat virus (RaTG13).
**January 23** City of Wuhan goes into lockdown.[32]
**January 29** The Coronavirus Task Force[33] is publicly announced by the White House and charged with leading the U.S. Government response.
**January 30** The International Health Regulations Emergency Committee of the WHO declares the outbreak a global health emergency[34].
**January 31** President Donald J. Trump declares COVID-19 a public health emergency[35] in the U.S.
**January 31** A book entitled "Analysis of Wuhan Coronavirus: Déjà vu[36]" is published as a free download. It discusses the existence and implications of the Furin Cleavage Site found on the viral spike protein.
**January 31** The scientific paper, "Uncanny similarity of unique inserts in the 2019-nCoV spike protein to HIV-1 gp120 and Gag" by Pradhan et al.,[37]is uploaded to the pre-print server bioRxiv. Two days later, it is withdrawn[38] after heavy criticism.

**January 31** Anthony Fauci, director of NIAID (National Institute of Allergies and Infectious Diseases) and Jeremy Farrar (director of the Wellcome Trust at the time) discuss need[39] for an emergency teleconference with leading scientists and public officials to be held on Saturday February 1.
**Late January**- BioNTech initiates[40] BNT162 vaccine program to prevent COVID-19.
**February 1** Emergency teleconference[41] is held between leading scientists and public officials including: Sir Jeremy Farrar, Anthony Fauci, Robert (Bob) Garry, Andrew Rambaut, Mike Ferguson, Eddie Holmes, Sir Patrick Vallance, Christian Drosten and Kristian Andersen.
**February 2** The WHO publishes a report[42] that the 2019-nCoV outbreak and response has been accompanied by a "massive infodemic" and that their "technical risk communication and social media teams have been working closely to track and respond to myths and rumors."
**February 2** Moderna validates in-vitro expression of mRNA-1273[43].
**February 3** Second teleconference call with Gain of Function scientists, Trevor Bedford, Anthony Fauci, Tom Inglesby, Gigi Gronvall at the request [44]of Kelvin Droegemeier, Science Advisor for Trump and the director of the White House Office of Science & Technology Policy. The purpose of the event was to "combat misinformation" surrounding the origin of the virus.
**February 4** U.S. Health and Human Services (HHS) Secretary Alex Azar invokes the PREP Act[45], shielding all manufacturers, distributors, administrators, and prescribers of future COVID-19 medical countermeasures from virtually all liability. This is 35 days before the World Health Organization declares COVID-19 a pandemic.
**February 4** Vaccine Research Center vaccinates mice. Moderna ships pre-clinical drug product.[46]
**February 7** Wuhan doctor, Dr. Li Wenliang, who tried to ring early alarms about the cluster of infections, dies[47] after contracting the virus.
**February 11** WHO officially names novel coronavirus SARS-CoV-2 and the disease it causes COVID-19, which stands for Coronavirus Disease 2019.
**February 11-12** WHO R&D Blueprint's holds a global research and innovation forum in Geneva, Switzerland, co-chaired by Jeremy Farrar.
**February 15** Study in *The Lancet* [48]suggests the first case of a man infected with 2019 novel coronavirus appeared on Dec 1, 2019, with no links to Huanan market.
**February 16** Kristian Andersen, Andrew Rambaut, Robert Garry, Eric

Holmes and W. Ian Lipkin upload[49] their first version of the "Proximal Origin of SARS-CoV-2"paper on virological.org.
**February 19** Jeremy Farrar, Christian Drosten, Peter Daszak and 24 other scientists co-author "Statement in support of the scientists, public health professionals, and medical professionals of China combatting COVID-19" published in *The Lancet*,[50] which declared "We stand together to strongly condemn conspiracy theories suggesting that COVID-19 does not have a natural origin."
**February 22** First elderly man in Northern Italy[51] is said to have died after being infected with coronavirus.
**February 24** Moderna ships the first batch[52] of mRNA-1973 to NIAID (part of National Institutes of Health, NIH), 42 days from sequence selection for use in their Phase 1 clinical study.
**February 25** The NIH begin their first clinical trial[53] in the U.S. for potential COVID-19 treatment, Remdesivir, an anti-viral drug originally developed to treat Ebola.
**February 28** Bill Gates writes an article for the *New England Journal of Medicine*[54] arguing for an immediate and comprehensive response to the threat posed by COVID-19.
**March 4** Lockdown extended to all of Lombardy, Italy.
**March 9** Lockdown extended to all of Italy.[55]
**March 10** Then-secretary of U.S. Health and Human Services (HHS), Alex M. Azar II, invokes [56]PREP Act immunity for the "manufacture, testing, development, distribution, administration, and use" of covered countermeasures against COVID-19.
**March 11** WHO declares COVID-19 a global pandemic.[57]
**March 11** The CDC COVID-19 risk assessment states:[58] "For the majority of people, the immediate risk of being exposed to the virus that causes COVID-19 is thought to be low."
**March 12** China official Zhao Lijian tweets[59] that the U.S. army may have brought the epidemic to Wuhan.
**March 12** UK Prime Minister, Boris Johnson, warns the British public:[60] "Many more families will lose loved ones before their time."
**March 15** UK's "Stay home, protect the NHS, save lives" campaign[61] is launched. States within the U.S. begin to implement shutdowns. The New York City public school system with 1.1 million students shuts down.[62]
**March 16** Phase 1[63] Moderna's clinical trial starts. A total of 63 days from sequence selection to first human dosing.

**March 16** BioNTech SE[64] provides further details on the company's R&D effort, "Project Lightspeed" to develop a potential vaccine. On the same day it announces a strategic alliance with Fosun Pharma to develop a COVID-19 vaccine in China.
**March 16** Prof Neil Ferguson of Imperial College COVID-19 response UK team predicts "approximately 510,000 deaths in GB and 2.2 million in the U.S." by May-June 2020 in an unmitigated pandemic in "Report 9."[65]
**March 17** "The Proximal Origin of SARS-CoV-2" by Kristian Andersen et al. is published in *Nature Medicine*[66] where the unnatural origin of the Furin Cleavage Site is rejected. W. Ian Lipkin is one of the cited authors along with Andrew Rambaut, Edward Holmes and Robert Garry.
**March 17** Pfizer signs a letter of intent[67] with BioNTech to co-develop a potential COVID-19 vaccine.
**March 19** UK's Health Security Agency issues statement:[68] "COVID-19 is no longer considered to be a High Consequence Infectious Disease (HCID) in the UK."
**March 19** Operation Rescript is formally activated[69] (the UK's military-led domestic response to the COVID-19 pandemic under the Military Aid to Civil Authorities (MACA) framework.
**March 23** England goes into its first ever lockdown.[70] Similar measures are implemented in Scotland, Wales and Northern Ireland.
**March 24** UK Ministry of Defense (MoD) formally authorizes the deployment[71] of the 77th Brigade (77X), a specialist British Army unit focused on information operations (Info Ops), media operations, and strategic communications to support Operation Rescript.
**March 27** Trusted News Initiative (TNI), a global network of news organizations, tech platforms, and fact-checkers expand[72] its operations to combat COVID-19 misinformation.
**Around April** Theories that the virus came from a laboratory[73] gain popularity. U.S. President Trump confident[74] coronavirus originated in a Chinese virology lab.
**April 29** First news reports of the U.S. government's Operation Warp Speed[75], jointly led by the Department of Defense (DoD) and the Department of Health and Human Services (HHS).
**April 30** Bill Gates[76] states: "I suspect the COVID-19 vaccine will become part of the routine newborn immunization schedule."
**May 1** WHO reiterates virus believed to be "natural in origin."[77]

**July 10** WHO specialists[78] visit China to lay groundwork for an international investigation.
**July 22** U.S. States Department Of Defense (DoD) awards[79] Other Transaction Agreement (OTA) to Pfizer to scale up manufacture of their BNT162b2 vaccine candidate. (An initial order of 100 million doses for $1.95 billion)
**October 31** UK's PM Boris Johnson announces a second lockdown in England.
**November 18** Pfizer reports 95% effectiveness[80] of their mRNA COVID-19 vaccine based on the analysis of a dataset that included 170 PCR test confirmed COVID-19 cases among the Phase 3 volunteers (162 in the placebo group and eight in the vaccinated group).
**December 2** UK's Medicines and Healthcare products Regulatory Agency (MHRA) grants[81] Emergency Use Authorization of Pfizer-BioNTech COVID-19 vaccine.
**December 10** *New England Journal of Medicine*[82] publishes pivotal study "Safety and Efficacy of the BNT162b2 mRNA COVID-19 Vaccine" by Polack et al.
**December 11** U.S. Food and Drug Administration (FDA) grants[83] Emergency Use Authorization (EUA) of Pfizer-BioNTech's COVID-19 vaccine (BNT162b2), later branded as Comirnaty, for individuals aged 16 and over.
**December 16** WHO announces an international team of experts[84] will travel to China to help investigate origins of the virus.
**December 18** Moderna's Spikevax (mRNA-1273) is granted Emergency Use Authorization[85] (EUA) by the U.S. Food and Drug Administration (FDA) for individuals aged 18 and over.
**December 21** European Medicines Agency (EMA) grants Conditional Marketing Authorization[86] (CMA) of Pfizer-BioNTech COVID-19 vaccine.

**2021**

---

**January 6** WHO experts arrive at China border and denied entry[87] visas
**January 6** England and the rest of the UK enter third national lockdown[88] which lasts until 19 July
**January 6** Moderna's COVID-19 vaccine (Spikevax) is granted Conditional Marketing Authorization[89] (CMA) by the European Medicines Agency (EMA) allowing the vaccine to be distributed and used across European Union member states for individuals 18 years and older.
**January 14** WHO experts allowed[90] into China

**February 9** WHO-led press conference[91] states, "it is extremely unlikely that this virus was a laboratory construct." WHO investigation ends with no new insights into the origins of the virus.

**May 14** 18 prominent biologists write an open letter in the journal *Science*[92] calling for a new investigation of all possible origins of the virus.

**July 5** Follow-up to February 2020, Lancet letter: "Science, not speculation, is essential to determine how SARS-CoV-2 reached humans" is published in *The Lancet*.[93]

**August 21** FDA posts infamous "You're not a horse, y'all"[94] tweet in relation to ivermectin

**August 23** Pfizer/BioNTech Covid vaccine under the brand name "COMIRNATY" gets full FDA approval.[95]

**August 26** Pentagon announces Covid vaccine mandate[96] for military.

**August 31** Drs. Marion Gruber and Philip Krause are forced out[97] of the FDA.

**September 1-2** CDC changes definition of a vaccine from "producing immunity"[98] to "producing protection."[99]

**September 9** Biden administration announces Covid vaccine mandates[100] for all federal employees.

**September 16** "The origins of SARS-CoV-2: A critical review" is published in *Cell*[101] by Farrar et al. The authors conclude: "There is currently no evidence that SARS-CoV-2 has a laboratory origin."

**September 20** DRASTIC group releases EcoHealth Alliance's DoD grant proposal (DEFUSE)[102] to introduce furin cleavage sites.

CHAPTER ONE

# LOCKING IN THE NARRATIVE

*"Using biological weapons under the cover of an endemic or natural disease occurrence provides an attacker the potential for plausible denial. Biological warfare's potential to create significant economic loss and subsequent political instability, coupled with plausible denial, exceeds the possibilities of any other human weapon."*

~Lt Col Robert P. Kadlec, MD, USAF, in the book *Battlefield of the Future: 21st Century Warfare Issues*,[103] 1998

The origin of SARS-CoV-2, a virus that precipitated the most disruptive health event in a century, remains shrouded in contention. From day one, governments, the World Health Organization, elite journals, and influential scientists emphasized a zoonotic hypothesis: a bat virus jumping the species barrier at Wuhan's Huanan wet market, a classic case of nature's mishap. However, examination of available evidence reveals a more complex picture involving laboratory research, gain-of-function experiments, and conflicts of interest that were not initially disclosed. Key to establishing this narrative were three major papers, penned by influential scientists and published in elite journals, that locked in the natural-origin view while alternative ideas were dismissed as conspiracy theories.

## The Three "Pillar" Publications

To cement the narrative that SARS-CoV-2 arose through natural evolution rather than laboratory intervention, three pivotal publications (authored by influential scientists and disseminated in prestigious academic journals), appeared to contribute to a concerted effort toward this end: *The Lancet's* "Statement in Support of the Scientists, Public Health Professionals, and Medical Professionals of China Combatting COVID-19"; *Nature Medicine's* "Proximal Origin of SARS-CoV-2"; and *Cell's* "The Origins of SARS-CoV-2: A Critical Review."

Firstly, in the joint statement dated February 19, 2020, authored by 27 prominent scientists from nine countries, which included notable figures such as Sir Jeremy Farrar (Former Director of Wellcome Trust, 2013-2023), Christian Drosten (whose team pioneered the diagnostic PCR test for COVID-19 in 2020 and for SARS in 2003), Peter Daszak (President of EcoHealth Alliance Inc.), and Mike Turner (Acting Director of Wellcome Trust's Science Division), and published in *The Lancet*,[104] the authors unequivocally expressed their unified stance in praising China and denouncing lab origin conspiracy theories. They stated, "We are public health scientists who have closely followed the emergence of 2019 novel coronavirus disease (COVID-19) and are deeply concerned about its impact on global health and wellbeing. We have watched as the scientists, public health professionals, and medical professionals of China, in particular, have worked diligently and effectively to rapidly identify the pathogen behind this outbreak, put in place significant measures to reduce its impact, and share their results transparently with the global health community. This effort has been remarkable... We stand together to strongly condemn conspiracy theories suggesting that COVID-19 does not have a natural origin." The statement concluded with a declaration of no competing interests, followed by a Chinese translation of the full text.

However, an investigation[105] revealed that 26 out of the 27 scientists who signed the joint statement/letter were either linked to Chinese researchers from the Wuhan Institute of Virology (WIV) or its funders. These findings are relevant since the debate over the origin of the virus has coalesced around two theories: the zoonotic hypothesis, where the virus evolved in nature (spilling over from animal to human) and the lab-leak theory, where the virus was genetically engineered and escaped a virological lab (either by intent or accident). Central to the lab-leak theory is the WIV, which houses China's only biosafety level-four super lab and other lower-level labs, where scientists have reportedly engaged in Gain of Function research (research that improves the ability of a pathogen to cause disease) on bat coronaviruses, located in the same city to first report on the "pneumonia of unknown cause." Therefore, the fact that the cosignatories of the letter/joint statement declared no competing interests has been criticized as potentially misleading, given that all but one had ties to the WIV.

In addition, the "Addendum: competing interests and the origins of SARS-CoV-2"[106] was later added to the letter in June 2021, well over a year after it was published in *The Lancet*, due to "some readers" questioning the "validity of this [non-competing interests] disclosure, particularly as it relates to one of the authors, Peter Daszak." The addendum revealed Daszak's recombinant virus work in China and his ties to the WIV, through his private charity, EcoHealth Alliance, the "global non-profit leading scientific research into the critical connections between human, animal and environmental health."

EcoHealth, has been a U.S. partner of the Wuhan Institute of Virology, which has funded the collaborative gain of function research, thanks to the generous grants it has received from the National Institutes of Health (NIH). From 2014 onwards, EcoHealth Alliance Inc. has received in total $60 million from the U.S. Department of Health and Human Services (HHS) with $4.3 million of U.S. taxpayers' money awarded to the NIH project "Understanding the Risk of Bat Coronavirus Emergence." The grant was suspended[107] in April 2020, by former President Donald Trump's administration cutting off money funneled to the WIV. However, it was later restored under the Biden administration, where the NIH went on to award EcoHealth with $650,000[108] in grant money to study bat coronaviruses and "assess their ability to infect humans" in October 2022 with a further grant worth $576,290,[109] awarded the following year.

In June 2023, three previously unreleased State Department cables, obtained by the U.S. Right to Know,[110] revealed that Wuhan Institute of Virology conducted classified research on behalf of the Chinese military since at least 2017. Over $2 million[111] in U.S. taxpayers' money reportedly went into funding what have been characterized as secret "(PLA) People's Liberation Army shadow labs[112] at WIV."

The third cable[113] revealed how Beijing authorities, rather than local officials, censored the critical early days of the pandemic. Explosive statements read: "Beijing knew earlier than they admit" and "Xi [Jinping] lied to obfuscate his role in the cover up." On the heels of these revelations the WIV was suspended[114] and later banned[115] from receiving U.S. grant money by the Biden administration. "It's past time that the Biden administration made this decision, but they deserve no credit for finally doing what the evidence and facts demanded. It is outrageous that it took them so long," Reps. Cathy McMorris Rodgers (R-Wash.), Brett Guthrie (R-Ky.), and Morgan Griffith (R-Va.) said in a joint statement.

Turning back to the overdue addendum to the open letter published in *The Lancet* on June 21, 2021, which highlighted the various competing interests of Peter Daszak, resulting in the British-born scientist having to recuse[116] himself the very next day from the UN-backed commission, led by the prominent scientific journal, to examine the origins of Covid, since it sparked a major outcry.

Nonetheless, Daszak's conflict of interests did not seem to bother the World Health Organization, who had invited Daszak to be part of their joint investigation with China, along with another controversial scientist, Marion Koopmans[117], a prominent Dutch virologist with strong ties to gain-of-function research through her institutional affiliations and collaborations.

The team visited Wuhan earlier that year with their report[118] concluding that the lab leak theory was "extremely unlikely." Their findings have been questioned by critics, given that China announced an additional $30 million in funding for the WHO in April 2020 to supplement the $20 million already donated a month earlier. Along with the third State Department cable revealing how Beijing authorities, rather than local officials, censored the critical early days of the pandemic. These circumstances raised serious questions about the independence and credibility of the WHO's joint investigation with China.

In addition, an email from Daszak revealed his involvement in organizing the conspiracy-theory-condemning joint statement, raising questions among critics about potential bias in favor of China. The February 8, 2020, email,[119] released under Freedom of Information Act, disclosed how Daszak wrote the letter (joint statement) after being asked by "our collaborators" in China for a "show of support". It is interesting how that "show of support" took the form of rushing to condemn the lab-leak theory, which he had a vested interest in suppressing because of his inconvenient ties to the WIV and gain of function research.

The cosignatories' categorical rejection of a non-natural origin for the virus mirrored the conclusions of "The Proximal Origin of SARS-CoV-2"[120] one of the most influential scientific papers in history. Authored by Kristian Andersen, Andrew Rambaut, W. Ian Lipkin, Edward Holmes, and Robert Garry, this seminal paper was published in *Nature Medicine* on March 17, 2020, a month after the statement's release. An earlier version of the Proximal Origin paper was uploaded to Virological.org on February 16 and was cited in the joint statement of scientists published in The Lancet three days later.

The authors concluded: "We do not believe that any type of laboratory-based scenario is plausible." Lead author, Kristian Andersen, an evolutionary biologist and associate professor of immunology and microbiology at Scripps Research, said in a press release:[121] "We can firmly determine that SARS-CoV-2 originated through natural processes."

On the same day, the Proximal Origin paper was published, João Monteiro, *Nature Medicine's* editor-in-chief, posted the following on social media.

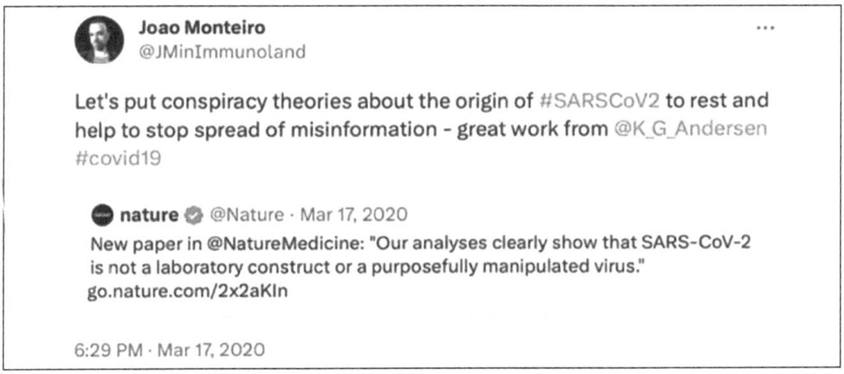
Joao Monteiro
@JMinImmunoland

Let's put conspiracy theories about the origin of #SARSCoV2 to rest and help to stop spread of misinformation - great work from @K_G_Andersen #covid19

nature @Nature · Mar 17, 2020
New paper in @NatureMedicine: "Our analyses clearly show that SARS-CoV-2 is not a laboratory construct or a purposefully manipulated virus."
go.nature.com/2x2aKIn

6:29 PM · Mar 17, 2020

A detailed analysis of the events leading up to the writing of the Proximal Origin paper will be covered later in this chapter.

In September 2021, the third scientific paper to further dispel the theory that the virus emerged through laboratory manipulation was published in *Cell*,[122] entitled, "The origins of SARS-CoV-2: A critical review" by Jeremy Farrar et al. The other authors happened to be the same ones who wrote the Proximal Origin paper: Kristian Andersen, Andrew Rambaut and Robert Garry.

The *Cell* paper concluded: "There is currently no evidence that SARS-CoV-2 has a laboratory origin. There is no evidence that any early cases had any connection to the WIV [Wuhan Institute of Virology], in contrast to the clear epidemiological links to animal markets in Wuhan, nor evidence that the WIV possessed or worked on a progenitor of SARS-CoV-2 prior to the pandemic. The suspicion that SARS-CoV-2 might have a laboratory origin, stems from the coincidence that it was first detected in a city that houses a major virological laboratory that studies coronaviruses."

## The Gain-of-Function Studies

Farrar et al.'s conclusion (19 months after *The Lancet* letter signed by leading scientists, of which Farrar was a cosignatory) can be viewed as highly flawed, considering the volume of circumstantial evidence known well before the paper was written. According to a U.S. intelligence report made public from May 2021, three researchers from the Wuhan Institute of Virology sought hospital care for an illness in November 2019, although no information was given on why they got sick. This was written about in a Wall Street Journal report[123] on May 23, 2021. Therefore, Farrar et al.'s Cell article, concluding in absolute terms: "there is no evidence that any early cases had any connection to the WIV [Wuhan Institute of Virology]" is highly refutable.

Furthermore, the authors' claim of there being no evidence that the WIV "worked on a progenitor of SARS-CoV-2 prior to the pandemic" is unsubstantiated given the extensive scientific work published from virologist, Dr. Shi Zheng-Li, director of the Center for Emerging Infectious Diseases at the WIV, (otherwise known as 'Bat Woman' because of her extensive research on SARS-like coronaviruses of bat origin) along with other notable US-based gain of function scientists with ties to the WIV.

It is noteworthy that on September 12, 2019, the Wuhan Institute of Virology's essential database suddenly went offline.[124] It was known to be the most important bat coronavirus database in China, holding more than 22,000 samples and sequence records from the WIV. The administrator of the database happened to be Dr Shi Zheng-li. This has led some to believe that it was possibly an act of coverup; to hide any incriminating evidence that tied the WIV to the emerging virus due to the plausibility that SARS-CoV-2 could have been among the viruses held in or derived from another virus in the WIV repository. It also points to the possibility that the novel virus was circulating well before the official reports.

On January 23, 2020, Zheng-Li released a report on bioRxiv stating the novel virus is 96.2% similar to a bat coronavirus (RaTG13). No detailed information on RaTG13 is given, other than her lab at the WIV had "previously detected [it] in Rhinolophus affinis [horseshoe bat] from Yunnan Province."

Her paper failed to mention the fact that in early April 2012, six miners cleaning bat feces from a copper mine shaft (where horseshoe bats were particularly present) in Mojiang, Yunnan province, fell seriously ill. All of them developed symptoms very similar to COVID-19 (cough, fever and breathlessness) but the virus was not transmitted any further. Three of them died of severe pneumonia. Viral samples taken from the Yunnan miners were taken to the Wuhan Institute of Virology, the only level 4 biosecurity (BSL-4) lab in China that was also studying bat coronaviruses. Interestingly, China's first ever purpose built BSL-4 lab was opened at the WIV in 2013. They were designed with the assistance of the U.S. Centers for Disease Control (CDC), the Pasteur Institute, and the French diagnostics firm, bioMérieux, which was then led by Stéphane Bancel, who later became the CEO of Moderna.

In 2013, Zheng-Li co-authored a paper with her team, including WIV partner, EcoHealth Alliance president, Peter Daszak, published in *Nature*,[125] entitled "Isolation and characterization of a bat SARS-like coronavirus that uses the ACE2 receptor." Their paper claimed a breakthrough in coronavirus research by successfully isolating three viruses from Chinese horseshoe bats. One was classified as WIV1, which had a S Protein that integrated with human ACE-2 receptors. This effectively demonstrated the direct human infection of SARS-like viruses to humans, without the need of an intermediate host. Their work was funded by grants from the U.S. NIAID (National Institute of Allergy and Infectious Diseases), NIH (National Institute of Health)/NSF (National Science Foundation) and the United States Agency for International Development (USAID) Emerging Pandemic Threats (EPT)/ PREDICT.

The U.S. government's Emerging Pandemic Threats program, known as PREDICT, was launched in 2009 and run by the CIA-linked USAID, costing the taxpayer $207 million. Inspired by the 2005 H5N1 bird flu scare, PREDICT sought to identify animal viruses that in the future could infect humans. In this way, the program's "predictions" were thought to head off new pandemics.

Notably, several months before 3/11, the U.S. government quietly shut down USAID's surveillance program. Peter Daszak told The New York Times at the time, "the end of the program is definitely a loss." It certainly was a loss for EcoHealth, which substantially benefitted from being a recipient of PREDICT's generous funding. In total, USAID gave a staggering $64.7 million to the New York-based charity through the years with the Pentagon directly giving a further $39 million. Federal grant data gathered by independent researchers has shown that EcoHealth received more than $123 million from the U.S. government in total. (Interestingly, another of PREDICT's partners- Metabiota, founded by virologist Nathan

Wolfe, went on to stir controversy for its work done in biolabs in Ukraine and the fact that it was funded by President Biden's son, Hunter Biden's investment firm, Rosemont Seneca. Nathan Wolfe also happens to serve on the editorial board of EcoHealth Alliance and is a member of DARPA's Defense Research Council.)

Turning back to Zheng-Li and her team at the WIV, including well known U.S. based gain of function scientists, Ralph Baric and Vineet Menachery of University of North Carolina, Chapel Hill, publish a further paper in the British journal, *Nature Medicine* in 2015, "A SARS-like cluster of circulating bat coronaviruses shows potential for human emergence." An extract reads: "To examine the emergence potential (that is, the potential to infect humans) of circulating bat CoVs [coronaviruses], we built a chimeric virus [a virus that contains genetic material derived from two or more distinct viruses] encoding a novel, zoonotic CoV spike protein from the RsSHC014-CoV sequence that was isolated from Chinese horseshoe bats in the context of the SARS-CoV mouse-adapted backbone." The authors discuss their creation of a synthetic virus, a self-replicating chimeric virus. This lab-manipulated virus had the original SARS, (which infected thousands in 2002-2004 and was linked to at least two documented lab escapes in Singapore and Beijing) as its backbone, with the key S protein replaced by the one they had found in a bat coronavirus (SHC014) mentioned in Zheng-Li's 2013 paper. This new virus demonstrated a powerful ability for cross-species infection. The mice infected with the lab-made virus revealed severe lung damage with no cure. Somehow, the authors of the NIAID/NIH funded study failed to acknowledge: "USAID-EPT-PREDICT funding from EcoHealth Alliance, to Z.-L.S" in the earlier version of the article, first published online. The initials Z-L.S match the name Zheng-Li Shi.

To combat the circulating "conspiracy theory" that the virus was engineered in a lab, on March 30, 2020, an editors' note was added to the article, stating: "We are aware that this article is being used as the basis for unverified theories that the novel coronavirus causing COVID-19 was engineered. There is no evidence that this is true; scientists believe that an animal is the most likely source of the coronavirus."

What makes this noteworthy is that on February 1, 2020, Dr. Anthony Fauci, who was director of NIAID at the time, forwarded the exact study in an urgent email, to his deputy, Hugh Auchincloss, classifying it as "IMPORTANT." It is noteworthy that Fauci used an alternative title for this scientific paper: "Baric, Shi et al- Nature medicine-SARS Gain of function." This suggests that "America's doctor," identified the work done on lab-engineered SARS-like coronaviruses as gain of function research. Furthermore, the fact that in early 2020, Fauci was urgently highlighting this study (which his agency helped to fund) in private, classifying it as important, raises questions about whether he believed this type of research was connected to the origin of the novel virus. This email and others sent by Fauci are discussed in greater detail later in this chapter.

A year after the *Nature Medicine* paper, Baric and Menachery go on to publish their study[126] conducted at the University of North Carolina at Chapel Hill, "SARS-like WIV1-CoV poised for human emergence" in 2016, giving special acknowledgment and thanks to "Dr. Zhengli-Li Shi of the Wuhan Institute of Virology for access to bat Coronavirus sequences and plasmid of WIV1-CoV spike protein."

This controversial gain of function study, like the others, was funded by the Fauci-led NIAID at the time. The paper showed how they had worked with SARS-like coronavirus sequences isolated from Chinese horseshoe bats. Based on these sequences they reconstructed the viruses to evaluate their potential to infect human cells and in humanized mice. They found that the newly identified virus, known as WIV1-CoV, could bind to the same receptors as SARS-CoV. They also showed that the virus readily and efficiently replicated in cultured human airway tissues, suggesting an ability to jump directly to humans.

In the paper, the co-authors wrote: "However, it remains unclear from the current policies and GOF [Gain of Function] environment if these types of studies will be permissible. Although limits and standards for these types of experiments must be established, erring on the side of caution is not without its own risks and balancing the benefits of these types of studies must also be weighed against the potential hazards." Their statement refers to the moratorium on the funding of gain of function research because of its capability to produce biological weapons. The pause was initiated under the Obama administration on October 17, 2014[127] and rescinded on December 19 2017,[128] when the U.S. National Institutes of Health (NIH) announced that they would resume funding these types of experiments involving influenza, Middle East respiratory syndrome coronavirus, and severe acute respiratory syndrome coronavirus.

Baric and Menachery's gain of function study was published in March 2016, meaning their controversial research would have violated the moratorium. However, in the article, the authors deny that any violation took place by stating: "These studies were initiated before the U.S. Government Deliberative Process Research Funding Pause on Selected Gain of Function Research Involving Influenza, MERS, and SARS Viruses and the current paper has been reviewed by the funding agency, the National Institutes of Health (NIH). Continuation of these studies has been requested and approved by the NIH." Their statement also highlights the fact that the NIH was content to continue the funding of this risky scientific work to increase the pathogenic potential of emerging viruses. It is paradoxical how these gain of function scientists acknowledged the "potential hazards" associated with "these types of studies" but believed that "erring on the side of caution" was somehow "not without its own risks" too.

When considering all the published gain of function studies, there is sufficient evidence to support the possibility that the WIV along with its U.S. based partners "worked on a progenitor of SARS-CoV-2 prior to the pandemic" leading to the further, highly plausible theory that the virus had a laboratory origin, despite the public display of condemnation and vehement dismissal of it by an elite group of scientists and officials representing highly influential funders of scientific research.

## Genesis of the Proximal Origin Paper

Besides the published scientific literature, a trove of highly confidential emails and Slack messages exchanged between a group of prominent scientists and health officials, only made public, thanks to a Freedom of Information Act lawsuit leading to its release[129] by the U.S. National Institute of Health (NIH), presents compelling evidence for the lab-origin of the virus. This is particularly noteworthy as many individuals within this group held the belief that such a scenario was plausible.

Take for instance, Sir Jeremy Farrar, former professor of Tropical Medicine at the University of Oxford and former director of the Wellcome Trust, (the world's richest medical research foundation based in the UK), who currently serves as Chief Scientist to the World Health Organization, believed in the lab-origin theory in early 2020, despite lending his name to *The Lancet* letter strongly condemning the "lab-origin conspiracy theory" around the same period.

Farrar admitted in his book *Spike: The Virus v the People*, published in July 2021, he was so concerned about the virus being man-made that he raised it with the former head of M15 and a Wellcome trustee, Eliza Manningham-Buller who advised him to get a burner phone and increase his security. Allegedly, further discussions with other researchers caused him to dispel those fears. However, in his "tell-all" book, Farrar failed to mention *The Lancet* letter or how instrumental he was in the prompting and 'micro-managing/editing' of *Nature Medicine's* "Proximal Origin" article (exhibited in court-ordered released emails), which concluded that "any type of laboratory-based scenario" was not plausible. The article went on to become one of the most influential scientific articles in history and was used as a critical tool in shutting down the debate over the origin of the virus. It was cited by many leading public officials, such as Dr. Anthony Fauci, and the mainstream media when condemning "right wing, lab-leak conspiracy theories." It also assured governmental officials and the broader scientific community that there was no need to scrutinize the labs at the pandemic's epicenter in Wuhan, China.

Notably, under Farrar's leadership, the Wellcome Trust, established in 1936 by the pharmaceutical magnate Henry Wellcome to "improve the health of everyone" also happened to be one of the major grant donors (along with the U.S. National Institutes of Health) for two of the key authors in the pivotal "Proximal Origin" paper: Andrew Rambaut and Kristian Andersen. It is also of particular interest that the Trust has maintained long-standing ties with the Chinese Center for Disease Control and Prevention (China CDC). Dr. George Gao, China CDC Director-General at the time, had previously served as a research assistant at the Wellcome Trust. Strikingly, Gao was reportedly the first to inform Farrar of the novel virus during a phone call on New Year's Eve 2019, while the British infectious disease researcher was waiting in an airport lounge. Interestingly, Gao himself was one of the key "players" in the high-level pandemic simulation Event 201, held on October 18, 2019, in New York City.

Turning to the highly confidential emails, which reveal how Farrar instigated the infamous Saturday, February 1, 2020, emergency teleconference of over a dozen international prominent public health scientists.

What could have been so urgent that needed to be discussed on that Saturday? Potential treatments to combat the novel virus, perhaps?

On the contrary, the private email exchanges and Slack messages[130] exchanged between leading scientists and public officials running up to the Saturday call and beyond, indicate its purpose was to ensure this elite group was to act in one accord over the origin of the virus. Certain explosive private messages exchanged between prominent scientists, indicate that no matter how plausible the lab theory was (that the virus was a product of risky gain of function research, which escaped from a Chinese lab funded by the U.S. taxpayer), it was not to be the one promoted by the group, given that politics was driving the science.

The significant collection of exchanges provides crucial insights into the genesis of the Proximal Origin paper, shedding light on the discussions that led to its formulation.

On Wednesday January 29, Farrar writes to Anthony Fauci, expressing that he "would be very keen" to hear Fauci's personal views about the virus.

On the Friday, Sir Jeremy Farrar is included in an email sent by Professor Kristian Andersen, who eventually became the lead author of the Proximal Origin paper, to Anthony Fauci, containing damning revelations.

**From:** Kristian G. Andersen (b) (6)>
**Sent:** Friday, January 31, 2020 10:32 PM
**To:** Fauci, Anthony (NIH/NIAID) [E] (b) (6)
**Cc:** Jeremy Farrar (b) (6)>
**Subject:** Re: FW: Science: Mining coronavirus genomes for clues to the outbreak's origins

Hi Tony,

Thanks for sharing. Yes, I saw this earlier today and both Eddie and myself are actually quoted in it. It's a great article, but the problem is that our phylogenetic analyses aren't able to answer whether the sequences are unusual at individual residues, except if they are completely off. On a phylogenetic tree the virus looks totally normal and the close clustering with bats suggest that bats serve as the reservoir. The unusual features of the virus make up a really small part of the genome (<0.1%) so one has to look really closely at all the sequences to see that some of the features (potentially) look engineered.

We have a good team lined up to look very critically at this, so we should know much more at the end of the weekend. I should mention that after discussions earlier today, Eddie, Bob, Mike, and myself all find the genome inconsistent with expectations from evolutionary theory. But we have to look at this much more closely and there are still further analyses to be done, so those opinions could still change.

Best,
Kristian

Andersen states that while on the surface the virus "looks totally normal" when one looks closely at the genomic sequences there are "unusual features" that make it "(potentially) look engineered." It is possible that Andersen was referring to certain unique features of the virus found on the viral spike protein, which is key to how the virus infects a human cell. The receptor binding domain (RBD) is part of the spike that binds to the human ACE-2 receptor cell. The novel SARS-Cov-2's spike binds very tightly to this type of human cell, 10 times[131] more than a SARS virus does. Furthermore, the furin cleavage site is a unique feature found in part of the spike protein that is made up of small amino acid sequences, which attract an enzyme called furin, which the human body makes in different tissues, in particular the upper and lower respiratory tract. This enables the virus to replicate easily in the human body, making it much more infectious.

Andersen's revelatory statement directly contradicts what he wrote as lead author in the "Proximal Origin" paper (the first version of the paper was uploaded online approximately two weeks after he wrote the January 31 email), where he and the other co-authors concluded: "We do not believe that any type of laboratory-based scenario is plausible." Andersen then goes on to write in his email to Anthony Fauci and Jeremy Farrar, "I should mention that after discussion earlier today, Eddie, Bob, Mike and myself all find the genome inconsistent with expectations from evolutionary theory." "Mike" referenced in the email is Michael Farzan, chair of the Scripps Research Department of Immunology and Microbiology, who has made key discoveries related to how SARS-CoV infects human cells. "Bob" and "Eddie" are Robert Garry (Professor of Microbiology and Immunology at Tulane Medical School) and Edward Holmes (evolutionary biologist and professor at University of Sydney). Holmes was part of the first Chinese team to upload the complete genome sequence of the novel virus on Virological as early as January 10. They also happen to be the co-authors of the "Proximal Origin" paper.

Although, Holmes, Garry and Andersen shared the same views (as stated in the email) that the virus's genome was inconsistent with the evolutional (natural origin) theory, their paper stated otherwise: "Our analyses clearly show that SARS-CoV-2 is not a laboratory construct or a purposefully manipulated virus."

On July 11, 2023, professors Kristian Andersen and Robert Garry, presented their testimonies[132] to the U.S. Oversight Subcommittee on the Coronavirus Pandemic at the hearing, "Investigating the Proximal Origin of a Cover Up." In the hearing, private slack messages between Prof. Andrew Rambaut, (professor of molecular evolution at the University of Edinburgh and co-author of the Proximal Origin paper) and Prof. Kristian Andersen, sent on February 2, 2020, (the day after the teleconference) were exhibited. These candid messages revealed how these scientists believed that "natural selection and accidental release" were both "plausible scenarios." Nevertheless, their paper published shortly afterwards concluded: "We do not believe that any type of laboratory-based scenario is plausible."

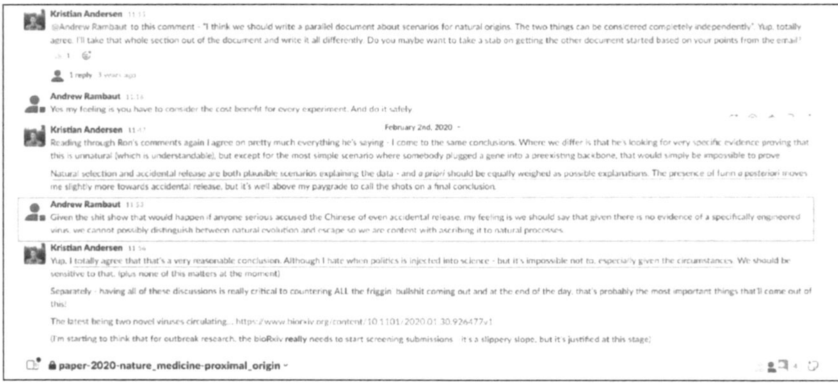

**Kristian Andersen**
@Andrew Rambaut to this comment - "I think we should write a parallel document about scenarios for natural origins. The two things can be considered completely independently". Yup, totally agree. I'll take that whole section out of the document and write it all differently. Do you maybe want to take a stab on getting the other document started based on your points from the email?

1 reply 3 years ago

**Andrew Rambaut**
Yes my feeling is you have to consider the cost benefit for every experiment. And do it safely

February 2nd, 2020

**Kristian Andersen**
Reading through Ron's comments again I agree on pretty much everything he's saying - I come to the same conclusions. Where we differ is that he's looking for very specific evidence proving that this is unnatural (which is understandable), but except for the most simple scenario where somebody plugged a gene into a preexisting backbone, that would simply be impossible to prove

Natural selection and accidental release are both plausible scenarios explaining the data - and *a priori* should be equally weighed as possible explanations. The presence of furin *a posteriori* moves me slightly more towards accidental release, but it's well above my paygrade to call the shots on a final conclusion.

**Andrew Rambaut**
Given the shit show that would happen if anyone serious accused the Chinese of even accidental release, my feeling is we should say that given there is no evidence of a specifically engineered virus, we cannot possibly distinguish between natural evolution and escape so we are content with ascribing it to natural processes.

**Kristian Andersen**
Yup, I totally agree that that's a very reasonable conclusion. Although I hate when politics is injected into science - but it's impossible not to, especially given the circumstances. We should be sensitive to that. (plus none of this matters at the moment)

Separately - having all of these discussions is really critical to countering ALL the friggin' bullshit coming out and at the end of the day, that's probably the most important things that'll come out of this!

The latest being two novel viruses circulating... https://www.biorxiv.org/content/10.1101/2020.01.30.926477v1

(I'm starting to think that for outbreak research, the bioRxiv **really** needs to start screening submissions - it's a slippery slope, but it's justified at this stage)

**paper-2020-nature_medicine-proximal_origin**

An explosive message from Rambaut particularly stands out:

"Given the shit show that would happen if anyone seriously accused the Chinese of even accidental release, my feeling is we should say there is no evidence of a specifically engineered virus, we cannot possibly distinguish between natural evolution and escape, so we are content with ascribing it to a natural process."

Andersen agrees, responding: "I hate when politics is injected into science- but it's impossible not to, especially given the circumstances. We should be sensitive to that."

Their exchange suggest that politics may have influenced these scientists, rather than science alone. But was there another critical factor influencing what they eventually wrote in their Proximal Origin paper? Perhaps, it had something to do with the emergency teleconference call, of which they were all participants, organized by Jeremy Farrar, who was Director of the Wellcome Trust at the time, which prompted the evolutionary biologists to write the paper.

The further exchange of slack messages between Ramabut and Andersen, a day after the call, shows that both these leading scientists were analyzing the plausibility of the lab-leak theory, with Rambaut suggesting they write the report (Proximal Origin Paper) "erring on the side of extreme caution." The lead-author of the Proximal Origin Paper's comments are particularly revealing, Andersen writes, "The main concern coming up reading through all these papers is the kind of stuff that is being done-getting MERS-like viruses to infect humans, getting SARS-like viruses to cause disease in mice and infect humans etc. There's a very strong focus on the spike protein for all that work…One important thing I came across though-for the SARS GoF [Gain of Function] studies they created a reverse genetics system for their bat virus on a whim. So Ron and Christian's argument (which I found to be the strongest) about that not being feasible is not true- they were already creating those."

"Ron and Christian" who participated in the confidential teleconference and referred to in Andersen's message are Ron Fouchier, a Dutch scientist behind some of the most controversial gain-of-function experiments and Christian Drosten, a German virologist and director of the Institute of Virology at Charité Hospital.

Drosten also happened to serve on a bat conference advisory committee with Ecohealth Alliance and Dr. Shi Zheng-li of the Wuhan Institute of Virology. Drosten, was the co-lead author of the controversial "Corman-Drosten paper,"[133] that was "peer-reviewed" in less than 24 hours. It laid the groundwork for the PCR test that would define COVID-19 diagnosis worldwide. Drosten's diagnostic PCR test for COVID-19 was remarkably shipped out the very day the genome sequence of SARS-CoV-2 became public. He was also "first past the post"[134] to develop a diagnostic test for SARS back in 2003. The many scandals of the WHO-adopted "gold standard" COVID-19 PCR test is written about in chapter 6.

It is not surprising that both these scientists had the strongest argument for the virus not having a lab origin, based on their connections with either directly being involved with gain of function studies or with those conducting the experiments.

Andersen references certain "papers" and specifically "SARS GoF studies" which refers to the risky gain of function experiments conducted by the WIV and its U.S. partners, mentioned earlier. He points out that the lab-origin theory is entirely feasible, which is why it is so remarkable that he along with the other "Proximal Origin" authors state: "It is improbable that SARS-CoV-2 emerged through laboratory manipulation of a related SARS-CoV-like coronavirus."

The evolutionary biologist asserts a striking paradox that the U.S. government's PREDICT program is in fact creating the very pandemics they are supposed to prevent. He humorously remarks: "One thing I find kinda funny here- all this work getting bat samples was supported by PREDICT. So if they're not able to predict the pandemics they themselves cause, then I'd say their program is in pretty bad shape.."

**Kristian Andersen** 22:35

One thing I find kinda funny here - all of this work getting bat samples was supported by PREDICT. So if they're not able to predict the pandemics they themselves cause, then I'd say their program is in pretty bad shape...

Sorry had to get that off my chest. Pandemic preparedness indeed.

February 3rd, 2020

So, what could have made the authors of the eventual 'Proximal Origin' paper do such an abrupt U-turn in a short space of time? Or perhaps their private opinions on Covid's origin did not change, just what they chose to write in published scientific papers, and could the emergency February 1 teleconference have been instrumental in that?

Andersen's January 31 email and subsequent slack messages shared just one day after the February 1st teleconference, point to the fact that the lab-origin theory would have been discussed during the call, and the group's agreed-upon strategy. From analyzing the emails and messages, one interpretation is that the promotion of the China-friendly, natural origin theory, may have been the "agreement on next steps," specified in Farrar's carefully worded email scheduling the teleconference, where he stressed the information and discussion was to be shared "in total confidence."

**Date:** Saturday, 1 February 2020 at 15:34

**1st February (2nd Feb for Eddie)**
**Information and discussion is shared in total confidence and not to be shared until agreement on next steps.**

**Dial in details attached.**
**Please mute phones.**
**I will be on email throughout – email Paul or I Paul if any problems**
**If you cannot make it, I will phone you afterwards to update.**

The teleconference was set for 7pm GMT. The participants were the following: Jeremy Farrar, Anthony Fauci, Francis Collins, Kristian Andersen, Robert Garry, Christian Drosten, Mike Ferguson, Ron Fouchier, Eddie Holmes, Marion Koopmans, Stefan Pohlman, Andrew Rambaut, Paul Schreier and Patrick Vallance.

The "back-slapping" and sense of relief in the exchange of emails that followed imply the group settled on the 'agreement' quickly and were grateful for Farrar's "leadership on this critical and sensitive issue," as stated by Francis Collins, director of U.S. National Institutes of Health (NIH) from 2009- Dec 2021.

**From:** Fauci, Anthony (NIH/NIAID) [E]
**Sent:** Sat, 1 Feb 2020 22:06:26 +0000
**To:** Jeremy Farrar;Collins, Francis (NIH/OD) [E]
**Subject:** RE: Teleconference

Thanks, Jeremy. We really appreciate what you are doing here. Pleasure to work with you.
Best,
Tony

**From:** Jeremy Farrar (b) (6)>
**Sent:** Saturday, February 1, 2020 4:00 PM
**To:** Collins, Francis (NIH/OD) [E] < (b) (6)>
**Cc:** Fauci, Anthony (NIH/NIAID) [E] (b) (6)
**Subject:** Re: Teleconference

We are altogether as you know! Conversations with you and Tony, and Patrick and others – always great working with you both

**From:** Francis Collins (b) (6)>
**Date:** Saturday, 1 February 2020 at 20:50
**To:** Jeremy Farrar (b) (6)
**Cc:** "Fauci, Anthony (NIH/NIAID) [E]" (b) (6)
**Subject:** Re: Teleconference

Hi Jeremy,
I can make myself available at any time 24/7 for the call with Tedros. Just let me know.
Thanks for your leadership on this critical and sensitive issue.
Francis

Sent from my iPhone

Farrar's remark, "We are altogether as you know!" indicates the unified purpose of the group, which appears to be the crafting of a narrative to undermine the lab-origin theory. The fact that half of the participants on the call (Jeremy Farrar, Kristian Andersen, Christian Drosten, Eddie Holmes, Robert Garry, and Andrew Rambaut) later became authors of influential scientific papers refuting this theory strongly suggests the coordinated nature of their efforts.

Indeed, Andersen's statement from his February 8th email provides further insight into the group's objective. He mentions, "Our main work over the last couple of weeks has been focused on trying to disprove any type of lab theory, but we are at a crossroad where the scientific evidence isn't conclusive enough to say that we have high confidence in any of the three main theories considered."

Interestingly, Andersen expresses his reluctance towards publishing "this document in a journal" and emphasizes the importance of gathering additional evidence, including awaiting the pangolin virus sequences and to "further scrutinize the furin cleavage site." This points to the scientist's original intention: to take a more cautious approach, "gather more evidence" and not draw conclusions prematurely. However, this turned out not to be the case as the Proximal Origin paper was published the following month in one of the most prestigious scientific journals.

> On 8 Feb 2020, at 22:15, Kristian G. Andersen (b)(6)> wrote:
>
> A lot of good discussion here, so I just wanted to add a couple of things for context that I think are important - and why what we're considering is far from "another conspiracy theory", but rather is taking a valid scientific approach to a question that is increasingly being asked by the public, media, scientists, and politicians (e.g., I have been contacted by Science, NYT, and many other news outlets over the last couple of days about this exact question).
>
> To Ron's question, passage of SARS-like CoVs have been ongoing for several years, and more specifically in Wuhan under BSL-2 conditions - see references 12-15 in the document for a few examples. The fact that Wuhan became the epicenter of the ongoing epidemic caused by nCoV is likely an unfortunate coincidence, but it raises questions that would be wrong to dismiss out of hand. Our main work over the last couple of weeks has been focused on trying to *disprove* any type of lab theory, but we are at a crossroad where the scientific evidence isn't conclusive enough to say that we have high confidence in any of the three main theories considered. Like Eddie - and I believe Bob, Andrew, and everybody on this email as well - I am very hopeful that the viruses from pangolins will help provide the missing pieces. For now, giving the lab theory serious consideration has been highly effective at countering many of the circulating conspiracy theories, including HIV recombinants, bioengineering, etc. - here's just one example: https://www.factcheck.org/2020/02/baseless-conspiracy-theories-claim-new-coronavirus-was-bioengineered/.
>
> As to publishing this document in a journal, I am currently not in favor of doing so. I believe that publishing something that is open-ended could backfire at this stage. I think it's important that we try to gather additional evidence - including waiting on the pangolin virus sequences and further scrutinize the furin cleavage site and O-linked glycans - before publishing. That way we can (hopefully) come out with some strong conclusive statements that are based on the best data we have access to. I don't think we are there yet.
>
> Best,
> Kristian

Furthermore, the pangolin virus sequences referenced in Andersen's email, which the scientist hoped would "provide the missing pieces," was in response to a prior email sent the day before by Farrar, who notified Fauci and Collins that new preliminary data had come in from China concerning coronaviruses found in pangolins. Farrar wrote: "Reports coming out overnight that Chinese group have pangolin viruses that are 99% similar. This would be a crucially important finding and if true could be the 'missing link' and explain a natural evolutionary link."

As it turned out the pangolin data was not the "missing link."[135] It neither offered an explanation for the furin cleavage site nor was it "99% similar" to the novel virus. In a Slack message[136] dated February 20th, Andersen wrote: "The more pango sequences I see the less likely I find that they are intermediate.." The following day, he wrote in an email: "There is no evidence on present data that the pangolin CoVs are directly related to the COVID-19 epidemic."

## Farrar, "Editor" of the Proximal Origin Paper

Further damning evidence reveals how Jeremy Farrar (representing one of the world's wealthiest organizations for funding scientific research, second to the Gates Foundation) organized not just the teleconference call, which led to the writing of the 'Proximal Origin' paper but also went so far as to edit it too. The email below shows the extent to which Jeremy Farrar was involved with the writing of the scientific paper.

**Date:** Monday, 17 February 2020 at 18:11
**To:** Jeremy Farrar [redacted]
**Cc:** [redacted] "Garry, Robert F" [redacted], Edward Holmes [redacted], Ian Lipkin [redacted]
**Subject:** Re: Connections COVID-19

Sure, attached.

K

On Mon, Feb 17, 2020 at 9:02 AM Jeremy Farrar [redacted] wrote:

Sorry to micro-manage/microedit!

But would you be willing to change one sentence?

From
It is unlikely that SARS-CoV-2 emerged through laboratory manipulation of an existing SARS-related coronavirus.
To
It is improbable that SARS-CoV-2 emerged through laboratory manipulation of an existing SARS-related coronavirus.

Farrar begins by apologetically writing "Sorry to micro-manage/microedit!" then proceeds to craft a statement later found in the published paper. His request for a change in the wording from "It is unlikely.." to "It is improbable.." is particularly telling as it changes the conveyed message from considering the lab-origin theory as plausible to rendering it not credible. Such direct involvement from a representative of a major organization funding scientific research raises significant questions about potential biases or conflicts of interest in the paper's conclusions.

Kristian Andersen's characterization of Farrar as the "father figure of the Proximal Origin paper" in his written testimony[137] to the U.S. Oversight Subcommittee on the Coronavirus Pandemic further underscores Farrar's significant contribution to the paper's development. Surprisingly, Farrar's name is absent from the published list of the paper's authors, which is interesting given his level of involvement. However, the authors did express gratitude to the Wellcome Trust for its "support."

## Conflicts of Interest

It is worth noting that Prof. Andrew Rambaut, one of the co-authors, is one of the Wellcome Trust's grant recipients of the Collaborative Awards in Science[138] in genomic surveillance worth totaling over £1.2 million.

At the June 11, 2023, U.S. subcommittee hearing, Andersen's grant application to the NIH was brought up and whether that influenced what he wrote in the Proximal Origin paper. Under oath, Andersen stated: "Excluding the possibility that somebody is a time traveler, no, that is just not possible given the timeline."

His response was centered around the fact that his NIH grant was issued before the Proximal Paper was written. However, Andersen failed to mention that an existing funding request from his lab, Scripps Research, was set before Fauci's NIAID, to the tune of $8.9 million.

The grant was not confirmed until May 21, 2020, indicating that it was still pending during the conference call. Andersen's laboratory, Scripps Research publicized the funding in August 2020, approximately nine months after his assertion that it was already settled. Even their press release characterized it as a "new $8.9 million grant."[139]

Turning back to the evening of January 31, 2020, Greg Folkers, Chief of Staff (1991-2023) of the National Institute of Allergy and Infectious Diseases (NIAID), forwards the Science article[140] "Mining coronavirus genomes for clues to the outbreak's origins" to Anthony Fauci, who in the early hours of Saturday morning forwards it on to Colonel Dr. Robert (Bob) Kadlec. Kadlec served as Assistant Secretary of Health and Human Services (August 2017 - January 2021) and was responsible for the creation of the COVID-19 vaccine development program, Operation Warp Speed.[141] He was the first Homeland Security Director of Biosecurity Policy under President George W. Bush and was involved with the eerily predictive "Dark Winter," a bio-terrorist attack simulation, just months before the September Anthrax-letter attacks and 2019's "Crimson Contagion," a pandemic event simulation of a respiratory virus originating from China, in the year preceding 3/11. (Kadlec and these events are discussed in detail in chapter 16.)

An extract from the Science article reads: "The role of Huanan Seafood Wholesale Market in Wuhan, China, in spreading 2019-nCoV remains murky, though such sequencing, combined with sampling the market's environment for the presence of the virus, is clarifying that it indeed had an important early role in amplifying the outbreak. The viral sequences, most researchers say, also knock down the idea that the pathogen came from a virology institute in Wuhan."

It is difficult to ascertain how Fauci reached his opinion that the article "gives a balanced view" as stated in his email, when it appears to dismiss one of the major theories about the origin of the virus- that "the pathogen came from the virology institute in Wuhan."

Notably, Peter Daszak of EcoHealth Alliance was quoted in the Science article, stating: "Every time there's an emerging disease, a new virus, the same story comes out: This is a spill over or the release of an agent or a bioengineered virus. It's just a shame. It seems humans can't resist controversy and these myths, yet it's staring us right in the face. There's this incredible diversity of viruses in wildlife and we've just scratched the surface. Within that diversity, there will be some that can infect people and within that group will be some that cause illness." He went on to comment: "If we don't find the origin, it could still be a raging infection at a farm somewhere, and once this outbreak dies, there could be a continued spill over that's really hard to stop. But the jury is still out on what the real origins of this are."

Peter Daszak's statements appear contradictory. He underscores the importance of determining the virus' origin, remarking that this question remains unresolved. However, his earlier remarks directly undermine one of the predominant theories: a laboratory origin, by labelling it a "myth" and later, as evidenced in the following March 2020 email, a "conspiracy theory." Critics have pointed to this contradiction as evidence of bias in the origins debate.

**To:** Baric, Ralph
**From:** Peter Daszak
**Sent:** Tue 3/17/2020 10:03:52 AM (UTC-04:00)
**Subject:** Follow up to the National Academies meeting we did in February
SC on EID and 21st Century Threats - One Pager.pdf
Standing Committee on EIDs and 21st C Health Threats. Details.pdf

Hi Ralph,

Just wanted to let you know that the National Academies did set up a Standing Committee as requested by the OSTP Director, who's on the President's COVID taskforce. It's called the "Standing Committee on Emerging Infectious Diseases & 21st Century Health Threats". The charge to the committee is attached. NASEM put out a call and I was nominated. I got some questions from NAM about my relationship to the Wuhan lab, but I explained that it's purely academic (no funds from China to me), and I offered to recuse myself from any discussions about the conspiracy theories re. lab release or bioengineering. The NASEM staff were ok with that and I joined the Committee. There was a meeting to discuss research agenda for COVID-19 and a doc has been written up on this for the OSTP. The meeting had a public session. I've attached the agenda, and details of who's on the committee (provisional, but we are prob now all approved).

Just wanted to let you know what's happening. I don't think this committee will be getting into the lab release or bioengineering hypothesis again any time soon – White House seems to be satisfied with the earlier meeting, paper in Nature and general comments within scientific community. National Security staff were in the room with OSTP on the first call.

Cheers,

Peter

**Peter Daszak**
*President*

EcoHealth Alliance
460 West 34th Street
New York, NY 10001
USA

Daszak's email to the NIAID-funded gain-of-function scientist, Ralph Baric, is highly revelatory as it speaks to his vested interests and lack of impartiality. Daszak updates Baric about his nomination to the Standing Committee on Emerging and Infectious Diseases & 21ST Century Health Threats[142] and his response to certain inconvenient questions: "I got some questions from NAM [National Academies meeting] about my relationship to the Wuhan lab but I explained that it's purely academic (no funds from China to me) and I offered to recuse myself from any discussions about the conspiracy theories re. lab release or bioengineering. The NASEM [National Academies of Science, Engineering and Medicine] staff were ok with that and I joined the Committee."

He characterizes his ties to the Wuhan lab as "purely academic" and states there were "no funds from China to me," a comment that critics have characterized as defensive and potentially misleading. He does not mention that his private organization channeled funds to the WIV, a lab that some sources have characterized as having ties to the Chinese military, via U.S. taxpayer-funded NIH grants. Questions arise about how recusing himself from any discussion about "conspiracy theories re. lab release or bioengineering" would render him an effective and unbiased Committee member and about how the NASEM staff were "ok" with that. Particularly, since the Committee was set up in March 2020 to "inform the U.S. federal government on critical science and policy relating to emerging infectious diseases" and one of the topics for discussion was "access to information, samples, and other materials to determine the origin and evolution of emerging infectious diseases."

Another revealing aspect of his statement is his indication that "this committee" is unlikely to delve into the theories of lab release or bioengineering "again anytime soon." Daszak's tone, marked by optimism and relief, strongly reveals his bias and intention to dismiss what he labels as "conspiracy theories." His reference to the "paper in Nature" (Andersen et al.'s Proximal Origin paper) as a key factor in appeasing the White House and dissuading further exploration of the lab-origin theory underscores the effectiveness of the strategy outlined during the teleconference.

CHAPTER TWO

# CRACKS IN THE NARRATIVE

*"Everything converges towards possible laboratory manipulations..."*

~ Professor Luc Montagnier (1932- 2022), "COVID-19, SARS and Bats coronaviruses genomes peculiar homologous RNA sequences," International Journal of Research GRANTHAALAYAH, July 2020

In the final days of January 2020, as the world still believed it was facing a mysterious pneumonia outbreak in Wuhan, China, an obscure Indian preprint landed like a grenade. It identified what appeared to be HIV-derived inserts in the spike protein of the new coronavirus (including a never-before-seen furin cleavage site of staggering infectious potential) only to be withdrawn by its authors within seventy-two hours amid widespread criticism.

Over the same frantic weekend (31 January- 2 February), a closed circle of the world's most influential virologists, funders, and senior government scientists held emergency teleconferences. They privately acknowledged that parts of the viral genome looked "engineered," sent frantic midnight emails invoking the possible need for FBI or MI5 investigations. Rapidly, they converged on a singular conclusion that critics argue served to protect gain-of-function research and the institutions that had funded it.

What followed suggests a departure from open scientific debate. Evidence indicates what appears to be a coordinated effort, executed through elite journals, major research funders (including some with government ties), and senior health officials, that effectively marginalized alternative data, undermined dissenting scientists, and established a singular narrative about the origin of a virus that would soon upend the world.

## The Curious Case of the HIV Inserts

Coincidentally, on the same day as the January 31 email exchange between Anthony Fauci, Robert Kadlec, Kristian Andersen, and Jeremy Farrar in reference to the Science article, an explosive scientific paper was posted on the preprint server, bioRxiv by Pradhan et al.[143] The paper, written by a group of Indian scientists, revealed the "uncanny similarity on unique inserts in the 2019-nCov spike protein to HIV-1 gp 120 and Gag." The authors of the Pradhan et al. paper concluded, "we identified 4 unique inserts in the 2019-nCoV spike glycoprotein that are not present in any other coronavirus reported till date. To our surprise, all the 4 inserts in the 2019-nCoV mapped to short segments of amino acids in the HIV-1 gp120 and Gag among all annotated virus proteins in the NCBI database. This uncanny similarity of novel inserts in the 2019- nCoV spike protein to HIV-1 gp120 and Gag is unlikely to be fortuitous. Further, 3D modeling suggests that at least 3 of the unique inserts which are non-contiguous in the primary protein sequence of the 2019-nCoV spike glycoprotein converge to constitute the key components of the receptor binding site. Taken together, our findings suggest an unconventional evolution of 2019-nCoV that warrants further investigation."

The Indian scientists went on to write: "To get structural insights and to understand the role of these insertions in 2019-nCoV glycoprotein, we modelled its structure based on available structure of SARS spike glycoprotein." The following image, taken from the Pradhan et al. paper, is a 3D model of the spike protein showing the 4 HIV inserts. "Insert 4"-QTNSPRRA is the one that codes for the furin cleavage site, which has never been seen before in a virus, and increases the ability of the virus to infect via the inhalation route.

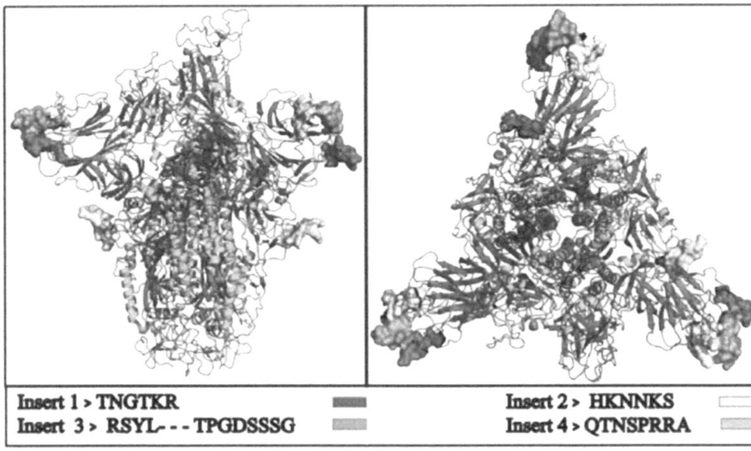


**Figure 3. Modelled homo-trimer spike glycoprotein of 2019-nCoV virus.** The inserts from HIV envelop protein are shown with colored beads, present at the binding site of the protein.

The Pradhan et al. paper triggered widespread condemnation[144] by the mainstream media. The morning after its publication, the co-founder of bioRxiv, John Inglis, took to social media to quell the storm, by highlighting how a special warning[145] had now been placed on all coronavirus papers: "bioRxiv is receiving many new papers on coronavirus 2019-nCov. A reminder: these preliminary reports have not been peer-reviewed. They should not be regarded as conclusive, guide clinical practice/health-related behavior, or be reported in news media as established information."

A further flurry of activity occurred into the late hours of that Friday with Fauci engaging in a call with Kristian Andersen, which evidently left him disturbed regarding Andersen's "concern about the Furin site mutation in the spike protein of the currently circulating 2019-nCoV." Just past midnight, Fauci wrote an alarming letter to Jeremy Farrar, copying in Kristian Andersen, relaying his fear.

From: Fauci, Anthony (NIH/NIAID) [E]
Sent: Sat, 1 Feb 2020 00:38:35 +0000
To: Jeremy Farrar
Cc: Kristian G. Andersen
Bcc: Conrad, Patricia (NIH/NIAID) [E],Mascola, John (NIH/VRC) [E],Conrad, Patricia (NIH/NIAID) [E]
Subject: RE: Phone call

Jeremy:
I just got off the phone with Kristian Anderson and he related to me his concern about the Furine site mutation in the spike protein of the currently circulating 2019-nCoV. I told him that as soon as possible he and Eddie Holmes should get a group of evolutionary biologists together to examine carefully the data to determine if his concerns are validated. He should do this very quickly and if everyone agrees with this concern, they should report it to the appropriate authorities. I would imagine that in the USA this would be the FBI and in the UK it would be MI5. It would be important to quickly get confirmation of the cause of his concern by experts in the field of coronaviruses and evolutionary biology. In the meantime, I will alert my US. Government official colleagues of my conversation with you and Kristian and determine what further investigation they recommend. Let us stay in touch.
Best regards,
Tony

Anthony S. Fauci, MD
Director
National Institute of Allergy and Infectious Diseases
Building 31, Room 7A-03
31 Center Drive, MSC 2520
National Institutes of Health
Bethesda, MD 20892-2520
Phone: (b)(6)
FAX: (301) 496-4409
E-mail: (b)(6)
The information in this e-mail and any of its attachments is confidential and may contain sensitive information. It should not be used by anyone who is not the original intended recipient. If you have received this e-mail in error please inform the sender and delete it from your mailbox or any other storage devices. The National Institute of Allergy and Infectious Diseases (NIAID) shall not accept liability for any statements made that are the sender's own and not expressly made on behalf of the NIAID by one of its representatives.

What could have prompted Fauci to write that an MI5 or FBI investigation might be warranted?

It probably stemmed from Andersen's email to Fauci on January 31, followed by a subsequent call between them. In the email (referenced earlier in this chapter), Andersen mentions that "the unusual features of the virus make up a really small part of the genome (<0.1%), so one has to look really closely at all the sequences to see that some of the features (potentially) look engineered."

This revelation would have undoubtedly raised serious concerns for Fauci about the origin and potential engineering of the virus. Additionally, he might have been worried about the serious allegations that could follow regarding the association of his agency, the NIAID, funding programs that might have led to the creation of an engineered virus.

On the same day as the scheduled emergency teleconference (Saturday, February 1), Fauci sent an email to Hugh Auchincloss, acting deputy director of NIAID at the time (until he succeeded Anthony Fauci as director in January 2023) with the attachment "Baric, Shi et al- Nature medicine- SARS Gain of function.pdf."

**From:** Fauci, Anthony (NIH/NIAID) [E]
**Sent:** Sat, 1 Feb 2020 12:29:01 +0000
**To:** Auchincloss, Hugh (NIH/NIAID) [C] (b)(6)
**Cc:** (b)(6)
**Subject:** IMPORTANT
**Attachments:** Baric, Shi et al - Nature medicine - SARS Gain of function.pdf

Hugh:
It is essential that we speak this AM. Keep your cell phone on. I have a conference call at 7:45 AM with Azar. It likely will be over at 8:45 AM. Read this paper as well as the e-mail that I will forward to you now. You will have tasks today that must be done.
Thanks,
Tony

Anthony S. Fauci, MD
Director
National Institute of Allergy and Infectious Diseases
Building 31, Room 7A-03

This email and the renaming of the *Nature Medicine* paper to "SARS Gain of Function" indicate Fauci's recognition of the association between gain-of-function studies and Ralph Baric, the lead author of the paper. This connection was previously mentioned in this chapter.

Fauci expresses urgency in his email, stating, "It is essential we speak this AM. Keep your cell phone on. I have a conference call at 7:45 AM with Azar." The "Azar" mentioned is Alex Azar, who was then the head of the U.S. Health and Human Services and former director of the pharmaceutical company Eli Lilly U.S.. Azar was also referenced in a series of leaked European Medicines Agency emails, which are discussed in a later chapter.

On Sunday February 2, Francis Collins, director of the NIH, writes to Anthony Fauci stating, "In case you haven't seen, attached is the Indian paper claiming HIV sequences have been inserted into 2019-nCov, which has been roundly debunked."

One would have thought that Fauci, a HIV expert, who later that year was given the Lifetime Achievement Award for his work fighting the global HIV/AIDS crisis, would not have been so quick to dismiss the paper as "really outlandish." In fact, his outright dismissal of it, could be interpreted as an effort to control the narrative around this topic. The question is, why? Critics have questioned whether concerns about his agency's funding relationships may have influenced his response.

**From:** Fauci, Anthony (NIH/NIAID) [E]
**Sent:** Sun, 2 Feb 2020 11:26:13 +0000
**To:** Collins, Francis (NIH/OD) [E];Tabak, Lawrence (NIH/OD) [E];Wolinetz, Carrie (NIH/OD) [E]
**Subject:** RE: More on evolution of coronavirus

The Indian paper is really outlandish. Agree about Jon Cohen's nice summary.

**From:** Collins, Francis (NIH/OD) [E] (b) (6)
**Sent:** Sunday, February 2, 2020 5:58 AM
**To:** Fauci, Anthony (NIH/NIAID) [E] (b) (6); Tabak, Lawrence (NIH/OD) [E] (b) (6)>; Wolinetz, Carrie (NIH/OD) [E] (b) (6)>
**Subject:** More on evolution of coronavirus

In case you haven't seen, attached is the Indian paper claiming HIV sequences have been inserted into 2019-nCoV, which has been roundly debunked.

I found Jon Cohen's piece in Science to be a pretty useful summary:

https://www.sciencemag.org/news/2020/01/mining-coronavirus-genomes-clues-outbreak-s-origins

FC

That same day, three days after the Pradhan et al. paper was posted (and one day after the teleconference), it was suddenly "withdrawn" by the Indian authors.

In April 2020, the late Professor Luc Montagnier (1932- 2022), French virologist and joint recipient of the Nobel Prize of Physiology or Medicine for his discovery of the human immunodeficiency virus (HIV), referenced the Pradhan et al paper in an explosive interview with news platform CNews.[146] He claimed: "We have arrived at the conclusion that this virus was created." He accused "molecular biologists" of having inserted DNA sequences from HIV into a coronavirus, "probably" as part of their work to find a vaccine against AIDS. Professor Montagnier made a further point that he was not the first to suggest the connection and added that "a group of renowned Indian researchers" had also tried to publish a study showing that the novel coronavirus includes HIV DNA, but were forced to retract their claims and had been "smothered."

A few months afterwards, Montagnier published a scientific paper[147] which showed "how 16 fragments (Env Pol and Integrase genes) from different strains, both diversified and very recent, of the HIV1, HIV2 and SIV retroviruses have high percentage of homology into parts of the genome of COVID-19."

The paper went on to state: "Through the 14 facts relating to each of the 14 paragraphs of this article, everything converges towards possible laboratory manipulations which contributed to modifications of the genome of COVID-19, but also, very probably much older SARS, with perhaps this double objective of vaccine design and of "gain of function" in terms of penetration of this virus into the cell."

A noteworthy investigative report[148] from April 2024, presented evidence of ongoing efforts to create an HIV vaccine in Wuhan, particularly through a joint German-Chinese virology project involving key members based at the Wuhan Institute of Virology. An extract from the article reads: "But the fact of the matter is that someone was trying to create an HIV vaccine in Wuhan. For this was precisely the aim of the longstanding German-Chinese cooperative virology project…which gave rise to a full-fledged joint German-Chinese virology lab right in Wuhan. Indeed, as I have shown, the joint German-Chinese lab, located at Union Hospital on the left bank of the Yangtze River, is not just in Wuhan, but is also – unlike the Wuhan Institute of Virology – right in the area of the initial outbreak of COVID-19 cases in the city. Furthermore, the Wuhan Institute of Virology is itself an official partner in the German-Chinese virology network.. key members of the network who were conducting experiments meant to facilitate the development of an HIV vaccine are based at none other than the WIV."

## Unredacted Email Exchanges

Following the emergency teleconference, unredacted email exchanges among the participants on Sunday, February 2,[149] were obtained by The Nation and The Intercept. These emails provide further evidence that the scientists involved were considering the lab leak theory as a plausible explanation for the origin of the virus.

In an e-mail to Fauci and Collins, Farrar wrote, "On a spectrum if 0 is nature and 100 is released—I am honestly at 50!"

Farrar proceeds to summarize the viewpoints of several other scientists including Michael Farzan of Scripps Research Institute, who expressed concerns about the furin site and found it difficult to explain as a natural event outside of a laboratory setting. Farzan leaned toward an "accidental-release" explanation, expressing a ratio of "70:30" or "60:40" in favor of that possibility.

Additionally, Farrar noted that "Bob," referring to Robert Garry, was surprised by the presence of a furin cleavage site in the virus with even going so far as to state how easy it would be to be generated in a lab.

"I really can't think of a plausible natural scenario where you get from the bat virus or one very similar to it to nCoV [novel virus] where you insert exactly 4 amino acids 12 nucleotide [reference to furin cleavage site] that all have to be added at the exact same time to gain this function-that and you don't change any other amino acid in S2? I just can't figure out how this gets accomplished in nature…it's stunning. Of course, in the lab it would be easy to generate the perfect 12 base insert that you wanted" Garry [Bob] noted.

What is particularly noteworthy are the remarks from Ron Fouchier, the Dutch gain of function scientist mentioned earlier, whose previous research involving the H5N1 influenza virus has stirred great controversy.

In early 2011, Ron Fouchier of Erasmus University Medical Center investigated how bird flu viruses could cause human pandemics. Fouchier serially passed H5N1 avian influenza in ferrets until it could spread through respiratory droplets. Serial passage means transferring a virus multiple times from one host to another to see how it changes. The virus adapted in the ferrets' lungs, enabling it to replicate in mammalian lungs and transmit through coughing or sneezing.

Fouchier's creation of a novel and contagious strain of H5N1 prompted several scientists to express their concerns about the risks of creating novel potential pandemic pathogens. They formed the Cambridge Working Group which engaged in public advocacy influencing the U.S. government to suspend funding gain of function work in December 2014.

It is noteworthy that the Erasmus University Medical Center, where Fouchier works as Deputy Head of the Department of Viroscience, is also where Marion Koopmans works as Head. She took part in the February 1 teleconference and was appointed as a team member of the World Health Organization's investigation into the origins of COVID-19. Koopmans was also a key author of the "Corman-Drosten paper."

Turning back to Fouchier's email, where he presented an opposing view to the other scientists and was quick to label the non-natural origin of the virus as a conspiracy theory. "It is my opinion that a non-natural origin of 2019-nCoV is highly unlikely at present. Any conspiracy theory can be approached with factual information. I have written down some of the counter-arguments" he wrote.

It is noteworthy that Fouchier went on to write: "further debate about such accusations would unnecessarily distract top researchers from their active duties and do unnecessary harm to science in general and science in China in particular."

This suggests that his primary motive for the lengthy email was to express concern about the potential consequences of a continued debate on accusations related to gain-of-function studies. His apprehension appears to revolve around the possibility that such debate could distract top researchers from their work and potentially harm the progress of science, especially in China. A significant implication which can be drawn from Fouchier's statement is how the threat of funding cuts and potential consequences scientists may face if their work is perceived as too risky, are valid enough reasons according to him, for any debate over the origin of the virus to be shut down. This reveals the highly conflicted position from one of the world's most controversial gain of function scientists, which failed to go unnoticed by other members within the "close-knit group." Kristian Andersen wrote in a private Slack message:[150] "It's unbelievable how conflicted Ron [Fouchier] is."

Fouchier's email also went on to highlight the Pradhan et al paper from India, which identified the HIV-like sequences in the spike protein of the virus. "The similarity between the inserts in 2019-nCoV spike and sequences of HIV-1" was entirely dismissed by him as "accidental." According to Fouchier, "such similarities are explained by pure chance alone."

> 1. The biorxiv publication by Prashant Pradhan and colleagues from Delhi ("Uncanny similarity of unique inserts in the 2019-nCoV spike protein to HIV-1 gp120 and Gag") has already been heavily debated on biorxiv and virological.org. The similarity between the inserts in 2019-nCoV spike and sequences of HIV-1 is accidental. These are very short insert sequences that are highly similar to many Genbank entries. Such similarities are explained by pure chance alone.

However, in a December 2021 article from "Arkmedic's blog"[151] the author analyzed the Pradhan et al. paper and wrote: "These were not just random sequences from HIV. In his paper, Pradhan went further and recreated the structure of the virus with the location of the four inserts. Lo and behold, these 'random' inserts - all from HIV - are all at binding sites of the coronavirus. What are the odds?" The odds of that eventuality occurring was later explained as close to zero.

An email[152] from the former NIH director, Dr. Francis Collins sent to Drs. Jeremy Farrar, Anthony Fauci and Lawrence Tabak, echoed Fouchier's concern for harms to science, if the lab leak theory was not shut down.

"I share your [in reference to Farrar's] view that a swift convening experts in a confidence inspiring framework (WHO seems really the only option) is needed, or the voices of conspiracy will quickly dominate, doing great potential harm to science and international harmony," Collins wrote.

**From:** Francis Collins (b)(6)>
**Date:** Sunday, 2 February 2020 at 10:27
**To:** Jeremy Farrar (b)(6)
**Cc:** "Fauci, Anthony (NIH/NIAID) [E]" (b)(6), "Tabak, Lawrence (NIH/OD) [E]" (b)(6)
**Subject:** RE: Teleconference

Jeremy,

(b)(5)

I'm available any time today except 3:15 – 5:45 pm EST (on a plane) for a call to Tedros. Let me know if I can help get through his thicket of protectors.

Francis

> ... Though the arguments from Ron Fouchier and Christian Drosten are presented with more forcefulness than necessary, I am coming around to the view that a natural origin is more likely. But I share your view that a swift convening of experts in a confidence inspiring framework (WHO seems really the only option) is needed, or the voices of conspiracy will quickly dominate, doing great potential harm to science and international harmony...

However, a further email sent by Collins on April 16, 2020, to Drs. Anthony Fauci, Lawrence Tabak, Cliff Lane, and Mr. John Burklow, is even more damning in exposing his desire to stifle "this very destructive conspiracy." He goes on to express his disappointment with the "Nature Medicine article" for failing to "settle this," i.e., squash the lab leak theory for good.

**From:** Collins, Francis (NIH/OD) [E] (b)(6)
**Sent:** Thursday, April 16, 2020 5:02 PM
**To:** Fauci, Anthony (NIH/NIAID) [E] (b)(6)
**Cc:** Tabak, Lawrence (NIH/OD) [E] (b)(6); Lane, Cliff (NIH/NIAID) [E] (b)(6); Burklow, John (NIH/OD) [E] (b)(6)
**Subject:** conspiracy gains momentum

(b)(5)

https://www.mediaite.com/tv/foxs-bret-baier-sources-increasingly-confident-coronavirus-outbreak-started-in-wuhan-lab/

(b)(5)

Francis

> Wondering if there is something NIH can do to help put down this very destructive conspiracy, with what seems to be growing momentum:
>
> https://www.mediaite.com/tv/foxs-bret-baier-sources-increasingly-confident-coronavirus-outbreak-started-in-wuhan-lab/
>
> I hoped the Nature Medicine article on the genomic sequence of SARS-CoV-2 would settle this. But probably didn't get much visibility.
>
> Anything more we can do? Ask the National Academy to weigh in?
>
> Francis

It is noteworthy that four years later, during a seven-hour closed-door session[153] with the House Select Coronavirus Subcommittee in January 2024, Dr. Collins concurred with Dr. Fauci's acknowledgment that the "lab-leak hypothesis is not a conspiracy theory," despite his previous efforts to refute it using the March 2020 "Proximal Origin" scientific paper. Additionally, Dr. Collins acknowledged that Dr. Fauci had invited him to participate in the February 1, 2020, conference call that prompted the writing of *Nature Medicine's* "Proximal Origin" publication.

What is clear is that throughout these exchanges, the scientists were keenly aware of the growing public interest in the origin of the virus and "voices of conspiracy" on social media. Fauci wanted the group to act quickly, he wrote: "Like all of us, I do not know how this evolved, but given the concerns of so many people and the threat of further distortions on social media, it is essential that we move quickly."

And move quickly they did. On March 17, "The Proximal Origin of SARS-CoV-2" by Kristian Andersen et al., was published in *Nature Medicine*, where the unnatural origin of the furin cleavage site was outright rejected.

One month after the scientific paper's publication, Fauci addressed the public during a presidential briefing.[154] He happened to cite a study conducted by "a group of highly qualified evolutionary virologists" indicating that the genetic sequences of the virus were consistent with a natural jump from an animal to a human- the Proximal Origin paper. However, Fauci omitted any mention of his involvement with the study or its authors, including the series of email exchanges, late-night calls, and the request for comment about the paper before its publication. Additionally, he did not acknowledge how he was thanked by the lead author for his "advice and leadership."

Fri, Mar 6, 2020 at 1:22 PM

Dear Jeremy, Tony, and Francis,

Thank you again for your advice and leadership as we have been working through the SARS-CoV-2 'origins' paper. We're happy to say that the paper was just accepted by Nature Medicine and should be published shortly (not quite sure when).

To keep you in the loop, I just wanted to share the accepted version with you, as well as a draft press release. We're still waiting for proofs, so please let me know if you have any comments, suggestions, or questions about the paper or the press release.

Tony, thank you for your straight talk on CNN last night - it's being noticed.

Best,
Kristian

## Fauci's NIAID Funding Gain-of-Function Research

The following year in May 2021, Fauci, who at the time was the director of the National Institute of Allergy and Infectious Diseases (NIAID), which is part of the National Institute of Health (NIH), told U.S. Congress[155] that the NIH "has not ever and does not now fund gain-of-function research in the Wuhan Institute of Virology."

However, the contents of a January 2020 email from Greg Folkers to Fauci directly contradict what Fauci testified to Congress. It reveals the connection between Fauci's NIAID and the funding of gain-of-function studies, involving Ralph Baric, Peter Daszak, and the Wuhan Institute of Virology. Specifically, it highlights the funding of Peter Daszak's EcoHealth Alliance "for coronavirus research in China over the past five years, involving collaborators such as the Wuhan Institute of Virology (currently studying nCov) and Ralph Baric."

**From:** Folkers, Greg (NIH/NIAID) [E] (b)(6)
**Sent:** Monday, January 27, 2020 6:25 PM
**To:** Routh, Jennifer (NIH/NIAID) [E] (b)(6); Fauci, Anthony (NIH/NIAID) [E] (b)(6)
**Cc:** Billet, Courtney (NIH/NIAID) [E] (b)(6); Stover, Kathy (NIH/NIAID) [E] (b)(6); Conrad, Patricia (NIH/NIAID) [E] (b)(6)Marston, Hilary (NIH/NIAID) [E] (b)(6); Lerner, Andrea (NIH/NIAID) [E] (b)(6)
**Subject:** RE: For review (due to HHS for White House by 8:30 tonight): press conference talking points

As a place folder looks good to me.
+ Andrea who is the lead on a CoV talk ASF is giving on Tuesday

Also --- when talking about CoV (not necessarily in this venue) we have on our team (Vincent and folks we fund, Peter Daszak, Ralph Baric, Ian Lipkin, etc.) probably the world's experts non-human coronaviruses.

From David M -- EcoHealth group (Peter Daszak et al), has for years been among the biggest players in coronavirus work, also in collaboration with Ralph Baric, Ian Lipkin and others

NIAID has funded Peter's group for coronavirus work in China for the past 5 years through R01 1R01AI110964: "Understanding the Risk of Bat Coronavirus Emergence". That's now been renewed, with a specific focus to identify cohorts of people highly exposed to bats in China, and work out if they're getting sick from CoVs. Erik Stemmy is the Program Officer. Collaborators include Wuhan Institute of Virology (currently working on the nCoV), and Ralph Baric. The results of the work to date include:

- Sampled 10,074 bats and ~2,000 other mammals at 47 sites across S. China
- Discovered 172 novel β-CoVs (52 novel SARSr-CoVs), >350 novel α-CoVs
- Discovered closest relative to Wuhan nCoV (92% homology)
- Discovered Swine Acute Diarrheal Syndrome Virus (SADS-CoV) killing >25,000 pigs in Guangdong Province (Published in *Nature*)
- Found SARS-related CoVs that can bind to human cells (Published in *Nature*), and that cause SARS-like disease in humanized mouse models.
- Found that clinical signs of bat SARSr-CoVs in mice were not prevented with a vaccine candidate against SARS-CoV, and were not treatable with most monoclonal therapies being developed
- Found serological evidence that 3% of people living at the wildlife-human interface in rural China are being exposed to these bat SARS-related coronaviruses

Also – prior to the above R01, Peter's folks worked under an R01 with Eun-Chung Park as Program Officer on viral discovery in bats, and originally identified SARS-CoV as having a likely origin in bats (published in *Science*)

This means that by January 27th, 2020, Fauci was aware of the financial relationship between NIAID, NIH, EcoHealth Alliance and the WIV.

Thanks to the detailed notes on NIH communication between agency staff and the head of EcoHealth Alliance obtained by *The Intercept*,[156] Fauci was also aware of the collaboration between NIAID and EcoHealth Alliance to develop a grant policy aimed at circumventing the moratorium on gain-of-function research. This policy, devised by EcoHealth and endorsed by NIAID, permitted EcoHealth to conduct potentially hazardous experiments on novel bat coronaviruses with minimal oversight. These experiments, which would have been prohibited by the moratorium, were facilitated by this new policy.

In March 2023, Dr. Robert Redfield, U.S. Director of the Centers for Disease Control and Prevention (CDC) from 2018-2021, testified[157] to the House Select Subcommittee on the Coronavirus Pandemic. He revealed that in the early stages of the pandemic, there was a predetermined decision to promote a specific narrative, and anyone who disagreed would be "sidelined." Redfield referenced the notable conference call of February 1, 2020, claiming that it was convened by Fauci and former NIH Director Francis Collins to discuss COVID-19 origins. Redfield stated that he was excluded from the call and only learned about it later in June 2021. Redfield stated: "They made a decision, almost a P.R. decision, that they were going to push one point of view only and suppress rigorous debate. They argued they did it in defense of science, but it was antithetical to science."

In October 2022, a Senate investigation into the origins of COVID-19 concluded that the virus likely originated from a Chinese laboratory. The interim report,[158] released by Republicans on the Senate Health, Education, Labor, and Pensions Committee, found insufficient evidence supporting the theory of animal-to-human transmission and identified China's Wuhan Institute of Virology as the probable source of the virus.

"Based on the analysis of the publicly available information, it appears reasonable to conclude that the COVID-19 pandemic was, more likely than not, the result of a research-related incident," the report read.

In June 2023, a US Intelligence four-page report was declassified, intelligence agencies said it was unable to discover the origins of the pandemic but said it could not rule out the possibility the virus came from a laboratory.

"The Central Intelligence Agency and another agency remain unable to determine the precise origin of the COVID-19 pandemic, as both (natural and lab) hypotheses rely on significant assumptions or face challenges with conflicting reporting," the report said.

The intelligence agencies did not find evidence of a specific incident at the Wuhan Institute (WIV) that could have caused the outbreak despite "extensive work." The report went on to state: "We continue to have no indication that the WIV's pre-pandemic research holdings included SARSCoV-2 or a close progenitor, nor any direct evidence that a specific research-related incident occurred involving WIV personnel before the pandemic that could have caused the COVID pandemic."

Notably absent from the intelligence report is any mention of a critical fact: how the WIV's key bat coronavirus databases were taken offline in September 2019.

## Interview with an Ecohealth Alliance Whistle-Blower

In September 2022, I interviewed[159] former EcoHealth Alliance Vice President, turned whistle-blower, Dr. Andrew Huff PhD, who discussed his tenure at the controversial non-profit organization. Huff, an expert in the field of bioterrorism and bio-surveillance, worked at EcoHealth Alliance from 2014-2016. He reviewed the infamous research grant proposal "Understanding the risk of Bat Coronavirus Emergence"[160] that was submitted to the NIH detailing gain of function work, which he attests led to the creation of SARS-CoV-2, even though a moratorium was put in place in the U.S. since October 2014 for this type of research. Huff spoke on the "grey areas" of the moratorium, for instance, how it didn't apply to existing applications.

A screenshot of the EcoHealth Alliance application can be seen below revealing the section on "Humanized mice for experimental infection" found on page 125 of the document.

> **Humanized mice for experimental infection for Specific Aim 3**: In order to understand whether bat coronaviruses that utilize receptors found in people have the potential to infect people, we will use Swiss albino mice (standard breed at Wuhan University) that have been genetically modified to have human receptors. We'll infect them with cultured bat coronaviruses and determine which organs become infected and whether these mice are capable of shedding infectious virus. Humanized mice will be genetically modified to carry human ACE2 or DPP4 gene will be used to evaluate pathogenesis of CoVs. We cannot anticipate exactly how many viruses we will find that are candidates for experimental models, however we estimate that we will use
> Principal Investigator/Program Director (Last, first, middle): Daszak, Peter
>
> Vertebrate Animals Page 125

Huff warned Dr. Peter Daszak, his former boss, about the biosafety and biosecurity risks, but Daszak showed little regard for his concerns. Additionally, Huff disclosed that EcoHealth Alliance lacked both a biological security officer and an institutional biosafety committee, which are mandated for select agent gain-of-function research and thus violated NIH guidelines.

Initially named Wildlife Trust, EcoHealth Alliance was described to Huff as focusing on conservation. However, upon joining, Huff was surprised to learn from Daszak himself that no such conservation work was actually being conducted. This revelation contradicted the organization's public statements, as their website declares: "EcoHealth Alliance is a global non-profit, leading scientific research into the critical connections between human, animal, and environmental health."

According to Huff: "Peter [Daszak] stuck his head in the door and said, 'I need your help building a presentation.' I said, 'sure Peter, who's the audience?' He said, 'In-Q-Tel,' because I came from the National Security world, I knew exactly who In-Q-Tel was. They are the Central Intelligence Agency (CIA)/ Department of Defense (DoD) or Defense Intelligence Agency's venture capital firm. So, this is how the U.S. government invests in advanced technology start-ups. Quite famously, In-Q-Tel invested in Google, so Google Maps is probably In-Q-Tel's biggest win that we know of in history. The content of that proposal was mostly the gain of function work that was being done at EcoHealth Alliance, which was a combination of us collecting samples through USAID- bat coronavirus samples. Then those samples went through a series of laboratory techniques to basically develop SARS-CoV-2 so then they could make a medical countermeasure, which was the mRNA platform. This is all laid out in the [2014] presentation."

In-Q-Tel's 2016 Winter quarterly issue, entitled, "Five Major Challenges for Pandemic Prediction and Prevention" penned by Peter Daszak. He writes: "Can we predict the pandemic potential of a newly discovered pathogen?...For close neighbors of known pathogens, sequencing their receptor binding domains may provide a rudimentary strategy to assess potential virulence. For example, the SARS-like coronaviruses (SL-CoV) identified by our group in bats in China have varying degrees of sequence homology to the SARS coronavirus (SARS- CoV). We have shown that some SL-CoVs can bind directly to the human cell surface receptor for SARS-CoV, ACE2. Others have now demonstrated that chimeric viruses

(SARS-CoV backbone expressing SL-CoV spike protein) can infect human cells and cause clinical signs in humanized mice. Importantly, there appears to be a lack of immune cross-reactivity between SARS-CoV and our SL-CoV, suggesting that our SL-CoV has significant pandemic potential."

Daszak goes on to highlight how investing in "targeted surveillance" offers a "substantial return." He explains: "Overcoming pandemics will require new technological solutions, better interdisciplinary collaboration, and significant funding. However, a simple economic assessment suggests they are likely to have a substantial return on investment. With the costs of pandemics rising (between $10 and $30 billion for SARS), the relatively moderate cost (less than $10 billion) of conducting targeted surveillance, identifying novel pathogens from key wildlife species, and analyzing their potential risk becomes more attractive."

Given Daszak's position at EcoHealth Alliance, a non-profit known for its controversial research partnerships with the Wuhan Institute of Virology, his push for targeted surveillance and demand for "significant funding" in this field could be perceived as self-serving, since organizations like his own would directly benefit from this type of investment.

## Ecohealth Alliance's DEFUSE Proposal

In my interview[161] with Charles Rixey, former U.S. Marine Corps, Weapons of Mass Destruction defense professional and author of "The Myth of the Blind Watchmaker,"[162] he spoke about the infamous 2018 Project DEFUSE[163] grant proposal "that basically laid out exactly how to make the virus." It was submitted to DARPA (Defense Advanced Research Projects Agency) by Peter Daszak's EcoHealth Alliance, requesting a grant worth $14,209,245.

Rixey explained how the controversial document was leaked personally to him, which he later published on DRASTIC's website (the online group of researchers, microbiologists, and geneticists who came together to unearth the origin of SARS-CoV-2) in the fall of 2021, placing it in the public domain. Since its publication, hundreds of news stories have been written about it. The $14 million grant proposal contained damning information pertaining to gain-of-function work in collaboration with New York City-based EcoHealth Alliance, China's Wuhan Institute of Virology and the well-known U.S.-based gain-of-function scientist, Ralph Baric, of University of North Carolina, Chapel Hill. DARPA ultimately refused funding for the intended project, which planned to engineer a virus that resembles SARS-CoV-2, deeming it "too risky."

The following is an extract of a transcript of the Rixey interview.

CH: They [DARPA] refused it and for a couple of reasons, one of which being it looked like gain-of-function research, which it was. And what's interesting is that the Department of Defense used that as a reason to deny it even though technically the gain-of-function pause or moratorium had been lifted already. I think that they knew it was risky and they didn't want to mess with it for that reason. The other reason that they denied it, that people have not picked up on at all, that I was trying to raise awareness about, was the fact that they were talking about vaccinating bats but DARPA rejected that because they said that you don't want to make a vaccine for any animal, human or otherwise, with a partial epitope coverage of a vaccine.

SE: Can you explain what "partial epitope coverage" means?

CR: A partial epitope means they only use a portion of the virus in the vaccine. In fact, the grant proposal, it wasn't a lipid nanoparticle, but it was a very similar method to what they ended up using with mRNA. Right, so basically what they said was, in 2018, this is a stupid idea. This won't work especially with coronaviruses which are more prone to mutation and recombination than regular viruses. So, the Department of Defense, 18 months before the pandemic, rejected something almost exactly like mRNA technology. That is just so crazy, isn't it? What's even worse, the same Department of Defense that rejected that, another 18 months later, had the same vaccines mandated to all of their forces by the President of the United States.

What is also noteworthy is that the 2018 DEFUSE document details how they were going to introduce furin cleavage sites and sites binding DC-SIGN into coronaviruses. This is explained in another detailed article from Arkmedic's Substack. The author writes: "If you look through the proposal you probably won't make much of it because it looks like they were actually trying to look at 'defusing' the threat of coronaviruses. The only problem is that they weren't doing that at all. This is what they said they were going to do. In their words (the yellow highlights are the most important bits)" to use human ACE2 and grow in human cells. *S2 Proteolytic Cleavage and Glycosylation Sites:* After receptor binding, a variety of cell surface or endosomal proteases[68-71] cleave the SARS-CoV S glycoprotein causing massive changes in S structure [72] and activating fusion-mediated entry[64,73]. We will analyze all SARSr-CoV S gene sequences for appropriately conserved proteolytic cleavage sites in S2 and for the presence of potential furin cleavage sites[74,75]. SARSr-CoV S with mismatches in proteolytic cleavage sites can be activated by exogenous trypsin or cathepsin L. Where clear mismatches occur, we will introduce appropriate human-specific cleavage sites and evaluate growth potential in Vero cells and HAE cultures. In SARS-CoV, we will ablate several of these sites based on pseudotyped particle studies and evaluate the impact of select SARSr-CoV S changes on virus replication and pathogenesis. We will also review deep sequence data for low abundant high risk SARSr-CoV that encode functional proteolytic cleavage sites, and if so, introduce these changes into the appropr ate high abundant, low risk parental strain. *N-linked glycosylation:* Some glycosylation events regulate SARS-CoV particle binding DC-SIGN/L-SIGN, alternative receptors for SARS-CoV entry into macrophages or monocytes[76,77]. Mutations that introduced two new N-linked glycosylation sites may have been involved in the emergence of human SARS-CoV from civet and raccoon dogs[77]. While the sites are absent from civet and raccoon dog strains and clade 2 SARSr-CoV, they are present in WIV1, WIV16 and SHC014, supporting a potential role for these sites in host jumping. To evaluate this, we will sequentially introduce clade 2 disrupting residues of SARS-CoV and SHC014 and evaluate virus growth in Vero cells, nonpermissive cells ectopically expressing DC-SIGN, and in human monocytes and macrophages anticipating reduced virus growth efficiency. We will introduce the clade I mutations that result in N-linked glycosylation in rs4237 RBD deletion repaired strains, evaluating virus growth efficiency in HAE, Vero cells, or nonpermissive cells ± ectopic DC-SIGN expression[77]. *In vivo*, we will evaluate pathogenesis in transgenic hACE2 mice. *Low abundance micro-variations:* We will structurally model and identify highly variable residue changes in the SARSr-CoV S RBD, use commercial gene blocks to introduce these changes singly and in combination into the S glycoprotein gene of the low risk, parental strain and test ACE2 receptor usage, growth in HAE and *in vivo* pathogenesis.

Source: 'Absolute proof: The Gp-120 sequences prove beyond all doubt that "COVID-19" was man-made'[164]

In January 2022, Project Veritas, obtained a significant memorandum[165] written by former DARPA Fellow, Major Joseph P. Murphy to the Inspector General of the Department of Defense. The August 13, 2021, memorandum stated: "SARS-Cov-2 is an American-created recombinant bat vaccine, or its precursor virus. It was created by an Ecohealth Alliance program at the Wuhan Institute of Virology (WIV), as suggested by the reporting surrounding the lab leak hypothesis. The details of this program have been concealed since the pandemic began. These details can be found in the Ecohealth Alliance proposal response to the DARPA PREEMPT program Broad Agency Announcement (BBA) HR00118S0017, dated March 2018- a document not yet publicly disclosed."

The document Major Murphy was referring to, was the DEFUSE proposal, eventually leaked to Charles Rixey of the DRASTIC group and published online around September 2021.

## Moderna's Fingerprint

A further striking finding reported in a December 2021 article[166] from "Arkmedic's blog," is how the fourth HIV insert coding for the unique furin cleavage site, encompasses a 19-nucleotide sequence that happens to match a reverse complement sequence from a Moderna patent[167] filed in February 2016. The biotech's CEO, Stéphane Bancel, is listed as one of the inventors. The author wrote: "In order for that sequence to have arisen in that virus, the virus, which was manufactured with its HIV inserts, had to have been infected into patented cell lines supplied by Moderna that had that unique sequence not seen in any other virus."

A few months later, the scientific study "MSH3 Homology and Potential Recombinant links to SARS-CoV-2 Furin Cleavage Site" was eventually published after much difficulty in *Frontiers in Virology*[168] noting this alarming discovery. The scientists wrote: "A BLAST search revealed that a 19-nucleotide portion of the SARS-CoV-2 genome encompassing the furin cleavage site is a 100% complementary match to a codon-optimized proprietary sequence that is the reverse complement of the human mutS homolog (MSH3). The reverse complement sequence present in SARS-CoV-2 may occur randomly but other possibilities must be considered. Recombination in an intermediate host is an unlikely explanation...The presence of the 19-nucleotide long RNA sequence including the FCS with 100% identity to the reverse complement of the MSH3 mRNA is highly unusual and requires further investigations." The team also claimed that there was a one-in-three-trillion chance Moderna's sequence randomly appeared through natural evolution. The UK's *Daily Mail*[169] newspaper covered the findings, and Fox News host Maria Bartiromo[170] questioned Moderna's CEO Stéphane Bancel, who responded: "My scientists are looking into that data to see how accurate they are."

It is noteworthy that Moderna, DARPA-funded[171] and partnered with NIAID's Vaccine Research Center (VRC), finalized the sequence for their vaccine candidate mRNA-1273 on January 13, 2020, just a few days after China publicly shared the SARS-CoV-2 genome. This is discussed in further detail in chapter 9.

## The French Connection and the Many Problems at the WIV

Before heading up Moderna, Stephane Bancel was the CEO of bioMérieux (2007-2011), a French diagnostics company with significant business operations in the People's Republic of China (PRC). After the 2003 SARS pandemic, the Chinese contacted the French company bio-Merieux, owned by Alain Merieux, to design a level 4 bio facility (BSL-4) at the now infamous WIV. The project was approved by then-President of France, Jacques Chirac, and his Prime Minister, Jean-Pierre Raffarin, despite concerns from the French Ministry of Defense and French intelligence services. Raffarin himself described it as "a political agreement."

It took a decade for the facility to be built, at which time Bancel was head of bioMerieux and oversaw its design. Construction was completed in 2015 at a cost of $44 million but due to delays the BSL-4 space did not become operational until early 2018.[172]

An 84-page memo[173] released by Republicans on the House of Foreign Affairs Committee in August 2021, revealed: "In 2016, the PRC requested dozens of the containment suits required to work in the lab. The French Dual-Use Commission, tasked with considering exports of sensitive equipment, rejected their request. According to French reporting, the request was 'well above the needs of the Wuhan [lab].' This continued to fuel concerns within the French Ministry of Defense that the PRC was seeking to engage in military research or open a second BSL-4 lab for military means."

It should be noted that the PRC's request for "dozens of containment suits" in 2016 was made at the time when the BSL-4 space was not operational.

Two years later the U.S. State Department officials sent cables to Washington, D.C. highlighting concerns with safety issues at the WIV. The cables reported that scientists at the WIV noted "a serious shortage of appropriately trained technicians and investigators needed to safely operate this high-containment laboratory."

Furthermore, there were significant "safety concerns expressed by top PRC scientists in 2019 and unusually scheduled maintenance and repairs projects at the WIV." The memo also stated: "that researchers at the WIV, in conjunction with U.S. scientists and funded by both the PRC government and the U.S. government, were conducting gain-of-function research on coronaviruses at the WIV, at times under BSL-2 conditions."

BSL-2 conditions are commonly compared to the level of safety observed in a dentist's office.

In addition, according to the memo: "Athletes at the Military World Games held in Wuhan in October 2019 became sick with symptoms similar to COVID-19 both while in Wuhan and also shortly after returning to their home countries." This gives credibility to the theory that the virus was circulating in the latter part of 2019.

## Confessions to Congress

After years of denial from the NIH that it had not spent U.S. taxpayer dollars on funding gain-of-function research at the Wuhan Institute of Virology in China, its Principal Deputy Director, Lawrence Tabak, finally admitted to U.S. Congress on May 16, 2024, that it had.

During a session with the Select Subcommittee on the Coronavirus Pandemic, Rep. Debbie Lesko (R-Ariz.) questioned Tabak directly: "Dr. Tabak, did NIH fund gain-of-function research at the Wuhan Institute of Virology through EcoHealth?"

Tabak responded: "It depends on your definition of gain-of-function research. If you're speaking about the generic term, yes, we did."

He went on to add: "This is research, the generic term [gain-of-function], is research that goes on in many, many labs around the country. It is not regulated. And the reason it's not regulated is it poses no threat or harm to anybody."

It is astonishing how the Deputy Director of the NIH could state that gain-of-function research "poses no threat or harm to anybody" considering the catastrophic damage inflicted on society over the past few years not just from Covid but the containment measures, such as the lockdowns.

Tabak's admission transpired after four years of denials and evasions from U.S. federal public health officials, including himself and former NIAID Director Dr. Anthony Fauci, referenced earlier in this chapter.

During a hearing on May 1 before the House Select Subcommittee on the Coronavirus Pandemic, EcoHealth Alliance president Dr. Peter Daszak testified that his organization "never has and did not do gain-of-function research, by definition."

Chairman Brad Wenstrup (R-Ohio) of the House Select Subcommittee concluded: "EcoHealth Alliance President Dr. Peter Daszak is not a good steward of U.S. taxpayer dollars and should never again receive funding from the U.S. taxpayer. Dr. Daszak and his organization conducted dangerous gain-of-function research at the WIV, willfully violated the terms of a multi-million-dollar NIH grant, and placed U.S. national security at risk. This blatant contempt for the American people is reprehensible. It is imperative to establish higher standards of oversight at the NIH. The Select Subcommittee's detailed and comprehensive report today holds Dr. Daszak and EcoHealth Alliance accountable and sheds light on severe shortcomings in our public health systems."

Following on from the hearings, on May 15, 2024, the Department of Health and Human Services suspended[174] all grant funding for EcoHealth Alliance and proposed debarment. EcoHealth went on to dismiss Daszak as president.

On January 18, 2025, HHS formally debarred EcoHealth Alliance and its former president, for five years. Meanwhile, the former director of the National Institute of Allergy and Infectious Diseases, Anthony Fauci, went on to receive a pardon, one day before President Joe Biden left office. "I appreciate the action that President Biden has taken today on my behalf," Fauci said in a statement.[175]

After a two-year long investigation, the House Select Subcommittee on the Coronavirus Pandemic finally released their 520-page congressional report on the origin of the virus, titled "After Action Review of the COVID-19 Pandemic: The Lessons Learned and a Path Forward,"[176] on December 2, 2024. The key takeaways of the report summarized[177] by the subcommittee concluded that: "COVID-19 most likely emerged from a laboratory in Wuhan, China. The five strongest arguments in favor of the 'lab leak' theory include:

1. The virus possesses a biological characteristic that is not found in nature.
2. Data shows that all COVID-19 cases stem from a single introduction into humans. This runs contrary to previous pandemics where there were multiple spillover events.
3. Wuhan is home to China's foremost SARS research lab, which has a history of conducting gain-of-function research at inadequate biosafety levels.
4. Wuhan Institute of Virology (WIV) researchers were sick with a COVID-like virus in the fall of 2019, months before COVID-19 was discovered at the wet market.
5. By nearly all measures of science, if there was evidence of a natural origin it would have already surfaced."

• • •

In the March 2023 interview[178] with comedian and political commentator Jimmy Dore, Robert F. Kennedy Jr. alleged how the former Chief Medical Advisor to the U.S. President, Anthony Fauci had been in charge of developing bioweapons for the Pentagon since 2002, and in 2014, three viruses escaped from U.S. labs, so he moved his bioweapons research to the Wuhan lab. He asserted: "They took the money that Cheney gave them [from the Patriot Act], $2.2 billion, and they funneled it through NIH, and it all went through Anthony Fauci. So beginning in 2002, Anthony Fauci got a 68 percent raise from the Pentagon for doing bioweapons development, and he got a raise of billions of dollars a year, and then he started doing all of this gain-of-function.

In 2014, three of those bugs escaped in high-profile escapes from different labs in the U.S. Congress held hearings on it. Everybody was angry, and 300 top scientists sent letters to Obama saying you got to shut down Fauci because he is going to create a pandemic. So, Obama ordered a moratorium, and at that time, Fauci had eighteen different gain-of-function experiments he was doing around the U.S. He instead moved his stuff offshore to Wuhan, where he could do it out of sight of these 300 scientists and nosy White House officials who were trying to shut him down. And he continued to do it with the same people he was funding here, Ralph Baric and Peter Dazak, and they moved their operation to the Wuhan lab."

In his written testimony[179] to the U.S. Select Subcommittee on the Coronavirus Pandemic, Prof. Kristian Andersen stated: "Unfortunately, the important scientific question of the origin of the COVID-19 pandemic has been contorted by politics, while scientific discourse has been abandoned in pursuit of a preferred, coordinated narrative. The attacks directed against science and scientists are reckless and the effects far-reaching."

The evidence presented in the first two chapters supports the view that scientific discourse on the origin of COVID019 was heavily influenced by politics and institutional pressures. The irony, however, is that the "preferred, coordinated narrative" was the natural-origin hypothesis, advanced through the papers Andersen co-authored, while scientists who raised the possibility of a laboratory origin faced significant criticism and censorship (discussed in detail later in the book).

The late and former Secretary of State, Henry A. Kissinger penned an opinion piece for the Wall Street Journal entitled "The Coronavirus Pandemic Will Forever Alter the World Order,"[180] published on April 3, 2020. In it, he ominously declared, "When the COVID-19 pandemic is over, many countries' institutions will be perceived as having failed. Whether this judgment is objectively fair is irrelevant. The reality is the world will never be the same after the coronavirus." How uncannily prescient Kissinger's words turned out to be.

CHAPTER THREE

# "EXPERT" TAKEOVER

*"Now, as we collectively face down a global pandemic, we need these experts more than ever. And we need their voices, and their advice, to be full, frank and honest – our approach to this virus will always be guided by the scientific evidence."*

~Sir Patrick Vallance in *The Sun*, March 15, 2020[181]

In March 2021, while Britain was still gripped by the third national lockdown, I wrote the three-part investigative series "SAGE's Covert Coup,"[182] for *TCW*. In my view, this highlighted the unprecedented influence of the Scientific Advisory Group for Emergencies (SAGE), an unelected advisory body. The series examined who influenced Britain's pandemic response, its funding sources, and the potential shaping of advice. It pointed to connections among academics and advisers involving substantial funding from the Bill & Melinda Gates Foundation and the Wellcome Trust, alleged undeclared conflicts with pharmaceutical interests, and behavioral-science strategies that critics argue heightened fear to coerce compliance. The mainstream media did not cover the investigation at the time.

However, in December 2025, long after the lockdowns had ended and the harms had become irreversible, the *Daily Mail*[183] ran a headline reading: "Scientists who advised government during Covid did not reveal they had received more than £200m in grants from one of the world's biggest pharma investors, report says."

The article, based on a report by the campaign group UsForThem,[184] revealed that twenty-six SAGE members and their institutions had received more than £200 million from the Wellcome Trust, a charity with a vast investment portfolio linked to pharmaceutical companies, yet failed to declare these grants when advising ministers, appearing on television, or giving evidence to the Covid Inquiry.

While the *Daily Mail* presented this as a significant new revelation, elements of these funding connections and potential transparency issues were highlighted in my March 2021 investigation series. Written at a time, when greater scrutiny might arguably have made a difference. What follows is an adaptation of that investigation with the benefit of everything we know now.

## SAGE's Covert Coup: Part 1

Never before in UK history, in my view, have teams of statisticians, mathematical biologists, psychologists, anthropologists, behavioral scientists and epidemiologists working under the umbrella of SAGE[185] exerted such significant influence on government policy as during the past year.

On March 25, 2020, the Coronavirus Act received Royal Assent and was fast tracked through the government in four days. This act contained emergency powers[186] to enable public bodies to respond to the COVID-19 pandemic. Critics argue that SAGE and its subcommittees became the de-facto key drivers of the response, and it was the turning point when the UK ceased to be governed by elected officials. As an advisory body, SAGE is not directly accountable to the public. They advise the government on COVID-related matters, and the government has cited this advice on implementing the most stringent lockdown measures in our nation's history. In my view, SAGE has staged a "covert coup" in our country and hardly anybody has taken notice, let alone the mainstream media.

Below is a list of attendees from one of the early March SAGE meetings just before the first lockdown: Patrick Vallance (GCSA), Chris Whitty (CMO), Jonathan Van Tam (Deputy CMO), Steve Powis (NHS), Charlotte Watts (CSA DfID), Angela McLean (CSA MoD), John Aston (CSA HO), Sharon Peacock (PHE), Graham Medley (LSHTM), Neil Ferguson (Imperial), Brooke Rogers (King's College), James Rubin (King's College), Jeremy Farrar (Wellcome), David Halpern (CO), Ian Diamond (ONS), Tom Rodden (CSA DCMS), Aidan Fowler (NHS), Maria Zambon (PHE), Phil

Blythe (CSA DfT), Wendy Barclay (Imperial), Peter Horby (Oxford), John Edmunds (LSTHM), Carole Mundell (CSA FCO).

A closer examination of key experts reveals connections, in various ways, to pharmaceutical companies. technology firms, or major non-governmental organizations (NGOs), such as GAVI-The Vaccine Alliance, WHO, World Economic Forum, World Bank, Wellcome Trust and the Bill & Melinda Gates Foundation. Many have received substantial funding from the Bill & Melinda Gates Foundation and the Wellcome Trust. Reports indicate the UK has been a major beneficiary of university grants[187] given by the Gates foundation with $744 million disbursed to 38 universities, the top beneficiaries being: Imperial College London, UCL, LSTHM, King's College and Oxford University.

Several key SAGE members have held senior positions in the pharmaceutical industry prior to taking advisory roles in government and some reportedly still hold shares in related companies.

In December 2020, the *BMJ*[188] highlighted "the conflicts of interest among the UK government's COVID-19 advisors." Regarding Sir Patrick Vallance (Government Chief Scientific Advisor), the report noted: "By July the UK government had signed a coronavirus vaccine deal for an undisclosed sum with GlaxoSmithKline, securing 60 million doses of an untested treatment that was still being developed. In September, media outlets reported[189] that Vallance had £600 000 (€661 000; $800 000) worth of shares in the company."

Valance served as president of R&D at GSK from 2012-2017. During that time, in 2013, a new partnership between GSK and the Gates Foundation was announced to "accelerate research into vaccines for global health needs."

In the 2017 *BMJ Opinion* blog post,[190] the epidemiologist, Tom Jefferson, director of the Cochrane Collaboration's acute respiratory infections group, expressed concerns about pharmaceutical industry figures like Vallance, Witty and Van-Tam, assuming key advisory roles in the UK government.

As a researcher at the LHSTM, Prof. Chris Whitty was principal investigator on a consortium that received £31 million[191] from the Bill & Melinda Gates Foundation for malaria research; in 2020 he became the UK's Chief Medical Officer and Chief Scientific Advisor.

Prof. Jonathan Van-Tam (Deputy Chief Medical Officer), joined the pharmaceutical industry as an associate director at SmithKline Beecham (now GSK) in 2000. Van-Tam was the former Head of Medical Affairs at

Roche in 2001 and then went onto work at Aventis Pasteur MSD as the UK medical director the following year in 2002.

Van-Tam chaired the ECDC expert advisory group on H5N1 vaccines and advised the WHO during the H5N1 influenza (Bird Flu) pandemic in 2009- 2010. The WHO in turn triggered countries around the world, including the UK to buy enormous quantities of the drug oseltamivir (brand name: Tamiflu) produced by the pharmaceutical companies Roche and GSK, former employers of Van-Tam.

A 2010 investigation[192] by the *BMJ* and the Bureau of Investigative Journalism noted that some key scientists advising the World Health Organization on planning for an influenza pandemic had "declarable financial ties with drug companies that were producing antivirals and influenza vaccines. As an example, WHO's guidance on the use of antivirals in a pandemic was authored by an influenza expert who at the same time was receiving payments from Roche, the manufacturer of oseltamivir (Tamiflu), for consultancy work and lecturing."

Four years later, a BBC[193] article stated: "Tamiflu: Millions wasted on flu drug, claims major report." It went on to state: "Hundreds of millions of pounds may have been wasted on a drug for flu that works no better than paracetamol, a landmark analysis has said."

This was based on The Cochrane Collaboration[194] (a global non-profit organization of 14,000 academics) review on Tamiflu. Prof. Carl Heneghan Director, Centre for Evidence-based Medicine, University of Oxford, stated that the side effects of Tamiflu "included serious psychiatric adverse events, renal and metabolic adverse events."

## Part 2: Project Fear

SAGE's key subcommittees are: SPI-M[195] (Scientific Pandemic Influenza Group on Modelling) and SPI-B[196] (Scientific Pandemic Insights Group on Behaviors).

At the heart of SAGE is SPI-M. It's been driving government policy ever since the "war on COVID-19" began. The man who ran the SPI-M, at the initial start of the pandemic, was Prof. Neil Ferguson. He is also acting director of Vaccine Impact Modelling Consortium (VIMC) based at Imperial College London, which is closely tied to GAVI-The Vaccine Alliance, funded by the Bill & Melinda Gates Foundation.

Neil Ferguson's prior modeling has faced strong criticism: during the 2001 Foot and Mouth Disease outbreak, his epidemiological models influenced the UK government to pre-emptively cull over 6 million animals, at an estimated £10 billion[197] cost to the UK economy. As a result, the British farming community was utterly devastated.

Later, Prof. Michael Thrusfield of Edinburgh University, an expert in animal diseases, described Ferguson's modeling during the Foot and Mouth disease period as "severely flawed"[198] and "not fit for purpose." Ferguson's predictions of the worst-case scenario were seen as grossly over-estimated.

Similar critiques arose for the 2005 Bird Flu predictions, when Ferguson claimed that up to 200 million[199] people worldwide would die during the outbreak and up to 750,000 in the UK. This led to the stockpiling of Tamiflu in the UK from 2006 and it was widely prescribed later in the Swine Flu pandemic. The WHO was only able to link 78 deaths worldwide to the Bird Flu virus.

In the 2009 Swine Flu pandemic, Imperial's model led by Ferguson gave rise to the prediction of 65,000 deaths[200] from Swine Flu in the UK. In fact, only 457 deaths were linked to the virus. Based on Ferguson's model, the government spent a staggering £1.2 billion[201] to prepare for the Swine Flu pandemic. As a result of the government's preparations, over 20 million unused doses of vaccines were left as a stockpile in England.

Once more, it was Ferguson's modeling prediction in the March 16, 2020 "Report 9"[202] from the Imperial College COVID-19 response team that gave the dire warning of approximately 510,000 deaths by the end of May 2020 in the UK, if the government continued with its herd immunity response to the pandemic. This catastrophic prediction caused Boris Johnson to make an abrupt U-turn[203] and steered the course for draconian restrictions and lockdowns ever since. It was only after Ferguson was caught flouting the rules[204] in May 2020 by visiting his mistress that he resigned from SAGE (but he is still a member of the UK government body NERVTAG). Despite serious questions raised about the accuracy of Ferguson's modeling, he has continued to advise the government on pandemic response. It's worth noting that he was also very influential[205] in Boris' Christmas U-turn.

Just as SPI-M provides the mathematical modeling that informed lockdown policies, SPI-B supplies the behavioral science insights. In my view, it formed a key component of what I describe as a "PsyOp." I use the term "PsyOp" in its literal sense, meaning[206] a psychological operation or psychological warfare defined as "any action which is practiced mainly by psychological methods with the aim of evoking a planned psychological reaction in other people." Critics argue that this contributed to the fear-based approaches underpinning the lockdowns, which can be described as inhumane and disastrous, with estimates from early reports suggesting indirect costs including up 200,000 lives[207] lost over time (from delayed treatments and other harms) and economic impacts reaching around £2.4bn a day.[208]

And what was the planned "psychological reaction" that needed to be evoked by SAGE? The reaction of fear. Some analyses suggest the aim was to induce widespread fear so the public would more readily accept restrictions. This pattern of using fear in crises has been echoed throughout history.

The Johnson government, drawing on SPI-B's behavioral recommendations, developed a large-scale messaging campaign for COVID-19. The government spent hundreds of millions of pounds, more than £184 million[209] in 2020 alone, according to Cabinet Office figures, of taxpaers' money funding messages like this.

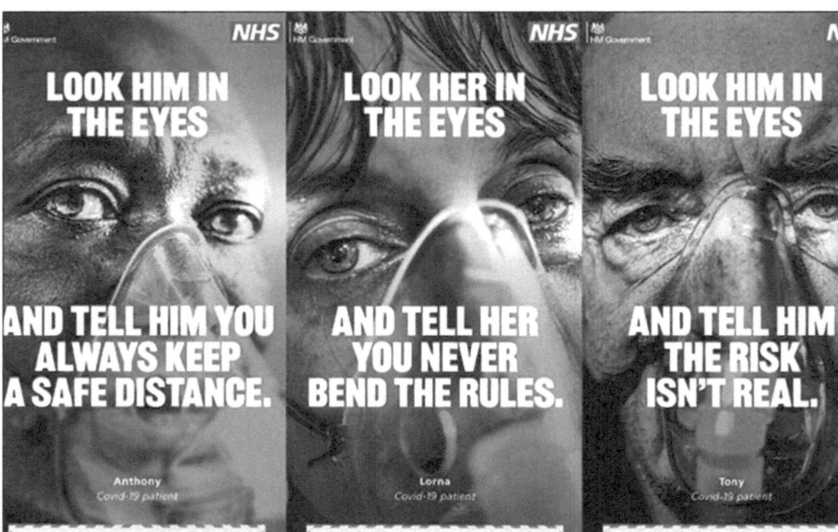
NHS
LOOK HIM IN THE EYES
AND TELL HIM YOU ALWAYS KEEP A SAFE DISTANCE.
Anthony
STAY HOME › PROTECT THE NHS › SAVE LIVES
NHS
LOOK HER IN THE EYES
AND TELL HER YOU NEVER BEND THE RULES.
Lorna
STAY HOME › PROTECT THE NHS › SAVE LIVES
LOOK HIM IN THE EYES
AND TELL HIM THE RISK ISN'T REAL.
Tony
STAY HOME › PROTECT THE NHS › SAVE LIVE

In order to understand the behavioral science behind the campaign of fearmongering- take a look at a screen shot from the March 22, 2020 SAGE meeting.[210]

| | | | | | | | |
|---|---|---|---|---|---|---|---|
| 2. | Use media to increase sense of personal threat | HIGH | HIGH | HIGH IF ACCOMPANIED BY OTHER OPTIONS | HIGH | COULD BE NEGATIVE | UNCERTAIN |
| 3. | Use media to increase sense of responsibility to others | HIGH | HIGH | HIGH IF ACCOMPANIED BY OTHER OPTIONS | HIGH | POSITIVE | UNCERTAIN |
| 4. | Use media to promote positive messaging around actions | HIGH | HIGH | HIGH IF ACCOMPANIED BY OTHER OPTIONS | HIGH | POSITIVE | UNCERTAIN |
| 5. | Tailor messaging | HIGH | HIGH | HIGH IF ACCOMPANIED BY OTHER OPTIONS | HIGH | UNCERTAIN | UNCERTAIN |
| 6. | Use and promote social approval for desired behaviours | HIGH | HIGH | COULD BE HIGH | HIGH | POSITIVE | UNCERTAIN |
| 7. | Consider enacting legislation to compel required behaviours | COULD BE HIGH IF EQUITY ISSUES ADDRESSED | DEPENDS ON TIMESCALE | COULD BE HIGH IF ACCEPTABLE AND ENFORCED | UNCERTAIN DEPENDING ON LEVEL OF ENFORCMENT | COULD BE NEGATIVE | COULD BE NEGATIVE |
| 8. | Consider use of social disapproval for failure to comply | UNCERTAIN | HIGH | COULD BE HIGH IF ACCOMPANIED BY OTHER MEASURES | HIGH | COULD BE NEGATIVE | COULD BE NEGATIVE |

Where I've circled, you can clearly see how the SPI-B subcommittee proposed the use of fear: "sense of personal threat" through the media and intimidation: "the use of social disapproval for failure to comply" against the trusting UK public. They even predicted that the overall effectiveness would be "HIGH." The only prediction they made with accuracy.

The report goes on to state, "There are nine broad ways of achieving behavior change: Education, Persuasion, Incentivization, Coercion, Enablement, Training, Restriction, Environmental restructuring, and Modelling."

Notably, "Coercion" is explicitly listed as an effective way of achieving behavior change in this report. The current government adopted the technique of coercion diligently through its 2020 Coronavirus Act and subsequent draconian laws- with the police handing out fines to people who illegally sat on a park bench, for example.

In summary, the SPI-B report highlighted the need for all three elements: fear, intimidation, and coercion. They were all incorporated into the production of a highly effective messaging/propaganda campaign against the public by the UK government, all paid for by the taxpayer.

## Part 3: The Mass Behavioral Experiment

A key SPI-B report[211] on "Increasing adherence to COVID-19 preventative behaviors among young people" was considered by SAGE on 22 October 2020. It provides an example, in my view, of how behavioral science was applied to encourage compliance amid reported declines in adherence among the 18-29 age group.

The report recommends various techniques to promote preventative behaviors. Some critics describe these as highly manipulative or ethically questionable. One such tactic is using "trusted" celebrities and commercial brands to influence the behavior of young people.

> - Communications targeting young people should where possible be **delivered by trusted**, non-governmental sources e.g. charities, celebrities, sports clubs, commercial brands.

Another suggests providing young people with "free mobile phones data, streaming and gaming," which is a form of inducement to encourage change.

Peer pressure and social conformity are central to other suggested approaches.

> - Communications should draw upon social norms of effective adherence by emphasising what other peers are doing *(descriptive* e.g. your peers are switching to socialising online) and approved perceptions of behaviours (*injunctive* e.g. your peers think you should start socialising online)

Key contributors to this and related papers (e.g., the March 22 SPI-B report) include Prof. Susan Michie, member of SPI-B, psychologist, professor of health psychology at University College London. Michie is director of UCL's Centre for Behavior Change and Health Psychology Research Group. Michie has been a political activist with the Communist Party of Britain for over 40 years and serves as a consultant advisor to WHO on COVID-19 and behavior. Her Human Behavior Change Project (HBCP) is funded by the Wellcome Trust.

Michie was reportedly among the prominent SAGE voices advocating school closures, describing them as "unsafe."[212] However, as noted in earlier analyses, a European Centre for Disease Prevention and Control (ECDC) report[213] (August 2020) found schools to be very low transmission settings for COVID-19, with significantly low child-to-child transmission and child to adult transmission.

The subsequent policy U-turn, cancelling Christmas plans and closing schools on the eve of the new school term, illustrates, in my view, the pattern of government responses during the crisis, with SAGE presenting stricter positions and the Prime Minister yielding.

Dr. David Halpern, psychologist, SPI-B member is head of the Behavioural Insights Team (BIT), unofficially known as the Nudge Unit, (since its formation in 2010) co-owned in part by Halpern, its employees, the Cabinet Office and the innovation charity Nesta. The group's revenues in 2017 climbed by a third to £14 million[214] and nearly 40% of that income came from overseas. Its worldwide offices have clients that range from government bodies to The World Bank.

BIT came under scrutiny when Private Eye criticized Halpern's high salary of £200,000 and for charging the government for work it used to do itself. It's worth noting, Halpern was a former member of Tony Blair's strategy unit and was the first to bring[215] "behavioral science" to Whitehall.

BIT is governed by "nudge" theory, conceived by Nobel Prize winning economist Richard Thaler that states governments can tweak people's behavior in subtle ways to avoid legislating and ordering.

In 2018, Halpern gave a video presentation[216] for the London Business Forum, explaining more about this "very light touch way of prompting human behavior." Some argue that this evolved from benign prompts to strong fear-based techniques during lockdown, culminating in campaigns like "Look into my eyes."[217]

Prof. Stephen Reicher, professor of psychology at the University of St Andrews, a fellow of the Royal Society of Edinburgh, a leading authority on crowd psychology is another member of SPI-B.

Reicher wrote in the *Guardian*[218] that "Covid has done much to further the study of behavior by bringing it into people's homes and day-to-day conversations." This candid statement, combined with the documented SPI-B recommendations to manipulate public perception through fear-based messaging and social pressure, raises profound ethical questions about the application of behavioral science techniques at population scale without explicit public consent or acknowledgment.

Reicher blamed the government for the spike in cases in September caused by the "Spanish variant" because lockdowns were eased during the summer. He was the author of the piece in the *Guardian*:[219] "Don't blame 'selfish covidiots.' Blame the government." He advocated strongly for the third lockdown, and in late December, called for a "five-point emergency plan"[220] beyond vaccination.

The justification for the third lockdown was a variant of SARS-CoV-2 said to have arisen in Kent (variant B117). SPI-M estimated that it was up to 70% more transmissible than the previously circulating form of the virus, and that it "may be more deadly."[221]

The modeling was compiled by Prof. Neil Ferguson, his close associate Dr. Erik Volz (Imperial College) and other members of NERVTAG (the New and Emerging Respiratory Virus Threats Advisory Group). This group assesses emerging respiratory virus threats.

Volz later noted that the model that produced the "70% more transmissible" statistic was flawed. In an online COG-UK showcase event[222] on Dec 18, 2020, hosted by Prof. Sharon Peacock, Executive Director and Chair of the COVID-19 Genomics UK (COG-UK) consortium (funded by the Wellcome Trust), Volz talked about the data for the new variant being "very noisy and overly-dispersed." He spoke of "lots of pitfalls you can fall into when analyzing the data."

He used the A222V variant (which arose after UK holiday makers returned from Spain last summer) as a reference, where high-fatality predictions did not materialize. "Trends don't always pan out," Volz noted in his presentation. Yet, it was this flawed modeling data for the new variant that Volz himself declared as "too early to tell, we don't have enough data" along with Wendy Barclays' (NERVTAG member) preliminary genomic characterization[223] of the new strain, that led to Johnson cancelling Christmas and the UK going into a third hard lockdown with schools, colleges and universities being closed from January 5-March 8.

A *Daily Mail*[224] report revealed that minutes from the Friday Dec 18, NERVTAG meeting showed that many members had "only moderate confidence" that the new strain was more transmissible. Most members concluded that there was "currently insufficient data" on the new strain and opposed drastic action. After the meeting, Witty and Valance presented the data to Johnson, showing the new variant to be highly transmissible. Around the same time, upon briefing Parliament on lockdown needs based on his modeling, Ferguson told *The Times*:[225] "I didn't even do biology O-level. I'd never even thought about using mathematics to study biological systems. And there's something very nice about pandemics in particular, the way they behave mathematically."

On commenting on China's lockdown measures Ferguson said: "It's a communist one-party state, we said. We couldn't get away with it in Europe, we thought and then Italy did it. And we realized we could."

In my view, SAGE and its subgroups' strong influence ultimately led to the suspension of Britain's fundamental freedoms for over a year.

The letter[226] from GP, Anne McCloskey, to BMJ editor, highlights the dangers of the lack of public scrutiny of the advice given by these advisors. She writes: "Governments were advised in this course of action by scientists and medics whose identity, qualifications and aptitude for this work was largely hidden from public scrutiny. Even now, the conflicts of interest of these people on whose advice our futures depend are not publicly available."

It's high time for an independent public inquiry to investigate SAGE's modeling data and the conflicts of interest of the scientists and indeed our politicians.

• • •

As evidenced above, from March 2021, I called for a full independent public inquiry to investigate the UK government's response to Covid. It took until June 2022 for an official UK COVID-19 Inquiry,[227] Chaired by Baroness Heather Hallett, a former Court of Appeal judge, to be set up, with the first public hearing held on 4 October of that year. The TaxPayers' Alliance[228] estimates that the Covid Inquiry is projected to be almost £277 million (£70 million higher than the original December 2023 estimate). The inquiry is widely described as one of the most expensive in UK history.

## The Questioning of the Experts

Critics have argued that the Covid Inquiry has been nothing more than a "vast white-washing exercise"[229] with its soft-line of questioning aimed at those whose decisions resulted in highly damaging lockdowns and manipulating the public with scare tactics. It has also enabled certain experts to use it as a platform to assert that locking the country down should have happened sooner and their messaging was not aimed at frightening the public but of "empowerment."

Take for instance, Prof. Stephen Reicher who was referenced in Part 3 of my *TCW* report. In his witness statement[230] made on March 27, 2023, he stated: "It has been estimated that this delay [in lockdown] was highly consequential in terms of the size of the first wave of COVID. Had measures been taken a week earlier some 30,000 lives could have been saved, two weeks earlier and the number could have been over 40,000."

He then went on: "To quote New Zealand Prime Minister Jacinda Ardern, the key thing is to 'go hard and go early.' Her words are supported by evidence that shows that those countries which acted in this way performed better not only in terms of health but also in terms of the economy and civil liberties. If there is one lesson about strategy, then, it is that dither and delay are the very worst options."

Reicher's open admiration for New Zealand's response to Covid, under Jacinda Ardern's leadership, and his claim that it "performed better in terms of civil liberties" is quite astonishing, when New Zealanders suffered under the most severe lockdowns in the world, where civil liberties were prohibited not promoted. The country closed its borders and went into full lockdown (level 4) shortly after the first single case was reported.

According to an article in *The Sydney Morning Herald*: [231]"New Zealand knows how to do a lockdown. In fact, one of the defining characteristics of Ardern's 'go hard, go early' strategy has been the deployment of strict lockdowns that would make most Australians wince."

It is noteworthy that in 2008, Jacinda Ardern, former leader of New Zealand's Labour party was elected president of the International Union of Socialist Youth,[232] shortly after her stay in London as an advisor to the Cabinet Office under Tony Blair's premiership. Her role as the International Socialist Youth president also saw her spend time in China.

In 2014, Ardern was chosen to participate in and completed the World Economic Forum's (WEF) Forum of Young Global Leaders, established by Klaus Schwab.

In a 2017 interview, Klaus Schwab highlighted that several prominent leaders such as then-German Chancellor Angela Merkel and Russian President Vladimir Putin, had been part of the Young Global Leaders initiative. Schwab expressed pride in this "young generation," citing Canadian Prime Minister Justin Trudeau as an example, where "more than half of his cabinet" were Young Global Leaders.

Turning back to Reicher's statement: "This general approach, with an emphasis on building a sense of shared identity, on creating positive relationships with the public and of working with the public ran through the documents produced by SPI-B. Sadly, however, these principles were generally ignored by Government."

Yet, in March 22, 2020, a document entitled, "Options for increasing adherence to social distancing measures"[233] that was "prepared by SAGE's behavioral science sub-group SPI-B" of which Reicher was part of, the members wrote: "The perceived level of personal threat needs to be increased among those who are complacent, using hard-hitting emotional messaging." It is astounding to think that a document like this, crafted by SPI-B, employing such overt fear and manipulation tactics, could ever be considered as fostering "positive relationships with the public."

Furthermore, contrary to Reicher's claim, the Government did not ignore SPI-B's "principles"; rather, they fully embraced them by implementing a "Project Fear" campaign, with the sole purpose to "frighten the pants off everyone"[234] as epitomized by former UK Health Minister, Matt Hancock, in his leaked WhatsApp message to his advisor from December 2020.

## Defending the Indefensible

When asked by the Inquiry: "If the Government was sold on using fear, was this because of or despite the advice of SPI-B?" Reicher responded: "one sentence from one SPI-B paper" was taken "out of context." He asserted: "The evidence for arguing that it was because of SPI-B is based on one sentence from one SPI-B paper. The sentence reads: 'the perceived level of personal threat needs to be increased among those who are complacent, using hard-hitting emotional messaging.' At first glance this might seem persuasive. But that depends upon taking the quote out of context and misunderstanding the argument as a whole. The next sentence in the SPI-B document reads: 'To be effective this must also empower people by making clear the actions they can take to reduce the threat.' In other words, if you want people to act, you must first of all confront them with the real risks."

The controversial SPI-B paper most certainly confronted the public with the "real risks" whilst simultaneously establishing a culture of fear and panic. Reicher's testimony characterized the fear-based messaging recommendation as merely "one sentence from one SPI-B paper," taken out of context. However, examination of the March 22, 2020 document reveals that recommendations to increase fear, employ social disapproval, and utilize coercion comprised a substantial portion of the paper's strategic advice. Beyond the single sentence Reicher referenced: "the perceived level of personal threat needs to be increased among those who are complacent," the document explicitly identified "Coercion" as an effective method for achieving behavior change, and detailed multiple techniques for using fear and social pressure to ensure compliance.

Another expert, Professor Susan Michie from SPI-B (referenced in Part 3 of my report), was summoned to provide a witness statement[235] for the Covid Inquiry. Her testimony echoes Reicher's denial of employing overt fear tactics on the public, despite evidence to the contrary found in the March 2020 SPI-B report.

In her August 22, 2023, statement she claims: "I do not recall 'nudge theory' being used by SPI-B in its work or reports. I do not know if it was used by those charged with considering behavioral issues within the Cabinet Office or other parts of Government, as SPI-B was not informed about their work. I also do not agree with the assertion that SPI-B was responsible for driving a culture of fear and do not believe that SPI-B ever used the phrase 'culture of fear' in its work. Scrutiny of the published reports of SPI-B's work and advice should make it clear that any accusations that SPI-B promoted unethical psychological techniques to encourage behavioral change are unfounded. SPI-B was certainly not undertaking a psychological experiment on the British population, as has been suggested."

Michie went on to reference the SPI-B document "Options for increasing adherence to social distancing measures" (March 22, 2020), which advised: "The perceived level of personal threat needs to be increased among those who are complacent, using hard-hitting emotional messaging." In her evidence (including oral testimony during Module 2 hearings), she noted that she did not recall any specific contributions she may have made to the meeting that produced this document. She maintained that she would not view the advice contained in it as "unwise or unethical." She further characterized the recommended messaging as designed to "empower people to act, not to scare them."

Yet this portrayal of behavioural messaging as primarily "empowering" rather than fear-driven was far from unanimous even within SPI-B. Strikingly, in a May 2021 *Telegraph*[236] report, fellow committee member Gavin Morgan (a psychologist who contributed to the group's work) expressed deep regret over the tactics, describing the deliberate use of fear as unethical and reminiscent of totalitarian methods: "Clearly, using fear as a means of control is not ethical. Using fear smacks of totalitarianism..It's not an ethical stance for any modern government. By nature I am an optimistic person, but all this has given me a more pessimistic view of people."

In sharp contrast, Professor Susan Michie concluded her witness statement to the UK COVID-19 Inquiry by asserting: "I have seen no evidence that the population as a whole was overly fearful of COVID-19, let alone that this was because of government communications exaggerating the risks. At the start of the pandemic the Westminster government was arguably overly complacent, reassuring the public that COVID-19 was mild for most people."

This claim invites scrutiny, particularly given the irony: Michie faults the government for early complacency in downplaying severity for the majority, yet that very reassurance aligned with contemporaneous evidence. On March 19th the UK's Health Security Agency announced "COVID-19 is no longer considered to be a High Consequence Infectious Disease (HCID) in the UK."[237] Early data further reinforced this perspective. Stanford epidemiologist Professor John Ioannidis' comprehensive 2022 analysis[238] of pre-vaccination national seroprevalence studies estimated the infection fatality rate (IFR) for those under 70 at a median of 0.095% (with even lower figures for younger subgroups, e.g., 0.034% median for 0-59 years).

What prompted the UK government to pivot so decisively from its initial "herd immunity" approach to imposing nationwide lockdowns in March 2020? A key catalyst is presented in the following chapter.

It is astonishing that the Professor of Health Psychology and Director of the Centre for Behaviour Change at University College London stated in her witness evidence to the UK COVID-19 Inquiry that she had seen "no evidence that the population as a whole was overly fearful of COVID-19, let alone that this was because of government communications exaggerating the risks." This assertion contrasts sharply with substantial evidence of widespread psychological impacts during the pandemic. Research has documented a marked rise in mental health difficulties, including heightened anxiety, depression, and specific fear-related syndromes, often linked to perceptions of risk amplified by public health messaging and restrictions. A notable example is COVID Anxiety Syndrome,[239] characterized by symptoms like health anxiety and compulsive behaviors such as frequent handwashing.

David Halpern, referenced in Part 3 of my report and head of the Behavioral Insights Team (BIT), also known as the Nudge Unit, (which incorporates the very "Nudge theory," a concept Susan Michie appeared unable to recall during questioning) stated in an interview with *The Telegraph*[240] that the government's use of fear tactics during the pandemic was warranted. He asserted, "There are times when you do need [fear] to cut through... particularly if you think people are wrongly calibrated."

In January 2022, MPs launched an investigation into the "grossly unethical tactics to scare public into Covid compliance." This was prompted by a letter written by a group of psychologists to Parliament's Public

Administration and Constitutional Affairs Committee. They warned that civil servants and Government scientists used frightening imagery to change public behavior during the pandemic, in a way they say was "unaccountable and unethical."

According to *The Telegraph*:[241] "The letter's 40 professional signatories - led by Dr. Gary Sidley, a retired clinical psychologist - said they opposed the use of dramatic adverts, which included slogans such as: "If you go out you can spread it, people will die."

Nevertheless, against the backdrop of the widespread condemnation of SAGE's fear tactics, the UK Government Resilience Framework[242] praised SAGE's "expert sub-groups," stating how their "high-quality science advice" played and "will continue to play a vital role in supporting government decision makers during active emergencies."

## Programming Fear and Compliance

The UK government's messaging was not limited to advertising campaigns. It also pushed for prescribed narratives to be incorporated into popular TV programs, such as EastEnders and Coronation Street.

In June 2025, in response to British independent journalist, Lewis Brackpool's Freedom of Information request, a disturbing series of redacted emails and "Official Sensitive" documents[243] from the UK's Department for Culture, Media and Sport (DCMS) revealed repeated government engagement with broadcasters (ITV, BBC, Channel 4, etc.) to promote specific COVID-19 messages, such as "stay at home."

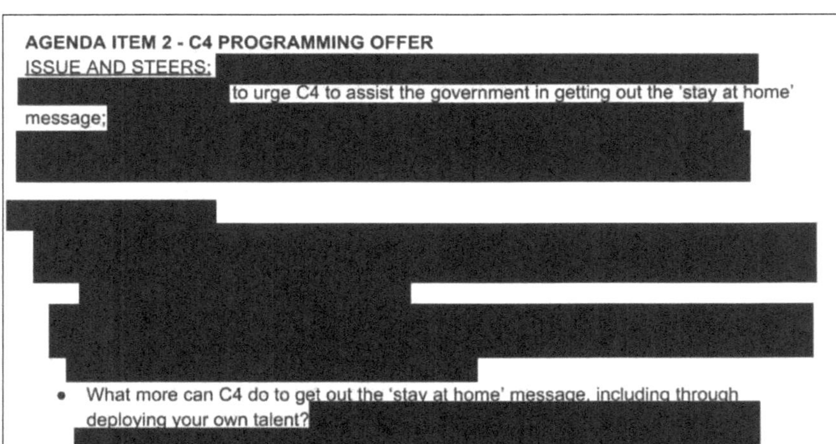

**AGENDA ITEM 2 - C4 PROGRAMMING OFFER**

ISSUE AND STEERS:

to urge C4 to assist the government in getting out the 'stay at home' message;

- What more can C4 do to get out the 'stay at home' message, including through deploying your own talent?

The 26 March and 1 April 2020 secret roundtables urged broadcasters to create "national unity" content and amplify government messages. The Minister for Media and Data (MMD) specifically asked about incorporating health messages into soap opera storylines.

> MMD asked if there were plans to introduce health messages into soap stories. ITV and BBC noted these had been filmed previously and filming had now ceased, however ITV have included voiceovers to episodes now to clarify govt messaging re social distancing. BBC committed to report back re other shows.

Government messaging, later changed to "encourage" Covid vaccine uptake. The following screenshot of a document reveals the Department of Health (DH), in coordination with the Department for Culture, Media and Sport (DCMS) brazen desire to use vaccine propaganda, by considering sending a joint letter to ITV to encourage the inclusion of "pro-vaccine messaging" in their soap opera storylines. Government officials specifically wanted to target "hard to reach groups" such as lower socio-economic and BAME communities.

> - **Vaccines:** Officials at the Department of Health have been in contact with DCMS to query whether ITV would be willing to assist with pro vaccine messaging in their content. As well as re-iterating public health messages about the safety of vaccines, DH are keen to engage with hard to reach groups (eg. lower socio economic and BAME groups). In particular DH has proposed writing to ITV (joint DH/DCMS letter) to ask them to consider including vaccine storylines in their soaps. Whilst we do not think it would be appropriate to write to ITV on this matter given the importance of broadcasters' operational and editorial independence, you may wish to explore with them whether they already have plans to develop content related to this area. An initial readout from ITV's meeting with BEIS indicates that they are planning soap storylines related to the environment and climate change and therefore they may be amenable to the idea of something similar in relation to vaccine messaging.

*The Telegraph*[244] covered these Freedom of Information requests, reporting that "Pro-vaccine messaging did end up in soaps. In one episode of EastEnders in April 2021, Patrick Trueman told Suki Panesar he felt like he had 'won the lottery' after getting his second vaccination. In the same clip, Karen Taylor was accused of being an 'anti-vaxxer' for worrying that they had developed the vaccine too quickly."

Notably, during the 1 April 2020 roundtable, ITV's CEO Carolyn McCall complained about the "unique issue of having large viewer numbers but low advertising revenue." This financial strain, combined with government requests for specific messaging, raises concerns about whether broadcasters felt compelled to comply with government suggestions to secure financial support.

Lewis Brackpool, the journalist who secured the damning FOI documents, offered me his perspective on their revelations: "The findings won't shock anyone who's noticed the recurring pattern of government storylines being embedded into fictional television. But to have it confirmed, especially when written evidence on the subject is so scarce, is still a jolt to the mind. These subtler methods of shifting public perception would make the Soviets blush. And yet, stepping into the shoes of a government institution, it's frustrating to admit that it does make sense if the aim is to seed a particular message or agenda."

## Where Are the Experts Now?

Since the publication of my investigative series in 2021, the influential experts in the Government's response to Covid have moved on to greener pastures. Take for instance, Sir Jonathan Van Tam, the UK's former Deputy Chief Medical Officer who became a household name during the pandemic. He stepped down from his government position in March 2022 and in a "revolving door" move went on to take the role of senior medical consultant[245] with COVID-19 vaccine developer, Moderna, in August 2023.

It must be noted that a Daily Sceptic article[246] authored by Drs. Carl Heneghan and Tom Jefferson reported that: "AstraZeneca declared a payment of £5,892 in 2022 to Jonathan Van-Tam, the former Deputy Chief Medical Officer for England and member of the U.K.'s Vaccine Task Force – a payment which Van-Tam has not declared as a potential conflict of interest in academic work such as this SARS-CoV-2 study."

In July 2022, Prof. Susan Michie was appointed[247] Chair of the WHO's Behavioral Advisory Group to advise the United Nations agency on how to increase adherence to vaccination campaigns and other initiatives that influence national health policy.

Sir Jeremy Farrar, former Director of the Wellcome Trust, participant of the UK government's Vaccine Task Force and Scientific Advisory Group for Emergencies (SAGE) was appointed[248] Chief Scientist of the World Health Organization (WHO) in 2023.

Sir Patrick Vallance, former Chief Scientific Adviser and chair of SAGE, who reportedly held £600,000 worth of shares in GSK (the same pharmaceutical company contracted by the UK government to develop a coronavirus vaccine), was appointed[249] Minister of State for Science, Innovation, and Technology under Sir Keir Starmer's new Labour government in July 2024. To circumvent the fact that he was an unelected Member of Parliament, Sir Patrick received a life-long peerage enabling him to sit in the House of Lords.

At the time of this book's publication, Chris Whitty remains the Chief Medical Officer (CMO) for England, continuing to advise the UK government on public health matters.

The COVID Inquiry has already cost taxpayers over £210 million (up to December 31, 2025, per the latest official financial report),[250] yet it avoids the one question that matters most: whose interests were they really serving when they demanded Britain be locked down?

CHAPTER FOUR

# LOCKDOWNS IN LOCKSTEP

*"Lockdown was an extreme and unprecedented response to an ancient problem, the challenge of epidemic disease. It was also something else. It marked one of the gravest governmental failures of modern times."*

~Former British Supreme Court Justice,
Lord Jonathan Sumption, *The Times*,
August 28, 2022

This chapter explores the global rollout of lockdowns, implemented by nations in near-synchronous lockstep. Governments insisted this non-pharmaceutical intervention was temporary, evidence-based, and essential to "flatten the curve" and prevent hospitals from being overwhelmed. However, it was an unproven, population-wide experiment that originated in post-9/11 U.S. biodefense planning and was first tested in Wuhan. The measure inflicted profound harm on society. The chapter exposes the deeply flawed modeling paper governments relied on to justify shutting down the world. It also highlights the stark hypocrisy of wine-and-cheese parties in Downing Street and the drug-fueled sex parties held by New York City's senior public health advisor, all while the public was barred from visiting dying relatives in care homes and hospitals. The chapter spotlights the resistance: Italian and Polish restaurateurs who defied closure orders; the scientists, doctors, and citizens who signed the Great Barrington Declaration; and the millions who took to the streets to reclaim their freedoms. Above all, more than five years later, it confronts the question that still haunts us. How did so many democracies surrender their liberties so swiftly and on the word of so few?

## "Thank you, China"

On 23 January 2020, the Chinese government imposed the world's first complete lockdown of a major modern city: Wuhan, a metropolis of more than 11 million people. Within days, the measure was extended across nearly all of Hubei province, confining roughly 58 million residents.

During the 2003 SARS outbreak, China had pioneered the first large-scale quarantining of healthy, unexposed individuals, locking tens of thousands inside their homes for weeks at a time. Yet in 2003, those measures remained targeted; the rest of Beijing and other cities continued to function. However, in January 2020, for the first time in recorded history, an entire major city (and soon an entire province) was placed under total lockdown. Virtually all residents, the overwhelming majority of them healthy and with no known exposure to the virus, were prohibited from leaving their homes. Public transport was suspended, private vehicles were banned from the roads, and movement between neighborhoods was forbidden. Disturbing footage circulated on social media of hazmat-suited workers welding apartment-block doors shut from the outside, with residents left screaming for help from high-rise balconies.

A certain influential person who chose not to condemn China's actions but thanked them instead, was Sir Jeremy Farrar, then-director of the Wellcome Trust. He took to social media to praise China for "setting a new standard for outbreak response."

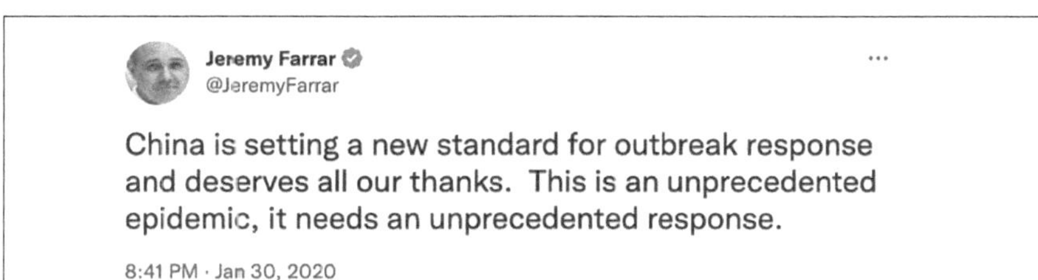
Jeremy Farrar
@JeremyFarrar

China is setting a new standard for outbreak response and deserves all our thanks. This is an unprecedented epidemic, it needs an unprecedented response.

8:41 PM · Jan 30, 2020

Unlike Farrar's abrupt U-turn on Covid's origin discussed in the previous chapter, his advocacy for lockdowns has remained steadfast.

In 2014, Sir Farrar co-authored a scientific paper along with Dr. Christopher Whitty (Chief Medical Officer to England since 2019), Prof. Neil Ferguson (the same epidemiologist who authored the infamous COVID-19 modellng paper triggering the UK Government to order its first ever lockdown) and Prof. John Edmunds (epidemiologist and member of New and Emerging Respiratory Virus Threats Advisory Group (NERVTAG) and of the Scientific Advisory Group for Emergencies (SAGE), which was published in *Nature*,[251] entitled, "Infectious disease: Tough choices to reduce Ebola transmission."

An abstract of the paper reads, "Whitty and colleagues explain why the United Kingdom is funding many small community centers to isolate suspected cases [of Ebola] in Sierra Leone." The authors went on to explain the UK government's proposal to build and support centers where people can self-isolate voluntarily, if they suspect they could have the disease. It could be argued that their paper acted as a progenitor of the UK's response to Covid. Only those "tough choices to reduce transmission" were made that much tougher, such as ordering the entire population (the healthy and suspected cases) to stay in their homes or face criminal charges if they "broke the rules."

Farrar has served on several UK government committees. In May 2020, he was appointed member of the UK's Vaccine Taskforce and SAGE, co-chaired by Sir Patrick Vallance (Chief Scientific Advisor to the UK Government from 2018-2023). Sir Jeremy was not only an early proponent of lockdowns but also pushed for the "vaccine plus" strategy-i.e.. more mask wearing and greater Covid testing.

In early November 2021, Farrar resigned from his role as a member of SAGE because of his frustration with the government's delay in introducing a further lockdown (the second of three). He even lamented about this in his book, *Spike: The Virus v The People* and how he had considered resigning from SAGE as early as September 2020 due to the rise in cases from the newly opened economy.

It is highly notable that from 2020-2021, the Wellcome Trust reaped the highest investment returns since the charity's creation. Its investment portfolio grew by almost £10bn[252] in just a single year. What stands out as the best investment pick was the U.S.-based food delivery company, DoorDash, which generated more than £1bn for the Trust because it happened to be such an early investor. It is widely acknowledged that food delivery businesses benefited substantially from the lockdowns. During this period, Jeremy Farrar, Director of the Wellcome Trust and a member of the UK's SAGE advisory group, was a vocal advocate for lockdown measures as part of the government's COVID-19 response. This overlap raises questions about potential conflicts of interest in pandemic policymaking.

On March 23, 2020, the UK's then-Prime Minister Boris Johnson announced[253] the country's first-ever lockdown, initially set to last three weeks "to flatten the curve." In stark reality, a series of extended lockdowns and stay-at-home orders spanned from March 2020 to June 2021. During this period, large parts of the economy were shut down, and "non-essential services." Shockingly schools, colleges, and places of worship were closed. Even sitting on public park benches was prohibited in post 3/11 Britain.

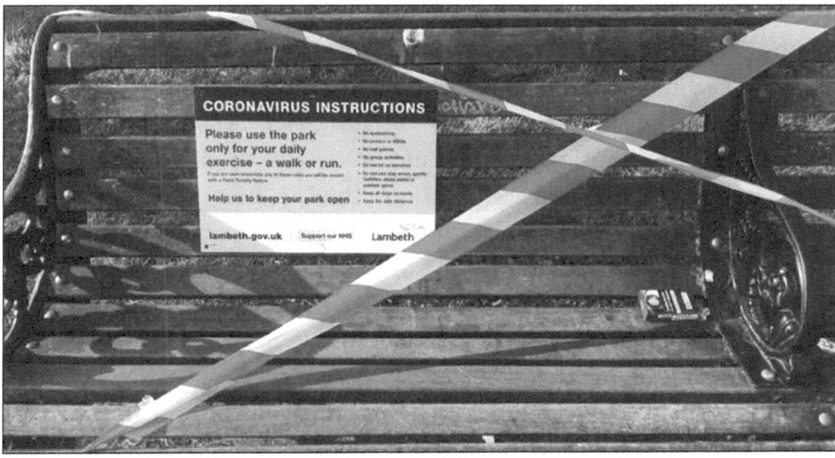
CORONAVIRUS INSTRUCTIONS
Please use the park
only for your daily
exercise – a walk or run.
Help us to keep your park open
lambeth.gov.uk
Lambeth

Source: Twitter @Rod_Porteous

However, emulating the People's Republic of China's coercive measures was not the UK government's initial strategy in dealing with the virus. The original plan was to achieve herd immunity by allowing it to spread through the population. On March 13, Sir Patrick Vallance, the UK government's Chief Scientific Adviser, told Sky News about the aim of building "herd immunity" by letting "enough of us who are going to get mild illness to become immune."

Justification for this measured approach was further reinforced by the UK Health Security Agency's (HSA) statement declaring[254] on March 19: "COVID-19 is no longer considered to be a High Consequence Infectious Disease (HCID) in the UK." A Freedom of Information Act release[255] revealed that the UKHSA's decision was based on the following factors: "In March, having several tests available to confirm cases and with more reliable data available to indicate a relatively low mortality rate (in comparison to other HCIDs), the scientific advice was that, whilst COVID-19 met some of the HCID criteria, it did not meet all of them and should no longer be regarded as an HCID."

So, what occurred then for the UK government to do such an abrupt U-turn from its herd immunity strategy and by declassifying Covid as a HCID?

The likely answer is the publishing on March 16th of Imperial College London's modeling paper predicting catastrophic hospitalizations and deaths, if various Non-Pharmaceutical Interventions (NPIs), such as the closure of schools and social distancing, were not implemented.

The paper entitled "Report 9"[256] by Prof. Neil Ferguson et al. stated: "In total, in an unmitigated epidemic, we would predict approximately 510,000 deaths in GB and 2.2 million in the U.S., not accounting for the potential negative effects of health systems being overwhelmed on mortality." Worldwide, Ferguson and his Imperial College London team predicted that in the "unmitigated" absence of interventions, COVID-19, "a virus with a comparable lethality to H1N1 influenza in 1918," could infect 7 billion, resulting in 40 million deaths.

This white paper sent shock waves around the world with the media playing a significant role in the spreading of its alarmist projections, greatly influencing public opinion and global government policies. The very next day, the UK media announced that the country was going to lockdown. In lockstep, the U.S. and other countries embraced the doomsday scenarios illustrated in Ferguson's modeling paper and triggered their own unprecedented lockdowns.

A March 16th 2020, New York Times article[257] reported: "Asked at a news conference with President Trump about what had led to the change in thinking by a White House task force, Dr. Deborah Birx, one of the task force leaders, said new information had come from a model developed in Britain."

The article went on to state: "The lead author of the study, Neil Ferguson, an epidemiology professor, said in an interview that his group had shared their projections with the White House task force about a week ago and that an early copy of the report was sent over the weekend."

My "SAGE's Covert Coup" report highlighted in the previous chapter, discussed the extensive history of Imperial College London's colossally defective modeling led by Prof. Neil Ferguson. To remind the reader, Ferguson and his team predicted up to 150,000 deaths from CJD (Mad Cow Disease) which led to the culling of approximately 11 million cattle, resulting in significant economic losses for farmers and the agricultural industry. In stark contrast to Ferguson's dire prediction, the actual number of deaths attributed to CJD was 2,704. Ferguson went on to make even more dire predictions: claiming up to 200 million people would die from H5N1 avian flu (bird flu), resulting in the culling of millions of birds, devastating the poultry industry. The actual number of deaths reported worldwide was just 455.

Considering Ferguson's remarkably poor track record, it is astonishing how only a handful of individuals challenged the dire forecasts presented in "Report 9," hailed as "the most influential scientific paper," which prompted over a hundred countries to implement lockdowns in lockstep.

## Ferguson's Flawed Lockdown Paper

The day after Ferguson's paper was published, The New York Times reported,[258] "It wasn't so much the numbers themselves, frightening though they were, as who reported them: Imperial College London...Imperial College has advised the government on its response to previous epidemics, including SARS, avian flu and swine flu. With ties to the World Health Organization and a team of 50 scientists, led by a prominent epidemiologist, Neil Ferguson, Imperial is treated as a sort of gold standard, its mathematical models feeding directly into government policies."

However, the "gold standard" of modeling used in Report 9 was in fact heavily flawed. The authors of the paper based their calculations on lab-confirmed symptomatic cases rather than actual infection rates, greatly inflating projected deaths and hospitalizations. They ignored evidence from early data, such as the Diamond Princess cruise ship, which indicated a much lower infection fatality ratio (IFR). Instead, the Imperial College data relied on the case fatality ratio (CFR) in Wuhan and not from the other places where the CFR was much lower.

Shockingly, the computer code used in the model was not publicly available nor peer reviewed, a crucial step in validating scientific findings. The code contained thousands of lines of "undocumented" code, making it difficult for others to understand or verify the model's assumptions and calculations. In addition, a senior software engineer from Google found the code riddled with amateurish errors, including giving different answers depending on the number of CPUs in the specific computer running the model, making the results unverifiable, and therefore completely unusable.[259]

Another key flaw with Ferguson and his team's modeling calculations is that they relied on the presumption of exponential growth of the virus.

What is noteworthy is how a number's man and winner of the 2013 Nobel Prize for Chemistry, the biophysicist, Michael Levitt, Professor of Structural Biology at the Stanford School of Medicine, began analyzing the number of COVID-19 cases from China in early January 2020. He noticed a crucial fact: the data was not supporting the "dire scenario" of millions of deaths predicted by many health experts, fueled by Ferguson's paper.

As early as February 2, Levitt published his "Analysis of nCov-2019 Data."[260] Among the most important of his observations was the data expressed in "Panel (E), which shows that the number of cases is growing more and more slowly. Specifically, the ratio of Deaths Today divided by Deaths Yesterday is decreasing. This decrease is monotonic for Total Deaths and Hubei Death since 1/25/2020 and linear for them both since 1/29/2020. This suggests by linear extrapolation that the number of new deaths will decrease very rapidly over the next week."

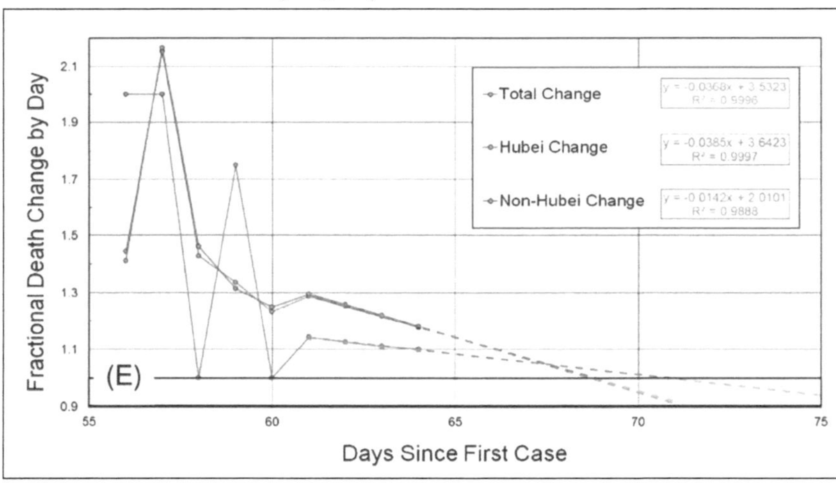


Source: Analysis of nCov-2019 Data, Panel E

On March 6, Levitt's critical and timely analysis was placed under the radar of Drs. Anthony Fauci and Francis Collins but it took a further 11 days for Fauci to forward it on to Dr. Andrea Lerner, an infectious diseases physician and medical officer in the Office of the Director of the National Institute of Allergy and Infectious Diseases of the NIH—and ask her opinion on the matter, coinciding with the time that Ferguson's paper was published.

**From:** Fauci, Anthony (NIH/NIAID) [E]
**Sent:** Tue, 17 Mar 2020 02:59:48 +0000
**To:** Lerner, Andrea (NIH/NIAID) [E]
**Subject:** FW: Modeling of COVID-19 from Mike Levit
**Attachments:** 1.Analysis_of_Coronavirus-2019_Data_Michael_Levitt-v1.pdf, 1.The_Corona_Chronologies. Part II - Rest of the World. Michael_Levitt,Stanford.pdf, 30.The_Corona_Chronologies. Part I - China. Michael_Levitt,Stanford.pdf

Please take a look and see what you think.

**From:** Tabak, Lawrence (NIH/OD) [E] (b) (6)>
**Sent:** Friday, March 6, 2020 8:46 PM
**To:** Collins, Francis (NIH/OD) [E] (b) (6); Fauci, Anthony (NIH/NIAID) [E] (b) (6)>
**Cc:** Lauer, Michael (NIH/OD) [E] (b) (6)>
**Subject:** Modeling of COVID-19 from Mike Levit

Francis, Tony –
Mike Levitt (Nobel prize in Chemistry, 2013) sent the attached modeling of the COVID-19 epidemic to Mike Lauer. I don't know if this will prove useful but wanted to pass it along in case.

He indicated that he was amazed to see how an Excel level analysis could allow him to predict the China epidemic would end as early at 2-Feb and get what he considers the best estimates for case fatality ratio. His first report from 2-Feb is attached as well as his most recent two-part report.

Larry

Source: FOIA-released Fauci emails

Notably, at the time, even the mainstream media reported on Levitt's findings. *The Los Angeles Times*[261] ran the headline: "Why this Nobel laureate predicts a quicker coronavirus recovery: 'We're going to be fine.'."

The article went on to state: "Here's what Levitt noticed in China: On Jan. 31, the country had 46 new deaths due to the novel coronavirus, compared with 42 new deaths the day before. Although the number of daily deaths had increased, the rate of that increase had begun to ease off. In his view, the fact that new cases were being identified at a slower rate was more telling than the number of new cases itself. It was an early sign that the trajectory of the outbreak had shifted.

Think of the outbreak as a car racing down an open highway, he said. Although the car is still gaining speed, it's not accelerating as rapidly as before.

"This suggests that the rate of increase in the number of deaths will slow down even more over the next week," Levitt wrote in a report he sent to friends on February 1 that was widely shared on Chinese social media. And soon, he predicted, the number of deaths would be decreasing every day.

Three weeks later, Levitt told the China Daily News that the virus' rate of growth had peaked. He predicted that the total number of confirmed COVID-19 cases in China would end up around 80,000, with about 3,250 deaths. This forecast turned out to be remarkably accurate: As of March

16, China had counted a total of 80,298 cases and 3,245 deaths — in a nation of nearly 1.4 billion people where roughly 10 million die every year."

Later in an interview with *Unherd*,[262] the Nobel laureate highlighted a key flaw in reference to Ferguson's paper: "In a footnote to a table it said, assuming exponential growth of 15% for six days. Now I had looked at China and had never seen exponential growth that wasn't decaying rapidly."

As real-world data emerged, actual outcomes diverged notably from Ferguson et al.'s "gold standard" predictions, rendering them grossly inaccurate. This became glaringly evident in countries that chose not to implement strict lockdowns, like Sweden, Taiwan, and Japan, which experienced significantly fewer deaths than projected in Ferguson's doomsday paper.

**Imperial College model's "unmitigated" COVID-19 predictions vs. actual deaths as of May 12, 2020**

| | Canada | US | UK | Sweden | Korea | Japan | Taiwan |
|---|---|---|---|---|---|---|---|
| Projection, March 26, 2020 | 326,000 | 2,654,000 | 600,000 | 85,000 | 381,000 | 1,400,000 | 212,000 |
| Actual, May 12, 2020 | 5,169 | 83,718 | 32,692 | 3,313 | 258 | 657 | 7 |

Source: The Flawed COVID-19 Model That Locked Down Canada[263]

It is undeniable that the purpose of the multi-country model in Imperial College's infamous Report 9 paper was to justify lockdowns and guide government policy as it was clearly stated by Ferguson et al. The authors wrote: "To help inform country strategies in the coming weeks, we provide here summary statistics of the potential impact of mitigation and suppression strategies in all countries across the world. These illustrate the need to act early, and the impact that failure to do so is likely to have on local health systems."

It is astonishing how Dr. Anthony Fauci (and other leaders of the White House task force) who were all fully aware of Prof Michael Levitt's analysis (which was based on actual real-world data) outright rejected it and instead followed the grossly flawed modeling predictions of Ferguson et al., resulting in lockdowns.

In March 2021, a peer-reviewed paper in *The Lancet*[264] admitted that Report 9's worst-case "unmitigated" scenarios were intended to prompt "action", acknowledging the projections were overly pessimistic: "Initial projections built worst-case scenarios that would never happen as a means of spurring leadership into action."

On October 17th 2023, Neil Ferguson (who became known as "Professor Lockdown") told the UK Covid Inquiry[265] that he did not tell officials to plunge the country into lockdown. He stated: "I don't think I stepped over that line to say, 'we need to do this now.' What I tried to do was at times, which was stepping outside the scientific advisory role, to try and focus people's minds on what was going to happen and the consequences of current trends."

## The Great Barrington Declaration

At a time when many countries were plunged into lockdowns, a group of leading public health scientists and infectious disease epidemiologists from around the world were calling on governments to take a very different and measured approach, one of "focused protection." They proposed the scientific theory of herd immunity and for only the vulnerable in society to shield.

On October 4th, 2020, they gathered in Great Barrington, Massachusetts, to draft and sign an open letter in response to the pandemic and restrictive lockdowns. It was published the following day.

"As infectious disease epidemiologists and public health scientists, we have grave concerns about the damaging physical and mental health impacts of the prevailing COVID-19 policies, and recommend an approach we call Focused Protection," the open letter reads. "Current lockdown policies are producing devastating effects on short and long-term public health."

The open letter came to be known as the Great Barrington Declaration,[266] authored by Drs. Sunetra Gupta of Oxford University, Jay Bhattacharya of Stanford University, and Martin Kulldorff of Harvard University.

Notably in March 2024, Kulldorff announced that Harvard had dismissed him for his opposition to the U.S. government's Covid control measures: the mask and vaccine mandates, also the lockdowns. He wrote in *City Journal*,[267] "I am no longer a professor of medicine at Harvard. The Harvard motto is Veritas, Latin for truth. But, as I discovered, truth can get you fired. This is my story—a story of a Harvard biostatistician and infectious-disease epidemiologist, clinging to the truth as the world lost its way during the Covid pandemic."

The Great Barrington Declaration was sponsored by the American Institute for Economic Research (AIER). It went on to amass close to one million signatures from scientists, medical practitioners, and concerned citizens from around the world.

In response to their open letter, the WHO was quick to condemn it as a "dangerous strategy and lacked sound scientific basis" with Tedros Adhanom Ghebreyesus, WHO Chief declaring it as "unethical."[268]

In the same month that the letter was published, the three doctors met with the then-Secretary of the U.S. Health and Human Services (HHS), Alex Azar, to discuss their declaration, resulting in the Trump White House to embrace it at the time when the former President was pushing to reopen[269] the U.S. economy.

However, dozens of scientists and public health authorizations called it "dangerous and deadly,"[270] and "a fringe idea." Fourteen public health groups, including the American Public Health Association wrote in an open letter:[271] "The declaration is not a strategy, it is a political statement. It ignores sound public health expertise. It preys on a frustrated populace. Instead of selling false hope that will predictably backfire, we must focus on how to manage this pandemic in a safe, responsible, and equitable way."

Critics of lockdowns could easily argue how broad economic shutdowns, school closures, and stay-at-home orders could possibly be "safe, responsible and equitable," given their documented harms to mental health, education, and livelihoods.

It is particularly striking that just three days after The Great Barrington declaration was published, Dr. Francis Collins then-Director of the National Institutes of Health (NIH) emailed[272] Dr. Anthony Fauci and Dr. Cliff Lane of the National Institute of Allergy and Infectious Diseases (NIAID) calling for "a quick and devastating published take down" of the Great Barrington Declaration's premises. In the message, Collins expressed concern over the document's growing traction, noting it had even garnered support from Nobel laureate Michael Levitt of Stanford University.

This email, later released via Freedom of Information Act (FOIA) requests, supports the inference that Collins played a pivotal role in initiating the coordinated backlash and public criticism that quickly intensified against the Declaration and its authors. These "three fringe epidemiologists" from the world's most prestigious universities and their evidence-based approach was systematically suppressed across media and academic platforms. These repercussions are later discussed in chapter 15.

**From:** Collins, Francis (NIH/OD) [E] (b) (6)
**Sent:** Thursday, October 8, 2020 2:31 PM
**To:** Fauci, Anthony (NIH/NIAID) [E] (b) (6); Lane, Cliff (NIH/NIAID) [E] (b) (6)
**Cc:** Tabak, Lawrence (NIH/OD) [E] (b) (6)
**Subject:** Great Barrington Declaration

Hi Tony and Cliff,

See https://gbdeclaration.org/ This proposal from the three fringe epidemiologists who met with the Secretary seems to be getting a lot of attention – and even a co-signature from Nobel Prize winner Mike Leavitt at Stanford. There needs to be a quick and devastating published take down of its premises. I don't see anything like that on line yet – is it underway?

Jeffrey Tucker, who served as editorial director at the American Institute for Economic Research (AIER) from 2017 until spring 2021, when he departed to found the Brownstone Institute,[273] co-sponsored the Great Barrington Declaration.

In a late 2024 interview, Tucker spoke to me about the isolation and censorship he experienced during lockdown, as well as its obscure but highly notable origins. The concept of lockdowns was born in post 9/11 bioterrorism planning, then quietly repurposed, becoming the blueprint for a synchronized global lockdown regime post 3/11, that demanded near-total compliance from billions of people.

Tucker's lockdown awakening came early, in March 2020. "My own expectation was that these things would last a few days, and people would realize the error of their ways... that you can't beat a virus with government coercion," he recalled. But as weeks turned to months, the extensions felt deliberate. By summer, amid U.S. riots and shuttered businesses, Tucker found himself "writing frantically... felt very much alone." Unbeknownst to him, Big Tech had severed his networks: "Millions of accounts... everything was much more censored than we knew at the time."

Traditional media, from The New York Times to The Wall Street Journal, celebrated the shutdowns, demonizing dissenters as reckless. "The fear was not just of the virus," Tucker said, "it was a sense of martial law." This intellectual vacuum birthed the Great Barrington Declaration.

In September 2020, AIER hosted epidemiologists Martin Kulldorff, Sunetra Gupta, and Jay Bhattacharya for a "tutorial for journalists;" a bid to educate the press on natural immunity and therapeutics. When invitations to top outlets went unanswered ("I must have sent 50 emails and not one person answered"), they pivoted to a public statement. Drafted overnight, the declaration went live within 36 hours: a website, a domain, and a moral stand against "fringe epidemiology." Within days, it amassed

15,000 signatures from scientists and doctors. Voices silenced for months. The backlash was swift and savage.

Great Barrington's town council accused AIER of "promoting evil" by borrowing their name, firing off a certified letter branding the declaration a scourge. Fauci and NIH insiders fumed privately, viewing it as a threat to their control. Tucker later realized why: lockdowns were not a panic response; they were a preparation.

He explained: "It took me two years to fully understand why the GBD (Great Barrington Declaration) enraged Fauci, the NIH, and the establishment so much. The lockdowns and fear campaigns weren't really about flattening the curve. They were about keeping the population terrified of the virus until the mRNA shots arrived. The whole point was to block natural immunity and force everyone into the new injection. The GBD offered the traditional, century-old public health alternative: focused protection and letting low-risk people live normally to build immunity. That was the real threat to their plan." It pierced the veil, exposing the injections as the endgame - not a savior, but a mandate. "You can't vaccinate your way out of a pandemic," Tucker noted. "The mRNA technology has never been tried before."

Tucker's own probe into lockdowns uncovers a genesis not rooted in science, but rather security state alchemy. He explained: "The real origin is post 9/11 bioweapons paranoia. After the anthrax scare, the Bush administration became obsessed with a possible bioweapons attack. George W. Bush was never the same after 9/11; he suffered a constant psychological meltdown. His bioweapons security team in the White House, led by a guy named Rajeev Venkayya, set out to overthrow the old public health establishment and they wanted some splashy, epic plan for dealing with a bioweapons attack. They put out contracts looking for ideas. A computer scientist at Sandia National Labs, Robert Glass, and his 14-year-old daughter Laura came up with the idea of closing schools and telling people to stay home. It started as her middle-school science fair project using a simple computer model. The idea got picked up and presented[274] in 2005–2006, and by 2006–2007 the CDC and U.S. government had officially adopted school closures, business closures, and travel restrictions for the first time ever in pandemic planning. It was never about public health science. It was bioweapons people with no epidemiology training reinventing pandemic response because they needed a dramatic plan on paper."

Tucker affirmed that "it was the bioweapons vaccine industry that was really behind the whole thing." Glass's model was a "smokescreen" seized by DHS (U.S. Department of Homeland Security) contractors, like Rajeev Venkayya, who shopped it as a "viable" non-pharma fix, while greasing rails for the shots. Funded by Project BioShield[275] (a $6 billion post 9/11 slush fund for countermeasures after the Anthrax attacks), which funneled billions to a vaccine industry on life support. (Project BioShield and the biodefense-industrial complex are discussed in greater detail in chapter 16.)

Notably, in one of Tucker's articles, he reflects[276] on his personal encounter with Venkayya. "In April of 2020, I got a call from Rajeev Venkayya. He credits himself with coming up with the whole idea of lockdowns back in 2006 while working for the biodefense desk as part of the George W. Bush administration. He then moved on to the Gates Foundation, then started a vaccine company. He told me on the phone to stop writing about lockdowns, which I found to be a ridiculous request. I asked him what the end game of these lockdowns was. He said plainly to me: there will be a vaccine. I was astounded that anyone could believe such a thing. No vaccine could be safely distributed to the population in time to keep society from falling apart. Moreover, there had never been an effective vaccine for a fast-mutating coronavirus."

Returning to my interview with Tucker, he lamented how "the pandemic response is dictating... our politics, our technology, our information flows." Five years on, with port strikes echoing lockdown-fueled inflation ($7 trillion printed, real wages gutted), he sees no endgame. "There is no moving on... it is all around us."

## Cost of Lockdowns

In a November 2022 debate in the UK parliament on "COVID-19: Economic Impact of Lockdowns,"[277] Taiwo Owatemi shared some staggering figures in relation to the vast waste of taxpayers' funds on lockdowns, including the hundreds of millions spent on building new hospitals that were barely used. The Labour MP for Coventry North-West stated: "The Government has spent in the region of £400 billion on the COVID-19 response, which has taken the national debt to over £2.1 trillion. To make matters worse, we know vast sums of money were wasted. For example, seven Nightingale hospitals were built in England, which was an impressive achievement completed in record time. However, most of them were hardly used in the way intended and they cost more than £530 million. The Yorkshire Nightingale closed before ever seeing a patient. Elsewhere, an eye-watering £673 million was spent on unusable personal protective equipment items. The £70 billion spent on furlough and £84 billion on business support schemes softened the blow for a while. However, the Federation of Small Businesses still warned of a ticking time-bomb, with 500,000 owners of small businesses—the backbone of our economy—at risk of going bust within weeks."

According to the systematic review by Vardavas et al.[278] on the "Cost of the COVID-19 pandemic versus the cost-effectiveness of mitigation strategies in EU/UK/OECD", the researchers found: "In the USA, the cost of the COVID-19 pandemic has been estimated at US$13 trillion for the first 20 weeks of the pandemic (90% of the country's annual Gross Domestic Product (GDP)) when drastic NPIs were predominately implemented, and approximately half of that figure corresponds to the projected 10-year decline in GDP attributable to the pandemic. Additionally, the global cost of the COVID-19 crisis has been estimated at 14% of the 2019 GDP (around US$12 206 million), while for Europe, it is even higher: 16% for the Eurozone and 19% for the UK."

## The Resistance

While much of the world lay crushed beneath the weight of lockdowns in 2020-2021, a series of public protests ignited across several countries. Outraged by the profound erosion of their basic civil liberties, the collapse of their businesses, and the lack of access to essential healthcare, people reached a breaking point. They took to the streets in protest.

I wrote about these extraordinary "acts of civil disobedience" that went virtually ignored by the mainstream media. My report, "It's high time Europe's lockdown rebellion spread to Britain," published by *The Conservative Woman*[279] (*TCW*) on February 12, 2021, stands today as a testament to the brutality of lockdowns and the resilience of the human spirit in the face of tyranny.

An excerpt from the article reads:

"It's almost a year since the pandemic disrupted our lives, creating a dystopian 'new normal.' Governments around the world have implemented strict lockdowns, stripping away their citizens' most basic freedoms. Businesses, schools and places of worship have all been forced to close.

In many countries it's become illegal even to protest. In the UK, gatherings of more than two people outside your household are banned on pain of fines of £200, doubling for further offences up to a maximum of £6,400. Businesses which refuse to close are being fined up to £10,000.

Countries across Europe have been handing out similarly draconian fines.[280] But on the continent a rebellion has emerged under the hashtag #IoOPRA (#IamOpen) around the notion of individuals combining to open up their businesses regardless. It started in Italy against the backdrop of anti-lockdown protests[281] in Naples and spread to most of the nation's major cities in October 2020, after the government announced further lockdown measures.

Italy was the first European country to be hit by the COVID-19 pandemic. It's hard to forget the images of the overwhelmed hospitals in Lombardy. After a year, small business owners have simply had enough of the restrictions and the devastating impact on their livelihoods. The initial welfare payments from the government to offset the loss of income have been stripped back to almost nothing, a lack of economic support which has played a key role in the protests with many Italians holding signs reading 'If you close us down, you pay up!'

By mid-January, 50,000 restaurants were open across Italy.[282] Police have been ejected by restaurant owners and angry customers shouting: 'Get out! Get out! We pay your wages from our taxes!'[283] These Italians have made it very clear that the risk to their future livelihood far outweighs the possibility of death by Covid.

This lockdown-defying movement has spread to other parts of the EU. The Poles, too, have had enough of life under lockdown. Poland's mass civil disobedience campaign was launched under the hashtag #OtwieraMY. Sebastian Piton,[284] leader of what has become known as the 'highlander veto' movement said: 'The entrepreneurs are this determined because they realized they won't survive another month, so they have no choice.'

The ski resorts of the Tatra mountains in northern Poland reopened as part of an anti-lockdown protest which began on February 1. In response the government announced a support package worth £195million for the region.

In the Czech Republic,[285] pubs and restaurants have refused government orders to shut.

The UK government has spent £280billion[286] to mitigate the economic impact of Covid. Despite these measures, some UK businesses have chosen to stay open. Steve Todd, owner of Reps Gym in Preston,[287] refused to close even after being given 11 fines for breaching the restrictions. Todd says his gym 'is a sanctuary for people struggling with isolation during the pandemic.' Two men were arrested at a Christian tea room,[288] which refused to close during the second lockdown. Hair salon owner Sinead Quinn has been fined a total of £27,000 because she refused to close."[289]

The piece closed by wondering just how widespread unreported defiance might actually have been and why Britain's resistance paled in comparison to Europe's. It then turned to Simon Dolan, founder of 'Keep Britain Free' and 'Fighting Back for Business', who offered a candid explanation in an exclusive interview.

"How many more open businesses go unreported and unpoliced may be higher than the media bother to find out, but perhaps because of Rishi's comfort blanket (then-Chancellor Rishi Sunak's furlough and support schemes) the protest movement in the UK has not gathered the momentum it has on the Continent.

Simon Dolan, UK businessman and founder of the 'Keep Britain Free' and 'Fighting Back for Business' movements, explained why in an exclusive interview with The Conservative Woman.

'Right from the start, the "stay home, protect the NHS, save lives" messaging was completely drilled into the minds of the UK population,' he said. 'Britons have been terrified by what I can only describe as government propaganda. I think this collective fear, along with British politeness, is what's preventing initiatives like this from taking off.

'Britain has ceased to be a free country and we must do everything in our power to get our freedoms back. Is it right to comply with laws which are so damaging and wrong? If enough businesses are to take a stand and open, the rules would have to change, as they have done in other countries.'

Dolan champions SMEs (small and medium-sized enterprises) which make up 'the lifeblood of our economy' and he is heavily critical of the government's Covid loan scheme. The general public may be unaware but these loans have sky-high interest rates of up to 35 per cent. He reiterated the plea he made to the Chancellor in The *Conservative Woman*[290] two weeks ago: SMEs should have their Covid loans written off.

Yet the prospect of loan repayments seems insufficient to galvanise British businesses into protest even though the hospitality sector in particular is being devastated.

Dolan is one of the few openly dissenting business voices. He said: 'The government's yo-yo restrictions and lockdowns are completely nonsensical and disproportionate to the threat. How else are we going to stop this nightmare if we don't speak up against it? There will come a point, very soon, where the dam will burst and I believe we will see widespread civil disobedience – indeed, that is inevitable in my mind.'

• • •

Notably, Simon Dolan launched the most high-profile private legal challenge[291] to the UK government's COVID-19 lockdown measures.

In May 2020, represented by barrister Francis Hoar, he filed for judicial review against then Health Secretary Matt Hancock, arguing that the March–July 2020 lockdown regulations were unlawful, irrational, disproportionate, and breached human rights. The case was crowdfunded and raised over £410,000.

In July 2020, Mr. Justice Lewis refused permission at the High Court, ruling the claim "unarguable" and that the measures had a legitimate aim. Dolan renewed his application to the Court of Appeal. On 1 December 2020, the Court of Appeal dismissed the claim,[292] primarily because it was filed too late (two months after the first lockdown regulations expired) and because a "rolling" judicial review that kept adding new regulations was impermissible. The court accepted that some of Dolan's arguments raised important constitutional issues but still ruled against him.

## The Lockdown Parties

On 30 November 2021, the *Daily Mirror*[293] broke the explosive "Partygate" scandal. Leaked photos revealed UK government staff, including then Prime Minister Boris Johnson, indulging in festivities at 10 Downing Street and other government buildings during 2020 and 2021, right in the thick of lockdowns.

*ITV News*[294] reported that a surprise birthday bash was arranged for Johnson by his wife Carrie during the first lockdown in June 2020. Family and friends were hosted in the Johnsons' private residence above Number 10, just nine days after Johnson solemnly urged the public "to continue to show restraint and respect the rules which are designed to keep us all safe."

While the public languished under harsh restrictions unable to mix outside their household or "bubble," Johnson and his cronies, including the then Chancellor and future PM Rishi Sunak, socialized at wine and cheese parties. As grieving family members were forced to sit six meters apart at their loved one's funeral, Conservative campaigners backing the then Conservative mayoral candidate for London, Shaun Bailey, cozied together enjoying canapés. While husbands were barred from visiting their dying wives in care homes to offer a final embrace, the then Health Secretary Matt Hancock, was caught on camera[295] fondling his top aide and married mistress Gina Coladangelo in a blatant breach of his own Covid rules.

Hypocrisy was not limited to the Conservative party. Labour leader, Sir Keir Starmer and Deputy Leader, Angela Rayner allegedly enjoyed beer and curry at a Durham social event in April 2021. The scandal came to be known as "Beergate."

Across the Atlantic, Dr. Jay Varma, who served as New York City's senior public health advisor from 2020-2021 was caught on secret camera[296] in September 2024 divulging details about his drug-fueled sex parties during lockdown. "I had to be kind of sneaky about it...I was running the entire Covid response for the city…we rented a hotel...we all took like, you know, molly [Ecstasy/MDMA] … 8 to 10 of us were in a room...like just being naked with friends…" the former senior public health advisor boasted.

These clandestine gatherings during lockdown did more than simply unveil a stark hypocrisy: they were a glaring signal that government officials were aware the virus posed less of a threat than their alarmist campaigns would have us believe.

Furthermore, while political elites "partied," hefty, fixed penalty notices were issued to the public who breached Covid regulations (as referenced in my earlier *TCW* article) by refusing to close their businesses, churches or for simply not wearing a face mask in a supermarket. By May 2020, these fines were increased.

Official Sensitive MA/FM/1624/20

**ADVICE**

**Background**

1. The UK Government increased the fine amounts for breaches of its Health Protection (Coronavirus, Restrictions) (England) 2020. The increases came into force on Wednesday 13 May. The table below shows the amounts of fines that can now be issued.

| First Offence | £100[1] |
|---|---|
| Second offence | £200 |
| Third Offence | £400 |
| Fourth Offence | £800 |
| Fifth Offence | £1600 |
| Upper limit | £3200 |

Source: *UK COVID-19 Inquiry*[297]

As of February 2022, police in England and Wales processed a total of 118,978[298] Fixed Penalty Notices (FPNs) for breaches under the Health Protection (Coronavirus, Restrictions) Regulations 2020 and subsequent amendments.

Notably, official reviews and parliamentary reports revealed systemic issues, including high error rates, incorrect legal application, and disproportionate impacts. This led to findings that all charges and a significant portion of fines issued under the Coronavirus Act 2020 were "unlawful."[299]

However, as recently as June 2024 (several years after restrictions had ended), Dr. Anne McCloskey[300] appeared at Northern Ireland's Londonderry Magistrates' Court in connection with an unpaid Covid fine of £255, imposed in 2022 for a "breach of Covid regulations." She was given an immediate warrant to pay the amount or go to prison for 14 days. As a point of principle, she refused to pay, resulting in Dr. McCloskey being sent to Hydebank Wood Prison. This is the same Dr. McCloskey, whose detailed critique of lockdown policy was published as a rapid response in *The BMJ* (noted in chapter 3).

CHAPTER FIVE

# LOCKING DOWN HARMS

*"Of all tyrannies, a tyranny sincerely exercised for the good of its victim may be the most oppressive."*

~C. S. Lewis

In the spring of 2020, governments across the world launched an unprecedented and untested experiment: nationwide lockdowns. Presented at the time as the only way to "flatten the curve" and "protect the vulnerable." These measures were imposed with near-universal political and media support.

Yet, as the dust settles more than five years on, a stark truth emerges: what was sold as salvation became a slow-motion tragedy, inflicting wounds far deeper and more enduring than the pathogen it sought to contain. From school closures, which caused a "generational catastrophe," to care homes where the elderly were quietly dispatched under "just in case" protocols. This chapter indicts the lockdown legacy as catastrophic overreach. A policy imposed without robust evidence, sustained by fear, and protected by the suppression of legitimate debate.

## Science's Damning Verdict

Several years on, the academic research has systematically demolished the claim that lockdowns were a net public-health success. A 2023 Johns Hopkins-linked meta-analysis[301] by Herby, Jonung and Hanke (covering every available stringent lockdown study at the time) concluded that lockdowns reduced COVID mortality by an average of only 0.2 % while inflicting catastrophic social and economic damage.

The Herby-Jonung-Hanke meta-analysis found that, "Lockdowns prevented relatively few deaths compared to a typical flu season – in England and Wales, 18,500–24,800 flu deaths occur, in Europe 72,000 flu deaths occur, and in the United States 38,000 flu deaths occur in a typical flu season. These results are pale in comparison to the Imperial College of London's modeling exercises (March 2020), which predicted that lockdowns would save over 400,000 lives in the United Kingdom and over 2 million lives in the United States."

They went on to conclude that COVID-19 lockdowns were "a global policy failure of gigantic proportions...The draconian policy failed to significantly reduce deaths while imposing substantial social, cultural, and economic costs."

A larger 2025 systematic review by Taylor et al.[302] examined 132 peer-reviewed studies on lockdown and school-closure effects. It found detrimental outcomes in over 90 percent of mental-health, child-development, obesity, and economic indicators, with the harm falling most heavily on the poor, minorities, and the disabled. The authors stated plainly: "Lockdowns and school closures were associated with detrimental health effects in the majority of outcomes analyzed."

The individual studies that these meta-analyses later synthesized were being published from mid 2020 onwards. Sweden's open-schools policy data, the falling infection curves before the March 2020 lockdown, the early signals of collateral harm: all of it was available, yet it was dismissed or suppressed.

A perfect illustration of this is the damning revelation that even when the country was being asked to surrender fundamental freedoms "for the greater good," an official ethics advisory group, formally commissioned to ensure that lockdown measures remained proportionate and respectful of civil liberties, was effectively "silenced" and sidelined by England's Chief Medical Officer, Professor Sir Chris Whitty.

A *Telegraph* investigation[303] published on 6 December 2025, revealed key findings about the Joint Biosecurity Centre Ethics Advisory Group (chaired by respected bioethicist Professor Sarah Chan). The group produced detailed reports throughout 2020 and 2021. These repeatedly warned that:

- Open-ended restrictions and the erosion of basic rights risked causing greater harm than the virus itself.

- Decisions were often driven more by modeling than by balanced moral reasoning.

Their reports were either buried, circulated only to a handful of officials, or delivered long after irreversible decisions had been taken, such as the launch of the much-criticized NHS COVID-19 contact-tracing app. Members described the experience as "deeply demoralizing," with one stating they had been used as a token gesture while ethical scrutiny was treated as an irritant to be managed away.

## School Closures

On March 4, 2020, the UK government's own behavioural scientists in SPI-B issued a clear warning[304] about school closures. They described the measure as highly disruptive and likely to impose an unequal burden on society. They ranked it among the least socially acceptable options available. Instead, SPI-B recommended a more targeted approach: isolating symptomatic cases and shielding the vulnerable, not blanket school closures. The group spelled out the foreseeable harms in stark terms:

- Grandparents would be unable to provide childcare, hitting working parents hardest, especially single parents and low-income families.
- The poorest children would lose access to free school meals, after-school clubs, and other essential social services.
- Household bills (heating, food delivery) would soar at the same time as incomes collapsed.
- Reduced adult oversight of children could create "risk of unintended consequences."
- Full household isolation would fall disproportionately on the least well-off and on the 7.5 percent of adults with no internet access.

Finally, SPI-B stressed that schools must not be overlooked in a crisis because they provide emotional support for children, free school meals, well-being monitoring, and act as community hubs for public-health messaging.

Astoundingly, on March 18th, the UK Government announced[305] that every school, college, and early years setting in the country was to close, recklessly disregarding the consequences of such drastic actions outlined in their own government paper published only two weeks prior.

In the UK, like in many other countries, schools were closed intermittently over an 18-month period between March 2020 and September 2021, derailing the education of an entire generation. I wrote about this extremely devastating Government measure in my debut piece for *TCW*[306] first published on February 8th, 2021. It chronicled the grinding toll of school closures: the "new normal" that turned parents into makeshift educators, while children endured screen-bound "remote learning."

The following is an excerpt from my article:

"The ECDC [European Centre for Disease Prevention and Control] report[307] on 'COVID-19 in children and the role of schools in transmission,' concludes that children are much less likely to contract the virus. In fact, less than 5% of COVID cases are reported among EU/EEA and the UK amongst children (aged 18 and under). Just as important, the report states that children were less likely to transmit the virus to adults. A survey, where 15 European countries took part, 10 replied that they did not have strong indications of child-to-adult transmission, whether in schools or other settings in their country.

In Sweden, where there were no school closures for children aged 16 and under. The Public Health Authority found that teachers were at no higher risk of COVID-19. This evidence counters the claim that teachers are at higher risk of contracting the virus from their students.

There's no doubt that school closures have disrupted the daily lives of families. It's also in no child's best interest to sit for hours in front of screens to access their 'remote learning.' Forbidden from properly interacting with their peers and from taking part in any organized extra-curricular group activity, the social and emotional development of children has been stunted.

Currently, 1 in 6 children in the UK have mental health issues brought on by the pandemic and school closures. This somber statistic is based on a recent report from the children's commissioner, Anne Longfield. She has strongly urged the government to work on a road map for the reopening of schools.

In the ECDC report, it stated that school closures should only be used as a measure of last resort. As a country, did we reach that level of last resort? Are schools really COVID hotspots and are our children the super-spreaders? I find no hard evidence to tell me so. UN Secretary General,

Antonio Guterres, stated that school closures have caused a 'generational catastrophe.' I find it very hard not to agree with him."

## A Child Psychologist Speaks Out

In March 2022, I interviewed[308] Dr. Zenobia Storah, a clinical child and adolescent psychologist. When asked if she had seen an increase in demand for her clinical services following school closures, she responded:

ZS: In terms of my personal practice, I've received so many referrals. I can't see all the children that are referred to me. It became quite apparent since about January last year. I was getting double, sometimes triple of what I could see. In my NHS work, commissioned by CCGs to assess and intervene for children, I saw the same trend. The children I've been seeing, those with learning disabilities or complex needs, neurodevelopmental conditions, were especially concerning at the start, as school closures hit them hardest. Special schools shut too, leaving families without respite care or face-to-face support. Services stopped overnight; distress spiked, manifesting in challenging behaviors. Parents struggled to manage, exacerbating everything. I saw school refusal and dropouts: kids unable to return once reopened. In private practice, referrals for OCD and health anxiety soared, worsened by lockdown stress and isolation. What I've seen mirrors reports: the government reinforced a state of fear; "if you leave the house, people can die." That's psychologically damaging.

SE: Did any of the children you saw have this inflated sense of fear?

ZS: Quite a lot. Parents said, "I've struggled to get them out of the house. They're fixated, so anxious about COVID." Children's behavior mirrors adults': fear at home amplifies it. News and messaging targeted kids too, which I think was particularly abhorrent. For example, the mother of one of the children that I came across over the pandemic, when the children came in from school, all their clothes were immediately taken at the door. They were put in the washing machine straight away. The children were straight away in the shower and this was still going on a year into the pandemic. Cognitive therapy helps, but if that's home life, it doesn't touch the root.

## A Headteacher Speaks Out

Very few educational professionals actively spoke out against school closures during the pandemic, likely out of fear of professional repercussions. One of the few who did, and perhaps the only headteacher in the UK, was Mike Fairclough. He not only opposed the closures but also raised alarms about the rollout of COVID-19 mRNA vaccines for children. In September 2022, Fairclough joined Drs. Clare Craig, Tony Hinton, and Renee Hoenderkamp in an open letter[309] to then Prime Minister Liz Truss, urging her to pause the Covid vaccine program for children.

During my interview[310] with Fairclough that month, he emphasized: "We have a legal duty to safeguard children against harm." By then, he had already faced two formal investigations sparked by complaints over his outspoken views on the risks of COVID mRNA vaccines. These led his school's governing board to launch probes. Shockingly, Fairclough later learned from one of the governors that the complainant belonged to an organized group, later identified as the Government's Counter Disinformation Unit (CDU), whose explicit agenda was to target and oust teaching professionals who challenged the vaccine rollout for children. The CDU is discussed in greater detail later in this book.

When I asked about the backlash he endured, Fairclough's response was candid and revealing: "I've been investigated twice by my employer. Initially, back in May 2021, there was a complaint. Not from my community, my staff, or even anyone in East Sussex where I live. It came from somebody in the North of England, who complained to my employer that I was spreading medical misinformation and that I therefore should be removed from my position. My local authority has always been very supportive of me, but they traditionally ask my governing board to carry out an investigation. During that investigation, one of my governors had a conversation with the complainant, who turned out to be part of a group of people whose specific role, she said, was to remove professionals from the education system or the health profession who were speaking out either about lockdowns, masks, or vaccines. So, it was a targeted and very coordinated attack.

I spoke to various lawyers, and they said: 'Look, you have a right to an opinion and to express yourself, and you're also protected as a whistle-blower.' So anyway, I said all of this during the investigation, and the complaint was dropped. Then a few months later, another complaint was made about me on the same lines. Again, that one was dropped, but in this case, the local authority commissioned somebody from outside the school to carry out the investigation.

So yes, there was that backlash. Online, initially, there were a lot of things. I mean, I'm banned from Twitter now for saying exactly those four statements: children are at extremely low risk of serious illness from COVID; vaccines pose known risks; they have no long-term safety data; and a person can still catch and spread COVID when vaccinated. I was banned for that reason. I think it was also because *The Epoch Times*[311] ran a piece about me because I'm the only school leader in the UK speaking out about this, literally the only one! Then it was Dr. Peter McCullough, who endorsed that on Twitter. On that same day, they cut me out, and I can only think it's possibly because I might inspire others to speak up.

I think it's really important for people to realize and understand that when you do something that is true to your heart and you take a stand, you still feel the fear. I've had great concerns about losing my job. If I lose my job, I lose my house, lose my livelihood, all that kind of stuff. But there's something else that happens within you when you do the right thing. It's a kind of sense of empowerment which eclipses all that fear."

## Too Little, Too Late: Inquiry Confessions on School Closures

On 20 June 2023,[312]the UK's ex-Chancellor, George Osborne gave evidence to the official Covid Inquiry, where he queried whether schools should have closed their doors to children throughout the lockdowns pressed upon the nation.

During the Inquiry, Osborne appeared to question the UK Government's school closures. He stated: "I don't want to jump ahead of this inquiry, but should the schools have been locked down in the way they were?"

Why did Osborne choose to speak up three years too late? He could have raised his concerns during the midst of the Government's devastating school closures but instead he chose to remain silent on the issue.

Dame Sally Davies, the UK's ex-Chief Medical Officer also gave evidence[313] at the Inquiry. She stated how the full impact of lockdowns (including school closures) was not considered and emotionally acknowledged how it had "damaged a generation." Davies then went on to paradoxically state: "It's clear that no one thought about lockdown. I still think we should have locked down, although a week earlier."

As part of Module 8 (Children and Young People) of the UK's Covid Inquiry, former Education Secretary Sir Gavin Williamson testified[314] on October 14, 2025, where he admitted to "many mistakes" in school closure decisions. "This was, and I will accept fault on this, during that first lockdown, I saw, and we saw, not just with our own eyes, with our own children, with our friends' children ... that [they] had actually suffered as a result of not being at school. And we also saw that children from the most disadvantaged backgrounds, the ones that had no one to look after them, were going to be most disadvantaged."

## The Scottish COVID-19 Public Inquiry

During the June 6th, 2023 public hearing[315] of the UK Covid Inquiry, Mr. Jacobs, representing the Trades Union Congress, astutely likened the official Inquiry to "turkeys deciding whether to vote for Christmas."

I agree, particularly considering the Inquiry's glaring omission of investigating the lives lost not just to Covid but rather to the government's catastrophic response policies, notably the highly damaging lockdowns. Instead of addressing these critical issues, the inquiry's focus seems limited to debating if the country should have initiated lockdowns sooner; whether there was adequate Personal Protective Equipment (PPE) and chasing after the lack of disclosure of WhatsApp messages and emails exchanged between cabinet ministers.

In stark contrast, the Scottish Inquiry[316] has been far more transparent, with numerous testimonies shedding light on the mistreatment of the elderly in care homes during the lockdowns: the horrific neglect; the coerced end-of-life protocols involving medications like midazolam and morphine and the blanket Do Not Resuscitate (DNR) orders.

The extract below is from a submission statement[317] by solicitor, Aamer Anwar on behalf of the Scottish Covid Bereaved which was read out during a hearing held by the Scottish COVID-19 Public Inquiry.

"It should not have come as a surprise to our politicians that when problems arise in society, the weakest and most vulnerable are the most likely to be badly affected. It is submitted that those in hospitals or care homes clearly fall within those categories, yet time and time again the Inquiry was presented with evidence which made it clear that there had been no special consideration given to vulnerable groups and how their needs were to be properly met during a pandemic. As a result, seemingly nonsensical rules were put in place. For example, there was an apparent total lockdown of care homes to avoid infection of residents whilst allowing for the discharge of patients from hospitals into those same care homes without testing. No consideration appears to have been given to the realities of care home staffing, where members of staff frequently worked within more than one such establishment.

Scottish COVID Bereaved submit that those in authority-imposed rules in relation to care which could not possibly be obtempered. Policies which resulted in the isolation of those with mental health issues or dementia showed a lack of planning and forethought. A failure to consider how healthcare professionals should best communicate with relatives about their loved ones in hospitals, care, or prison meant that there were no proper systems in place to allow for such communication. Whilst some found that there were no such problems, others were greatly frustrated by the lack of formal structure in place for this vital part of the caring process. There is, it is submitted, no better example of this than the issues surrounding the implementation of DNACPR (Do Not Attempt Cardiopulmonary Resuscitation) notices, of which the Inquiry will doubtless hear much more in the future. It was further evidence that there was a lack of prior consideration for how infection control would work during a pandemic.

Many of the bereaved felt most keenly the seemingly inconsistent rules around visitation in hospital settings. These rules appeared to differ not only across health boards or hospitals but also within individual hospitals. This absence, coupled with a lack of communication, meant that many felt unable to properly advocate for their loved ones.

This was perhaps most vividly illustrated when it came to end-of-life care. There appeared to have been a blanket approach taken towards many elderly care home residents rather than a human rights-based approach. In some cases, especially within care homes, many had reached a point where quality of life was more important than duration. While lockdown was initially understandable as an effort to keep these vulnerable individuals safe, as time went on other fundamental rights became equally as important. The Inquiry has heard evidence that dying residents were not given the end-of-life care that they would normally have received and that in some cases there appeared to be a focus on providing end-of-life medication to residents."

In reference to the scandal of discharging hospital patients into care homes at the start of the first lockdown, an anonymized care worker from a private care home, gave evidence during a Health and Social Impact hearing[318] held by the Scottish Inquiry: "I remember a lot of residents being brought in not very well and then I remember that our death rate just kept going up and up. We would, you know, have residents in the home that would maybe pass away every couple of months but when these patients started coming in from the hospital, they were passing away in droves, it was like every week, one, two, three people a week!"

In tragic irony, government messaging, such as former Health Secretary, Matt Hancock's warning to young people: "Don't kill your gran,"[319] while critics contend that policies under his department ultimately contributed to the loss of lives among the older aged population.

Specifically, guidance allowing the discharging of untested hospital patients into care homes, was later ruled as "unlawful" by the High Court in 2022. This policy of clearing beds was implemented so hospitals could be ready to handle the expected "tsunami"[320] of Covid patients, which somehow never fully materialized. This is clear from the largely unused Nightingale hospitals and reports of many facilities operating at half-capacity.

At the same Health and Social Care Impact hearing on May 23, 2024 (referenced earlier), Glasgow Royal Hospital porter of 25 years, Neil Craig[321] offered a striking observation: "We were used to the wards being full to capacity... but then you'd go into the wards and they were, like, half-empty."

In December 2020, Debbie Hicks was arrested and convicted of a public order offence for filming[322] an almost empty hospital and posting it online. This was at a time when the UK public were told repeatedly that the hospitals were "overwhelmed."

In January 2021, likely in response to the widely viewed video, the BBC[323] ran a piece: "Covid: The truth behind videos of 'empty' hospitals." In response to a question about empty hospital beds, NHS England chief executive Sir Simon Stevens said: "When people say that, that is a lie."

Lest we forget: during lockdowns, the phenomenon of the dancing nurses[324] in TikTok-style videos shot in empty hospital wards, suddenly proliferated across social media. This was mentioned in former MP Andrew Bridgen's speech to parliament (discussed later in this chapter).

If hospitals and frontline staff were truly overwhelmed, how could these workers find time to rehearse and film such choreographed dance routines?

## Dr. Burns' Witness Statement

In her witness statement[325] Dr. Jennifer Burns (former President of the British Geriatric Society, 2020-2022) reflected on lockdown harms to older people. Key sections from Dr. Burns' witness statement were read out during the closing statement of Stuart Gayle QC at the Scottish Inquiry's Health and Social Impact hearing on June 27, 2024.

An extract from her statement follows: "The Age UK survey is interesting, and I don't know if Age Scotland also something similar but one of the things I captured was that the term 'vulnerable' which was a blanket term used to apply to older people, is quite a shock for people who are happily living their lives. The report comments on anxiety related to the risks from the virus resulting in many being afraid to go out and resume previous activities even when restrictions had eased. Having to be isolated from family and close friends had an impact. We know that regular exercise, maintaining physical fitness, social interactions, and a sense of purpose all combine to build resilience and prevent disability. The lockdown affected many older people's ability to undertake these activities and the longer-term impact of this is likely to be negative for their physical and mental health.

Social isolation is harmful to care home residents and can result in low mood or cognitive or functional decline. We were restrictive for a lot of the pandemic for reasons that at the time I supported but on reflection and feedback from members, I consider that these restrictions were too prolonged."

## Midazolam and Morphine "End of Life" Protocols

A deeply troubling statement can be found in paragraph 81 of Dr. Burns' witness statement, where she refers to the "just in case medication" that was able to be given "ahead of time in preparation for changes as an illness such as Covid progresses." These medications include "Morphine or similar opiates for pain or breathlessness, Midazolam for agitation.."

This is particularly disturbing in light of the Midazolam scandal, which many allege contributed to excess deaths in UK care homes in spring 2020.

On April 18, 2024, Andrew Bridgen, then Independent MP for Northwest Leicestershire (formerly Conservative until 2023), delivered a blistering speech[326] in the House of Commons debate on "COVID-19 Pandemic

Response and Trends in Excess Deaths." He exposed the NHS' NG163 guideline as a "11-year sin" of systemic neglect.

Bridgen condemned the March 2020 consultation on DNRs (Do Not Resuscitate orders) for the elderly and disabled, which was circulated as policy and enacted by care homes and GPs amid hospital fears of being overwhelmed. "The result? People died who didn't need to die, while nurses performed TikTok dances," he lambasted. Standard protocols: steroids and antibiotics for excessive immune responses, were jettisoned, patients dispatched home with paracetamol "until their lips turn blue," then sedated, ventilated, and left to perish.

Turning to NG163 (NICE's April 3, 2020, "end-of-life" guidance), Bridgen severely criticized midazolam and morphine as "respiratory depressants" on the breathless: "It's hard to imagine... a more stupid thing to do than to give a respiratory suppression to somebody struggling to breathe... with symptoms of COVID-19." He contrasted this with cancer care, where such effects were deemed "reasonable."

"Can the minister explain why midazolam was removed from... NG191 on November 30, 2023?" he demanded, citing ministers' admissions that clinicians should have ignored the guideline for individual care. "If legal cases are brought for unlawful killing, can the minister tell us who's going to be taking the blame? Will it be NICE? Will it be NHS England or will it be the individual doctors and nurses who will be held to account?"

Bridgen highlighted NICE's removal of NG163 from their website: "Are they ashamed of the harm? They certainly should be."

Echoing this, Professor Emeritus Sam H. Ahmedzai and palliative medicine consultants warned in *The BMJ*[327] (April 20, 2020): "NG163 states: 'Sedation and opioid use should not be withheld because of a fear of causing respiratory depression'... [But for] people not previously known to be at the end of life, there is potential risk of unintended serious harm... without specialist palliative care advice." They urged revision "to prevent inadvertently adding to that suffering." NICE ignored their warnings.

## Care Home Horrors Exposed during Scottish COVID-19 Inquiry Hearing

The witness statement[328] by Gillian Grant, whose grandmother died at a care home from the "just in case" midazolam end-of-life protocol (the same scenario described in Dr. Burns' earlier statement), makes for a harrowing read. The BBC[329] even covered her testimony. Grant's grandmother represents the thousands of elderly who died in care homes during lockdown. Her death is noteworthy because it encompasses the many shocking scandals of that period: the administration of the controversial drug midazolam; the neglect experienced by a care home resident; and a DNR notice being obtained not just without consent but with a forged signature.

Grant was questioned[330] regarding her filed witness statement at the Scottish Covid Inquiry Impact hearing on Health and Social Care on 23 November 2023. She spoke about how her grandmother was admitted to the Mavisbank care home in the Autumn of 2020 and died on November 4th.

An extract from Grant's statement highlights the level of neglect that her grandmother endured: "I remember one time... they brought [her meal] in and banged it down in front of her. It was mince and chips... I could see the mince was raw... It was a horrible situation. I couldn't do anything other than let her eat it... There were other things too. She used to say... 'They took me for a shower today and... they just threw a big bucket of water over me.' ... Knowing what I know now, I wish I had seen that as the giant red flag it was."

After her grandmother's death, a DNR form was found by Grant's legal team with her name filled in and dated on the same day she categorically stated that she was not prepared to make any decision about a DNR on behalf of her grandmother. The only conclusion one can draw is that the signature found on her grandmother's DNR, the one she "did not even know existed," had been forged.

"I was provided with a document... the DNR but this had my name written on it. I was shocked as this was the first time I had seen this document... I had never authorized a DNR but this has my name on it... The DNR is incomplete... I was asked about a DNR but categorically stated that I was not prepared to make any decision... I think this conversation happened on the 2nd of November 2020 and this is the date of the DNR."

Grant's grandmother was given midazolam, the end-of-life protocol imposed by the doctor "just in case" her mild COVID worsened. "The other point is that the sedative they gave her is midazolam, which isn't a mild sedative... I don't understand why this was administered as we were at no point informed that she was end-of-life... From things I've read, midazolam can reduce your respiratory rate and I don't understand why they would have given her that? If somebody had told me it was midazolam, I would have said no."

## The Inquiry's Flawed Verdict

Reflecting on Nobel laureate Michael Levitt's prescient May 2020 UnHerd interview (referenced in chapter 4), his data-driven skepticism of lockdowns and alarmist models rings truer than ever: "There is no doubt in my mind that when we come to look back on this, the damage done by lockdown will exceed any saving of lives by a huge factor." Levitt was spot on. It may take decades to tally the full toll.

Four and a half years after the UK's first national lockdown, a September 2024 *Telegraph*[331] article captured the lingering shadow: "A growing body of evidence suggests we haven't truly turned the page on what now sounds more like a chapter from dystopian fiction. Instead, the effects of the Covid lockdowns endure, and will continue to be observed and charted for many decades to come. 'We'll probably be studying the impact of this for as long as we live,' says Adam Hampshire, professor of cognitive and computational neuroscience at King's College London."

Yet, on November 20, 2025, the UK COVID-19 Inquiry's "Module 2 In Brief"[332] report doubled down on the narrative, concluding the government's response was "too little, too late,"[333] with avoidable deaths and harm. It claimed an earlier lockdown on March 16, 2020 (one week before the actual date), could have saved up to 23,000 lives in England. The report relied heavily on a 2021 Imperial College paper by Neil Ferguson estimating a first-wave death toll drop from 48,600 to 25,600. But as David Spiegelhalter, emeritus professor of statistics at the University of Cambridge, told *The BMJ*:[334] "Modeling does not 'establish' anything—it is just an estimate based on numerous and challenging assumptions... And yet the models themselves estimate that daily infections were falling prior to lockdown on 23 March 2020, presumably due to the measures already in place. No doubt many lives would have been saved by earlier action, but this estimate from 2021 should be taken with caution."

In clinging to flawed models, the Inquiry perpetuates the very overreach it claims to scrutinize, ensuring lockdown's scars outlast even the virus.

CHAPTER SIX

# THE FLAWED "GOLD STANDARD"

*"It's just a process that is used to make a whole lot of something out of something. It doesn't tell you that you are sick and it doesn't tell you that the thing you ended up with was going to hurt you or anything like that."*

~Dr. Kary Mullis, inventor of the PCR (polymerase chain reaction) technique,1993

In the wake of the global response to 3/11, few scientific tools have wielded as much influence or sparked as much debate as the polymerase chain reaction (PCR) test. Originally developed by Nobel laureate Dr. Kary Mullis for genetic analysis, the PCR technique was never intended to diagnose infectious diseases. Yet, in early 2020, it became the cornerstone of global COVID-19 testing, shaping public health policies, justifying lockdowns, and driving economic and social upheaval.

While nations came under the heavy hammer of lockdowns to curb the virus' spread, the largest scale of mass testing the world has ever seen was rolled out. Targeting not only those who showed symptoms of the virus (symptomatic) but also those who did not (asymptomatic). It is estimated that hundreds of billions have been spent on global testing efforts. In the U.S. alone, around $81 billion[335] was allocated for COVID-19 testing.

In May 2020, the UK's NHS Test and Trace was set up with a budget of £22 billion with a further £15 billion being allocated-totaling £37 billion over two years. In February 2022, a question in Parliament was put forward to the Secretary of State for Health and Social Care: "What the amount (a) spent in 2020-21 and (b) of projected spend in 2021-2022 is on the purchase of (a) PCR tests, (b) lateral flow tests, (c) PPE and (d) other COVID-19 testing equipment?"

The then-Under-Secretary, former Conservative MP, Maggie Throup, responded[336] in writing: "We are unable to provide the amount spent in the 2020/21 and 2021/22 financial years on the purchases of PCR tests, lateral flow device tests and other COVID-19 testing equipment, as this information is commercially sensitive."

It has never been disclosed by the British government how much of taxpayers' money was spent on Covid testing. Their cited reason that "this information is commercially sensitive" is inexcusable.

At the heart of mass-testing and its unprecedented cost, lies the Corman-Drosten paper, published in Eurosurveillance on January 23, 2020, which established the real-time RT-PCR protocol as the "gold standard" for detecting SARS-CoV-2. However, before I introduce my three-part investigation on the PCR test, an underlying critical issue tied to the controversy of this test, must first be looked at.

## The Myth of Asymptomatic Spread

The big push to get everyone tested, particularly the asymptomatic stemmed from the headline-making German paper published in the *New England Journal of Medicine* (*NEJM*)[337] on January 30, 2020, entitled "Transmission of 2019-nCoV Infection from an Asymptomatic Contact in Germany."

This letter to the editor of the *NEJM* explained how in January 2020, a healthy German businessman contracted Covid after attending a meeting with his Chinese business partner, who had no symptoms at the time but fell ill on her flight back to China. Three additional colleagues also tested positive, with only one having direct contact with the Chinese business partner. All infected individuals were admitted to a Munich infectious diseases unit for isolation and monitoring. Despite high viral loads, none of the patients developed severe illness. The case outlined in the paper highlighted the potential for asymptomatic transmission and was used to justify the mass testing of the asymptomatic.

"There's no doubt after reading [the *NEJM*] paper that asymptomatic transmission is occurring," Anthony Fauci, director of the U.S. National Institute of Allergy and Infectious Diseases, told journalists at the time. "This study lays the question to rest."

Notably, Christian Drosten of Charité University of Medicine, Berlin, a co-author of the paper, declared no conflicts of interest[338] in the accompanying disclosure forms. However, Drosten led the development of the Charité PCR protocol for detecting SARS-Cov-2, which was accepted by the WHO on January 13, 2020, and became the "gold standard" for the mass testing of the asymptomatic. Critics have argued that this created a potential incentive to emphasize asymptomatic transmission. The many controversies tied to the PCR test can be read about later in this chapter.

As it turns out the *NEJM* paper was proven to be flawed.[339] In their paper, the researchers write "During her [Chinese business partner] stay, she had been well with no sign or symptoms of infection but had become ill on her flight back to China." They go on to conclude: "The fact that asymptomatic persons are potential sources of 2019-nCoV infection may warrant a reassessment of transmission dynamics of the current outbreak."

However, if the researchers had bothered to interview the woman before their paper was published, they would have been made aware of the fact that the businesswoman did feel unwell at the time. She showed symptoms. According to an article in *Science*[340] by Kai Kupferschmidt: "Officials at the Robert Koch Institute (RKI), Germany's federal public health agency, and the Health and Food Safety Authority of the state of Bavaria did talk to the Shanghai patient on the phone, and it turned out she did have symptoms while in Germany."

A document posted on the Public Health Agency of Sweden's website[341] critically stated: "The sources that claimed that the coronavirus would infect during the incubation period lack scientific support for this analysis in their articles. This applies, among other things, to an article in [*NEJM*] that has subsequently proven to contain major flaws and errors."

The Science article went on to quote Michael Hoelscher of the Ludwig Maximilian University of Munich Medical Center (one of the paper's researchers): "I asked the Bavarian Health and Food Safety Authority whether the information from that phone conversation called for a correction, and I was told that is not the case." The article disclosed: "(The Bavarian ministry of health, of which the agency is part, has not responded to a request for information from Science Insider.) But RKI disagreed. A spokesperson for the agency says RKI informed the World Health Organization (WHO) and European partner agencies about the new information."

"I feel bad about how this went, but I don't think anybody is at fault here. Apparently, the woman could not be reached at first and people felt this had to be communicated quickly" emphasized Christian Drosten, also quoted in the article.

What is particularly noteworthy is the information buried in a series of FOIA-released email exchanges between Dr. Anthony Fauci, then director of NIAID and the writer of that Science article, Kai Kupferschmidt.

On the day the Science article was published, February 3rd, Kai writes to Fauci asking for a further comment given that "the woman [in the German paper] did have symptoms."

> **From:** Kai Kupferschmidt (b) (6)
> **Sent:** Monday, February 3, 2020 11:47 AM
> **To:** Fauci, Anthony (NIH/NIAID) [E] (b) (6)>
> **Subject:** coronavirus quick question
>
> Tony,
>
> do you have 5 minutes for a quick phone call? Writing a story about the German paper claiming an asymptomatic case. Turns out the woman did have symptoms. You gave the paper a lot importance, so really wanted to get your reaction on this.
>
> Cheers
> Kai
>
> Kai Kupferschmidt
> contributing correspondent "Science"
> (b) (6)
> (b) (6)
>
> twitter: @kakape

The next day Fauci responds with the following email. He describes how "it is unfortunate that they did not interview the patient" but goes on to state how his comment was made based on talks with one of his colleagues in China and that he is "convinced that there is asymptomatic infection and that some asymptomatic people are transmitting infection." He makes a point of clarifying: "The *NEJM* paper may be incorrect, but according to reputable Chinese scientists, my statement is correct."

On 4. Feb 2020, at 01:29, Fauci, Anthony (NIH/NIAID) [E] (b) (6)> wrote:

Sorry that I got to this so late. I have been swamped. I just read your story in Science. It is unfortunate that they did not interview the patient. Obviously, this changes the conclusion of the paper. My comment: "There's no doubt after reading [the *NEJM*] paper that asymptomatic transmission is occurring" was made because there has been a lot of discussion among Chinese investigators that asymptomatic infection is occurring in Wuhan City and Hubei Province, yet no publication came out and said this. Since this was the first publication supposedly documenting this phenomenon, that is why I referred to the paper and made my comment. It is unfortunate that this error was published, but it still does not really change anything. Rather than rely on rumors, this evening I telephoned one of my colleagues in China who is a highly respected infectious diseases scientist and health official. He said that he is convinced that there is asymptomatic infection and that some asymptomatic people are transmitting infection. The NEJM paper may be incorrect, but according to reputable Chinese scientists, my statement is correct. Having said that, I have been saying for some time that even if asymptomatic infection occurs, it is very unlikely to be a major driver of the outbreak since most transmissions occur from someone who is asymptomatic.
Best regards,
Tony

His email ends with the highlighted text "most transmission occur from someone who is asymptomatic." However, the former chief medical advisor to the president quickly corrects himself in a subsequent email by writing "I meant to say that '...most transmissions occur from someone who is symptomatic'- not asymptomatic."

**From:** Fauci, Anthony (NIH/NIAID) [E]
**Sent:** Tue, 4 Feb 2020 01:08:37 +0000
**To:** Kai Kupferschmidt
**Cc:** Greg Folkers ( (b) (6));Billet, Courtney (NIH/NIAID) [E];Conrad, Patricia (NIH/NIAID) [E]
**Subject:** RE: coronavirus quick question

Kai:
Error in my statement to you. I meant to say that "......most transmissions occur from someone who is symptomatic" – not asymptomatic. I am really tired. Not much sleep these days.
Best,
Tony

This bombshell statement proves how Fauci knew that transmission was driven by the symptomatic not the asymptomatic in February 2020. Yet despite what he wrote in that private email, he went on to publicly advocate for the testing of the asymptomatic. In his speech as a keynote speaker for the American Association for Cancer Research's virtual meeting[342] on "COVID-19 and Cancer" in July 2020, Fauci stated: "The thing I'm most impressed with is, of all the viruses that I've been dealing with over the last several decades, COVID-19's extraordinarily wide spectrum of disease. Twenty to 45 percent of people are completely asymptomatic, while others can be pre-symptomatic in their spread." He went on to say: "The bottom line, common denominator is physical distancing. This can be accomplished by stay-at-home orders, closing or modifying school schedules, bans on public gatherings, and travel restrictions, followed by aggressive case identification and contact tracing."

• • •

My three-part investigation, "The Many Scandals of the PCR Test," published by *TCW*[343] in March 2021, examined and critiqued the controversial role of the "Corman-Drosten RT-PCR test", rapidly declared the "gold standard" for COVID-19 detection by health authorities such as the WHO.

Part 1 traces the rapid development and adoption of the Corman-Drosten RT-PCR protocol, highlighting criticisms regarding its scientific shortcomings as alleged by independent reviewers and the rushed peer-review process that cemented its global use. Part 2 discusses further criticisms, spotlighting a landmark Portuguese court ruling that declared PCR-based quarantines unlawful due to concerns over the test's reliability, alongside the UK's costly "Operation Moonshot," which has been criticized for squandered billions on a widely debated testing regime. Part 3 scrutinizes the authors of the Corman-Drosten paper, noting reported undisclosed conflicts of interest and alleged questionable ties to influential organizations. The following is an adaptation of my investigative series.

## Part 1

In 1993, the biochemist Dr. Kary Mullis won the Nobel prize for inventing the PCR[344] (polymerase chain reaction) technique. It was designed to analyse DNA in a cost-effective and expedient way by replicating a strand of DNA millions of times, allowing scientists to pinpoint a segment of the strand and amplify it. Polymerase is an enzyme which is essential for producing DNA and RNA. Mullis's revolutionary method was used to detect genetic mutations to identify genetic diseases such as sickle cell anemia. It was never designed to diagnose infectious diseases.

In a 1993 interview, Mullis candidly spoke about the dangers of the misuse of PCR testing. Perhaps not surprisingly, the video was removed from YouTube "for violating its terms of service." However, after some searching, I found it posted on archive.org.[345] In the video, Mullis candidly states: "It's just a process that is used to make a whole lot of something out of something. It doesn't tell you that you are sick and it doesn't tell you that the thing you ended up with was going to hurt you or anything like that."

Fast-forward to January 7, 2020. Authorities in China's Wuhan province announce that a novel coronavirus is the cause of cases of pneumonia detected around the end of December 2019. Remarkably, three days later, on January 10, a complete viral genome sequence is available on virological.org.[346]

Around this time in January, Professor Christian Drosten develops a RT (Reverse Transcription)-PCR test protocol for the novel RNA virus, SARS-Cov-2, in his lab in Berlin, based on Mullis's PCR technique. Drosten's testing protocol[347] is accepted by the WHO on January 13, 2020. This is almost two months before the World Health Organisation declares the novel coronavirus a pandemic on March 11, 2020.

On January 21, the Corman-Drosten paper[348] is submitted to the journal Eurosurveillance. A rushed peer review occurs the following day (this peer review has never been released despite repeated requests from international scientists). On January 23, the Corman-Drosten paper is published, laying the foundation for the RT-PCR test to be the gold standard for detecting SARS-CoV-2, later confirmed by the WHO.

Some of the authors of the research paper include: Victor M Corman, Christian Drosten (inventor of the RT-PCR protocol for SAR-CoV-2 who also happens to be the editor of Eurosurveillance), Olfert Landt (CEO of the Tib-Moblbiol biotech company), Jenna Ellis (Public Health England scientist), Maria Zambon (a member of the Government scientific advisory body SAGE, of the New and Emerging Respiratory Virus Threats Advisory Group and of the WHO International Health Regulations emergency committee). I will refer back to these authors and their reported conflict of interests in Part 2 of my investigative report.

The science journalist and geneticist Peter Andrews wrote an article[349] about an "external peer review"[350] of the RT-PCR test protocol conducted by the International Consortium of Scientists in Life Sciences (a group of 22 highly-experienced scientists from Europe, the USA and Japan) that was published on November 30, 2020. The group, led by Dutch molecular biologist Dr. Pieter Borger, found ten major flaws with the paper.

Andrews highlights some of the serious flaws of the Corman-Drosten PCR protocol, flagged by the group:

- Non-specific, due to erroneous primer design.
- Enormously variable.
- Cannot discriminate between the whole virus and viral fragments.
- Has no positive or negative controls.
- Has no standard operating procedure.
- Does not seem to have been properly peer-reviewed.

Dr. Mike Yeadon, one of the scientists who was part of the international review group, highlighted another major flaw with the PCR test in "its propensity to suffer from contamination, and the integrity of a PCR is very easily destroyed by invisible levels of contamination even in the hands of an expert, working alone and on a small handful of samples."

Critics argue that the limitations of RT-PCR testing extend further. The probability of a false positive result of COVID-19 arising from a PCR test is notably high, especially when a high cycle threshold (CT) value is used.

As I wrote earlier, the PCR test works by replicating strands of DNA or RNA in order for them to become large enough to identify. The number of cycles it takes to produce something identifiable is called the cycle threshold value. Anything above a CT value of 35 increases the chance of a false positive result.

Dr. Andrew N Cohen[351] co-authored a report as early as May 2020 warning of the dangers of false positive results generated from PCR testing. The research paper alarmingly states: "We derived a conservative estimate of the range of false positive rates that can reasonably be expected in SARS-CoV-2 testing. Findings: Review of external quality assessments revealed false positive rates of 0-16.7 per cent with an interquartile range of 0.8-4.0 per cent."

The paper goes on to state "the high false discovery rate that results, when prevalence is low, from false positive rates typical of RT-PCR assays of RNA viruses raises questions about the usefulness of mass testing; and indicates that across a broad range of likely prevalences, positive test results are more likely to be wrong than are negative results, contrary to public health advice about SARS-CoV-2 testing."

The implications of this are huge and lead to many questions as to why the UK government chose to implement Operation Moonshot[352] (the name given to the COVID-19 mass asymptomatic PCR testing scheme) with a targeted budget of £100 billion proposed by Johnson's former chief aide Dominic Cummings.

A staggering £12 billion was already spent by October 2020 until the Good Law Project stepped in[353] with the threat of legal action against the Government, claiming "that the Moonshot project was unlawful because it ignored scientific evidence and committed a vast sum of public money with no transparency as to how the decisions were made."

Additional concerns were raised about the awarding of contracts under the testing expansion efforts linked to Operation Moonshot, with some companies receiving large deals despite their scale or track record.

For example, a company called OptiGene was highlighted in a *Daily Mail* article[354] for being so small it doesn't even have to file full accounts. The article reads: "One deal – worth £387million – is with a firm based in Horsham, West Sussex, called OptiGene. Its 2019 accounts state it had assets of just £1.6million."

## Part 2

Here in Part 2, I discuss further criticisms surrounding this [Corman-Drosten] paper and its far-reaching influence on the worldwide draconian quarantines and social distancing policies that PCR test results have appeared to justify.

The turning point in questioning PCR reliability came on November 11, 2020, when a Portuguese appeals court ruled[355] that "the PCR process is not a reliable test for Sars-Cov-2, and therefore any enforced quarantine based on those test results is unlawful." An *OffGuardian*[356] article highlighted the decision: "In their ruling, judges Margarida Ramos de Almeida and Ana Paramés referred to several scientific studies. Most notably this study by Jaafar et al.,[357] which found that – when running PCR tests with 35 cycles or more – the accuracy dropped to three per cent, meaning up to 97 per cent of positive results could be false positives."

This groundbreaking ruling from a European appeals court raises significant questions about whether PCR, at high cycles, was sufficiently reliable as a standalone diagnostic tool for mandatory health measures.

Remarkably, the UK mainstream media did not cover the story, begging the question: Why was PCR testing not more thoroughly scrutinised in the UK judicial system, given the test's capacity for producing false positives when running 35 cycles or more?

In the months that followed, the public faced "unlawful" quarantining often based on PCR results, alongside taxpayer costs for programs like Operation Moonshot and NHS Test and Trace, which continued to rely heavily on PCR alongside lateral flow tests. (The NHS Test and Trace scheme and lateral flow tests are discussed in detail in the following chapter.)

On December 14, 2020, the WHO issued a medical product alert[358] warning that using a high CT value could potentially result in false positives. An extract from its statement reads: "When specimens return a high CT value, it means that many cycles were required to detect the virus. In some circumstances, the distinction between background noise and actual presence of the target virus is difficult to ascertain."

The report goes on to state that an "adjustment of the PCR positivity threshold is necessary to account for any background noise which may lead to a specimen with a high cycle threshold (CT) value result being interpreted as a positive result."

Dr. Thomas Binder MD, one of the 22 authors of the external peer review (mentioned in Part 1) of the Corman-Drosten research paper tweeted:[359] "It is madness to test with a hypersensitive unspecific RT-PCR test only, without consideration of CT & clinical findings. And it is the coronation of insanity to test even asymptomatic people in this way."

The WHO's technical data manager, Maria Van Kerkhove during the organisation's media briefing[360] in June 2020 stated: "Based on our data, it seems unlikely that an asymptomatic carrier will transmit the infection to someone else. We have a number of reports from other countries. They monitor asymptomatic carriers, their contacts, and do not detect further transmission."

This was further confirmed in an article in the *British Medical Journal* [361] by Professor Allyson Pollock, where she wrote: "A city-wide prevalence study of almost ten million people in Wuhan found no evidence of asymptomatic transmission."

So, who were key authors of the Corman-Drosten paper,[362] published in January, 2020 in Eurosurveillance that influenced such draconian quarantine and social distancing policies? The named are: Victor M Corman, Olfert Landt, Marco Kaiser, Richard Molenkamp, Adam Meijer, Daniel K W Chu, Tobias Bleicker, Sebastian Brünink, Julia Schneider, Marie Luisa Schmidt, Daphne GJC Mulders, Bart L Haagmans, Bas van der Veer, Sharon van den Brink, Lisa Wijsman, Gabriel Goderski, Jean-Louis Romette,

Joanna Ellis, Maria Zambon, Malik Peiris, Herman Goossens, Chantal Reusken, Marion P G Koopmans, Christian Drosten.

The paper underwent three revisions, the most significant of which concerned the conflict-of-interest disclosure. The updated statement clarified that "Olfert Landt is the CEO of Tib-Molbiol and that Marco Kaiser is a senior researcher at GenExpress and a scientific adviser to Tib-Molbiol." However, questions remain as to whether it was merely coincidental that Landt and his collaborator, Christian Drosten (the developer of the RT-PCR testing protocol) published their findings in the same journal for which Drosten served as editor, thereby reinforcing the global adoption of RT-PCR as the "gold standard" test for SARS-CoV-2.

On 10 June 2020, the editorial team at Eurosurveillance were contacted "about a perceived conflict of interest" concerning Olfert Landt, CEO of TIB Molbiol, resulting in them to issue an "Editorial note: possible undisclosed conflict of interest."[363] The editorial team stated: "We also received a detailed statement from the corresponding author, Christian Drosten, and from Olfert Landt, who explained that for the main reasons outlined above, they do not consider that being Tib-Molbiol's CEO constituted a conflict of interest with respect to the article in question at the time of submission."

Olfert Landt's Berlin-based biotechnology company, TIB Molbiol, was the first firm worldwide to manufacture and distribute RT-PCR testing kits for SARS-CoV-2. Strikingly, the first viable kits were prepared for shipment by 10 January 2020. An extraordinary head start highlighted by Bloomberg Business[364] in its article, "A Berlin Biotech Company Got a Head Start on Coronavirus Tests." This early advantage proved highly lucrative, with company profits reportedly tripling in February 2020 compared with the same month in 2019.

The German daily newspaper Der Tagesspiegel[365] also commented on TIB Molbiol's tripling of profits in February, along with some other interesting facts. See the English translation below.

> DER TAGESSPIEGEL
>
> His company had around 18 million in sales last year. This year it should be a multiple: In February alone, the company made three times as much sales as normal.
>
> He did not pursue any customer acquisition, nor did he advertise anywhere. But the operators of medical laboratories around the world know: Olfert Landt and team are usually the first to provide a test for viruses - experts speak of oligonucleotide synthesis.
>
> That was the case with the outbreak of the SARS pandemic in 2003, just like with the so-called avian influenza (H5N1) in 2006, with the swine flu (H1N1) and also with the coronavirus MERS from 2012.
>
> TIB Molbiol has no patent or the like on this technology. Other companies are now also producing test kits, but Landt's company is quick and thorough - and probably Berlin's most sought-after company at the moment. According to him, it has already produced three million tests since January and sent them to more than 60 countries. The first were airmailed to Hong Kong on January 10th. The leaflet wasn't even ready at that point. "We sent it afterwards by email".

The article highlights another noteworthy detail: Landt's company, TIB Molbiol, has also been "usually the first" to supply testing kits during the SARS, avian influenza (bird flu), swine flu, and MERS outbreaks.

Returning to the critical date of January 10, 2020. The Eurosurveillance-published Corman-Drosten paper stated: "A viral genome sequence was released for immediate public health support via the online community resource virological.org on 10 January."

This date coincides exactly with the day that TIB Molbiol reportedly sent its first testing kits for the novel virus "by airmail to Hong Kong." The fact that a diagnostic test capable of detecting SARS-CoV-2 was shipped on the same day the viral genome was publicly released raises important questions about the speed and circumstances under which the assay was developed.

## Part 3

The German virologist Professor Christian Drosten, one of the two lead authors of the Corman–Drosten (CD) paper, was among the first scientists to identify the SARS virus and to develop a diagnostic test for it in 2003. His long-standing collaborator and co-author, Olfert Landt, through his company TIB Molbiol, was the first to bring a SARS testing kit to market and later developed and distributed RT-PCR testing kits for SARS-CoV-2.

Another co-author of the CD paper, Marco Kaiser, serves as a senior researcher at GenExpress and also acts as a scientific adviser to TIB Molbiol. These professional relationships were not disclosed in the conflict-of-interest section of the original publication. Following correspondence with the Eurosurveillance editorial team regarding disclosure practices, the paper was revised on 29 July 2020 to include conflict-of-interest statements for Landt and Kaiser. However, Professor Drosten was not included in the revised conflict-of-interest declaration, consistent with the journal's stated editorial policies concerning editors who are also contributing authors.

> Go to section...
>
> In the article 'Detection of 2019 novel coronavirus (2019-nCoV) by real-time RT-PCR' by Corman et al. published on 23 January 2020, a conflict of interest statement was added for authors Olfert Landt and Marco Kaiser on 29 July 2020.

Drosten was turned into an overnight star after developing the real time RT- PCR test for SARS-CoV-2, which was accepted as the standard of testing by the World Health Organization. On March 17, 2020, the German weekly magazine *Stern*[366] published an article headlined, "This is how Christian Drosten became the most important man in Germany."

Drosten is the director of the Institute of Virology at Berlin's Charité hospital, one of Germany's largest university hospitals, a recipient of generous grants from the Bill & Melinda Gates Foundation. Dr Victor Corman,[367] the other lead author of the paper, also works at Charité's Institute of Virology. Drosten's evaluations have heavily influenced German government policy on mandatory mask wearing, school closures and lockdowns.

A review of Drosten's earlier work indicated that he played a prominent advisory role during Germany's swine flu controversy in 2009. At the time, he warned: "It is a widespread viral infection with side-effects far more severe than anyone could imagine from the most dangerous vaccine." At his urging, hundreds of millions of euros was spent on a rushed-through vaccine, GlaxoSmithKline's Pandemrix. His dire warnings though never came to pass. There were only 30 confirmed swine flu deaths[368] in Germany. However, Pandemrix[369] proved to have severe consequences, with links to narcolepsy in both children and adults. Drosten's predictions echoe that of Professor Neil Ferguson, detailed in my investigation into SAGE.

Another co-author of the Corman–Drosten research paper is Professor Maria Zambon, a British virologist who serves as a member of the

UK's Scientific Advisory Group for Emergencies (SAGE), the New and Emerging Respiratory Virus Threats Advisory Group (NERVTAG), and who also sits on the World Health Organization's International Health Regulations Emergency Committee. She is additionally Director of Reference Microbiology at Public Health England (now UK Health Security Agency). Through these roles, Zambon holds significant professional influence both nationally and internationally.

In Part 1 of my investigative report, I noted that the WHO adopted the Corman–Drosten RT-PCR testing protocol on January 13, 2020, despite the fact that the associated paper had not yet undergone formal peer review. The paper itself was subsequently reviewed and published in *Eurosurveillance* within 24 hours (an unusually rapid timeframe, with submission dated January 21 and publication on January 23). To date, the peer-review reports have not been made publicly available, despite multiple requests from independent researchers and international scientific groups.

It is also notable that the WHO did not formally declare COVID-19 a pandemic until March 11, 2020, nearly two months later. The speed of the protocol's acceptance and the institutional overlap between key authors and advisory bodies raises legitimate questions about governance processes and transparency standards.

Dr. Joanna Ellis, a key professional colleague of Professor Zambon in the Virus Reference Department (VRD)[370] at Public Health England (now the UK Health Security Agency) in London, also co-authored the CD paper. As the scientific lead for the Respiratory Virus Unit (RVU),[371] she oversees critical operations. The VRD functions as a WHO-accredited national laboratory, positioning it as a cornerstone of the UK's diagnostic response framework.

Given their senior scientific roles and institutional positions, both Zambon and Ellis were well placed to contribute expert guidance during the early phase of the pandemic. Their professional proximity to key advisory and laboratory networks highlights how a relatively small circle of experts played an extremely influential role in shaping the UK's rapid deployment of mass RT-PCR testing using the very Corman–Drosten protocol, in which they had direct involvement with developing.

As I discussed in Part 1, billions of pounds was spent by the UK government on the country's mass PCR testing program that has been ruled to be "unreliable" and critics argue to be "seriously flawed." However, in my view, what's even more tragic is the way it's been used to justify perpetual lockdowns which have devastated lives.

What is also interesting to note is that in the CD paper published in Eurosurveillance, the authors claimed "before public release of virus sequences from cases of 2019-nCoV, we relied on social media reports announcing detection of a SARS-like virus. We thus assumed that a SARS-related CoV is involved in the outbreak." They go on to report that "we downloaded all complete and partial SARS-related virus sequences available in GenBank by 1 January 2020." This appears to be a significant anomaly as the research paper begins by stating: "A novel coronavirus currently termed 2019-nCoV was officially announced as the causative agent by Chinese authorities on 7 January."

It is highly questionable why, more than a week before the Chinese authorities officially announced a novel coronavirus named 209-nCoV (later renamed SARS-CoV-2) as "the causative agent," the co-authors decided to rely on social media that a SARS-like virus had been detected. The next step they took was to download all the SARS related sequences by January 1 to develop an RT-PCR test designed to detect this new virus whose genome sequence had not officially been published until January 10.

Circling back to the 22-member International Consortium of Scientists in Life Sciences (ICSLS) who officially challenged the Corman-Drosten (CD) paper by submitting their own external peer review to Eurosurveillance (referenced in Part 1). The external peer review identified ten major scientific flaws of the RT-PCR test in detecting SARS-CoV-2. The scientists strongly criticized the CD paper for undergoing what they described as an inadequate peer-review process, containing "flawed science," and involving undisclosed "conflicts of interest." They called for a retraction of the paper. Eurosurveillance responded[372] several months later. An extract from their official statement reads: "An initial evaluation of the allegations was undertaken in collaboration with several board members, followed by a discussion at the annual editorial board meeting on 4 December 2020. This resulted in the decision that it was not necessary to publish an expression of concern with respect to allegation of scientific misconduct or fraud, and that there was no conflict of interest by the associate editors who co-authored the manuscript." The CD paper remains published to this day.

• • •

In October 2025, a peer-reviewed study published in *Frontiers in Epidemiology*[373] ignited widespread debate in Germany and beyond, due to its explosive implications for the COVID-19 pandemic response. The research, which analyzed official testing data from 2020–2021, concluded that the vast majority of positive PCR tests did not indicate active SARS-CoV-2 infections, suggesting massive overcounting of cases that justified lockdowns, mask mandates, and other restrictions. The researchers concluded: "only 14%—and possibly even fewer, down to 10%—of individuals identified as SARS-CoV-2-positive via PCR testing were actually infected, as evidenced by detectable IgG antibodies."

Germany's health authority, the Robert Koch Institute (RKI) "refused to comment"[374] over the study's findings of the staggering 86% false positive rate. However, Dr. Pieter Borger, lead author of "External peer review of the RTPCR test to detect SARS-CoV-2 reveals 10 major scientific flaws at the molecular and methodological level: consequences for false positive results" took to social media to express his response:[375] "In Germany, in most EU countries, a positive PCR was interpreted as infection with killer virus. Because of this non-science several real scientists stood up. They were excluded, demonized and attacked by Pharmaffia-driven politics and media. Free Science Now!"

CHAPTER SEVEN

# INNOVA: THE £4 BILLION VIP LANE SCANDAL

*"We had to buy before we knew they worked."*

~Professor Tim Peto,
chief investigator for lateral flow tests,
admitting the UK government's premature
procurement of Innova tests

In May 2021, I began an investigation that would unravel the web of a highly controversial public health procurement, costing the UK taxpayer billions. My investigation focused on the rapid antigen tests (also known as lateral flow tests), which were freely distributed through the UK's NHS Test and Trace program from May 2020 to April 2022.

This exploration culminated in a multi-part series for *TCW*,[376] published between June- September 2021, dissecting the widespread use of these Chinese-manufactured tests, exclusively licensed to Innova Medical Group (IMG), a fledgling California start-up at the time, uncannily founded around the time of 3/11.

Innova Medical Group, virtually unknown before the pandemic, "struck gold" with the UK government, securing colossal contracts amounting to nearly £4 billion within two years for its SARS-CoV-2 Antigen Rapid Qualitative Test. These deals were inked before UK government officials even knew whether they worked. In stark contrast, across the Atlantic, the U.S. Food and Drug Administration (FDA) issued an emergency recall of

Innova's rapid antigen tests, advising Americans "to throw them in the trash" that summer.

The UK government's spending on Innova accounted for over 12% of the £37 billion allocated in the NHS Test and Trace budget, only to be later criticized by the Chair of the Public Accounts Committee as having made "no measurable difference to the progress of the pandemic." It also speaks directly to the controversial procurement "VIP Lane" process used by the UK government during the COVID-19 pandemic to fast-track contracts for personal protective equipment (PPE), testing kits, and other critical supplies.

The following is an adaptation of Part 1 of "The Innova Scandal" series, first published on June 7, 2021.

## The Innova Scandal: Part 1

Mass testing of the UK's population has been key to the government's "war on COVID-19" for over a year now. It began with Boris Johnson's promise that it was the only way to avoid a second national lockdown,[377] an idea that has proved to be as ill-founded as it was ambitious.

Instead of freeing the country, this extortionately expensive rollout of millions of provenly inaccurate tests for Covid created a false sickness reality, characterized as early as October 20 last year as a "PCR test pandemic."[378]

Critics argue, this government created a pseudo-epidemic that traces back to the highly questionable PCR test, a diagnostic test for COVID-19 developed in Germany before the World Health Organization even declared a pandemic.

Originally hailed as the "gold standard" of testing for the novel virus, subsequent months revealed the PCR test to be highly flawed and unreliable. By January of this year the WHO itself was forced to admit that the test served only as an aid for diagnosis while at least one European court had ruled it to be unfit for purpose.

Operation Moonshot, the name given to this ambitious mass PCR testing scheme of the UK government, aimed to administer 10 million tests a day[379] by early 2021. Championed by the Prime Minister's former adviser Dominic Cummings and provided with an astronomical budget of £100bn, the scheme was abandoned after the Good Law Project (GLP) threatened legal action (referenced in an earlier investigation).

Instead of giving up on the mass testing idea, the government turned its attention to a different testing device and to spend further eyewatering sums of public money to purchase huge numbers of lateral flow tests (LFTs) from a newly formed start-up, Innova Medical Group, owned[380] by a little-known U.S. private equity house.

The Government subsumed Operation Moonshot under, and amalgamated it with, the NHS Test and Trace program, which had its own approved core budget of approximately £12.1 billion.[381] Yet, as with the PCR test, the government's investment in LFT could be described as another scandal in the making. This is the focus of my current investigation.

Despite the many failings of the PCR test, it was not abandoned and is still being used[382] as a confirmatory test for a positive result from a LFT under the NHS Test and Trace program.

In charge of this continuing and unprecedented mass screening program and collecting the data of millions of people was the head of Test and Trace, Baroness (Dido) Harding,[383] an Oxford University friend of former Prime Minister David Cameron and wife of Tory MP John Penrose.

In a former role as chief executive of the TalkTalk group in 2015 she had faced calls to resign after a cyber-attack in which the details of 4 million customers were accessed. The company admitted the incident had cost it £60 million and lost it 95,000 customers. Fining the company £400,000, the Information Commissioner Elizabeth Denham blamed the company's "failure to implement the most basic cyber security measures." Stepping down from TalkTalk in 2017, later that year Harding was made chair of NHS Improvement. Her subsequent appointment as head of Test and Trace by Matt Hancock remains a mystery, as does a further appointment as interim chief executive of the new Health Security Agency (HSA) which brought together NHS Test and Trace and Public Health England, a position Harding kept until Jennie Harries, former deputy CMO of England, took over in April 2021.

It was under Harding's aegis that the evaluation of several LFTs,[384] carried out by Public Health England's Porton Down laboratory and the University of Oxford, for the purposes of judging their accuracy and sensitivity, was published in November 2020.

Forty different lateral flow devices had been put forward. Nine met the criteria to continue to full evaluation, six made it to the third phase, but only the Innova SARS-CoV-2 Antigen Rapid Qualitative Test, the test that had been used in a Liverpool pilot scheme, with a specificity recorded as

99.68 per cent, won through. This was, in theory, critical. Specificity refers to the proportion of people without the disease that have a negative test, suggesting that the risk of false positives would be much lower than with the PCR test.

The Innova test was meant to be different in the rapidity of its results too. Working in a similar way to a pregnancy-style test a result could be delivered in 15-30 minutes. It was also portable, much cheaper than the PCR test, did not need to be processed in a laboratory, and could detect the virus directly without the amplification steps of the RT-PCR test. It sounded good. So thought Susan Hopkins, the chief medical adviser of NHS Test and Trace, who stated:[385] "These tests are proving to be accurate and reliable. And importantly they're able to detect COVID-19 in people without symptoms."

Sir John Bell, Regius Professor of Medicine at the University of Oxford, added his imprimatur: "The data in this validation report demonstrates that these inexpensive, easy-to-use tests can play a major role in our fight against COVID-19. They identify those who are likely to spread the disease and when used systematically in mass testing could reduce transmissions by 90 per cent."[386]

The task of ensuring "that the work is carried out to appropriate quality and timeliness standards," as set out in the protocol for the evaluation[387] of rapid SARS-CoV-2 antigen lateral flow devices, was given to Sir John, to whom progress was to be reported "at least weekly through an Oversight Group that he chairs."

With this endorsement from two of the UK's leading medical professionals, MHRA approval quickly followed, making Innova "the golden child" of COVID-19 self-test kits in the UK. The fact the government had to source them solely from the California-based start-up Innova Medical Group, which held the exclusive global rights to the tests (and was the only company able to supply the tests in such vast quantities), did not apparently bother those involved.

Sir John Bell, chairman of the New Test Approvals Group, which assesses virus diagnostic tests, and described as the government's "tests tsar" is a controversial figure. He is a former non-executive director of Roche (he stood down in 2020) and holder of shares worth £770,000 in the same pharmaceutical company that according to the *Daily Mail*[388] "sold us £13 million of 'pointless' antibody screening kits." Bell's controversial interests go back further.

In 2012 *The BMJ's* editor-in-chief published an open letter[389] to him regarding Roche's 2009 promise to release full reports from clinical trials of oseltamivir (marketed under the name Tamiflu) following an investigation by *The BMJ* and the Cochrane Collaboration. A subsequent comment revealed that Bell had received $420,000 from the company in 2011.[390]

An article[391] by Professor Peter Saunders accused Roche of "pushing an ineffective and costly drug" and concluded that Tamiflu worked "no better than paracetamol" after colossal expenditure by the UK government.

Sir John Bell, a member of SAGE, the chair of the global health advisory board of the Bill & Melinda Gates Foundation and a member of the Government's Vaccine Task Force, is no stranger to accusations of conflicts of interests between his various academic, government and industry roles.

In an article for *The BMJ*[392] earlier this year Paul Thacker asked why wouldn't either Oxford University or the government disclose the "long list" of financial interests of a high-profile researcher at the center of both? He was referring to Professor Bell. He also notes that since the COVID-19 outbreak began early last year, Bell has held high profile roles in the UK government's epidemic response while also working with AstraZeneca on the vaccine; yet both Oxford and the government refused to disclose Bell's financial interests even after *The BMJ* filed freedom of information (FOI) requests. More alarmingly, Thacker goes on, "it appears that the government is referring media enquiries about Bell through the Cabinet Office and is scrutinizing a reporter for *The BMJ* as it has other reporters it finds troublesome. *The BMJ* has been unable to gain either direct contact with Bell or contact through his employer, Oxford University, despite multiple attempts."

Innova Medical Group, the company benefiting from the UK Government's huge testing contract, is owned by the private equity group Pasaca Capital[393] which was founded by a Chinese investment banker, the enigmatic Dr. Charles Huang, in 2017. It has been revealed to be the single largest recipient of the Department of Health's Covid contracts after signing a £496million deal to supply LFTs last year. An earlier contract[394] with Innova cost the taxpayer £107million.[395]

More recently, this April the *Daily Mail* reported that Innova had raked in a total of £2.8billion to supply the UK with lateral flow Covid tests ahead of a plan to offer kits to everyone twice a week.[396] With more than a billion Innova tests bought so far by the UK government, a fierce debate is raging among scientists about their reliability, how they should be used and whether this is a responsible way to spend such huge sums of money.

On the heels of Part 1, the second installment examined the UK government's blind confidence in Innova despite mounting criticisms. Why did officials ignore warnings from top scientists? How did contracts totaling just under £1 billion precede full evaluation? And why was Innova, an obscure start-up, favored over competitors that passed the same screening process?

The following is Part 2[397] of the series, published on June 10, 2021.

## The Innova Scandal: Part 2

A joint report[398] by Public Health England (PHE) Porton Down and Oxford University published early last November gave the Government the green light to invest in and roll out the new lateral flow test (LFT). The "newly deployed lateral flow tests are highly reliable, sensitive and accurate in multiple settings" and "sensitive enough to be used in the community, including for asymptomatic people," they announced,[399] singling out the Innova Medical Group's SARS-CoV-2 Antigen Rapid Qualitative Test, selected for a Liverpool pilot scheme[400] starting that same week. This, they explained, was because only Innova's LFT was reported to be nearing completion of the 4-stage process at the time.

Led by an oversight group chaired by Sir John Bell, Regius Professor of Medicine at Oxford University, the evaluation program had begun a few months earlier in August. Of the 120-plus LFTs submitted for this review,[401] 40 passed phase 2 validation, 24 passed phase 3a validation and just four tests showed a sensitivity rate (the proportion of people who have the disease and get a positive result) of more than 70 per cent. The report focused on just one of these, Innova, and listed its attributes: a test specificity recorded as 99.68 per cent; an overall false positive rate of 0.32 per cent, and an overall sensitivity of 76.8 per cent for all PCR-positive individuals – "over 95 per cent of individuals with high viral loads" – and showing a 'minimal difference between the ability of the test to pick up viral antigens in symptomatic and asymptomatic individuals'.

These high sensitivity rates were recorded when the test was conducted by laboratory scientists. However, when used by trained members of the public, the rate dropped to 57.5 per cent. Surprisingly, this was not flagged as a problem by either Sir John Bell, who oversaw the report, or

Susan Hopkins from PHE. Both concluded that the Innova test had "sufficient sensitivity."[402]

Within days of the publication of the evaluation, other experts warned[403] in *The BMJ* that, to the contrary, the Innova lateral flow test was not fit for this "test and release" strategy as the tests "may miss as many as half of COVID-19 cases, depending on who is using them."

Jon Deeks, professor of biostatistics at the University of Birmingham and leader of the Cochrane Collaboration's COVID-19 test evaluation activities, could not have made his criticism clearer: "Independent evaluations for the World Health Organization have shown that other lateral flow antigen tests are likely to outperform Innova, but even those do not have high enough sensitivity to rule out COVID-19. The Innova test is certainly not fit for use for this purpose."

Another damning article in *The BMJ*[404] a few weeks later claimed the Innova lateral flow tests were "highly inaccurate." It reported "early results [of pilot studies] from students testing at the University of Birmingham and universities in Scotland showed that tests had a sensitivity of just 3 per cent and that 58 per cent of positive test results were false."

Their warnings might have proved a new blow to the UK government's ambitious plans for mass testing, but they were ignored. No brakes were applied. The use of the Innova Lateral Flow Test for the NHS Test and Trace scheme, to be rolled out to universities, hospitals, care homes and all secondary schools, was planned regardless.

Impervious to the critiques, a later PHE and Oxford University performance evaluation of the Innova LFT against the PCR test (co-authored by Susan Hopkins and published[405] in March 2021) found: "In phase 2 and 3a, where the same sample was used for both PCR and LFD specificity analyses, no false positives were detected." Such confidence as to the efficacy of the Innova tests curiously predates as well as postdates their UK clinical evaluation, and by some months. Examination of the government's purchase contracts for tests from IMG (Innova Medical Group) shows their first contract was agreed as early as September 2020 for £103.6million.[406] Subsequent contracts with IMG made before Christmas, before and after PHE and University of Oxford published the results of their evaluation, totaled just under one billion pounds.[407]

Here is a timeline of Government contracts with Innova Medical Group worth hundreds of millions of pounds.

**December 2020**

Department of Health & Social Care

SARS-CoV-2 Antigen Rapid Qualitative Test Kits
award: Innova Medical Group £226M

SARS-CoV-2 Antigen Rapid Qualitative Test Kits
award: Innova Medical Group £104M

**November 2020**

Department of Health & Social Care

SARS-CoV-2 Antigen Rapid Qualitative Test Kits
award: Innova Medical Group £496M

SARS-CoV-2 Antigen Rapid Qualitative Test Kits
award: Innova Medical Group £496M

**October 2020**

Department of Health & Social Care

Innova SARS-CoV-2 Antigen Rapid Qualitative Test Kits
award: Innova Medical Group £138M

Professor Tim Peto of Oxford University, chief investigator for lateral flow tests (overseen by Sir John Bell), admitted, "We had to buy before we knew they worked," arguing that "there was huge worldwide demand."

Officially the justification for using Innova as the sole supplier without a call for competition was that it was in accordance with Article 32 of the contract conditions: "Innova are the only available supplier of home use lateral flow tests for COVID-19 as there is currently no other supplier whose COVID-19 tests are authorized by the relevant regulator, the Medicines and Healthcare products Regulatory Agency (MHRA), for self-test use in the UK...No reasonable alternative or substitute exists: there is currently no other supplier of lateral flow devices that has MHRA authorization for the self-test use needed to satisfy DHSC's (Department of Health) requirement." (Notably, the source for that content has been deleted at the time of this book's publication.)

But why so many pre-orders for such huge numbers and amounts of money given the uncertainty surrounding them? The DHSC justification looked increasingly tenuous from January onwards when the Liverpool School of Tropical Medicine announced that the Excalibur Rapid SARS-CoV-2 Antigen Screening test, validated by LSTM, had been granted MHRA approval, stating:[408] "Now, following approval from the Medicines & Healthcare Products Regulatory Agency (MHRA), the Excalibur Rapid SARS CoV-2 Antigen Screening test can be deployed for widespread mass screening of populations to rapidly track down infectious individuals capable of spreading the disease."

It's striking that after January; further huge contracts were granted by the Government to Innova alone. The largest of these, for £1.2billion,[409] was agreed after Excalibur's MHRA approval; it stated a contract delivery date of 13 March to 28 April, and used the same legal justification for use of Article 32.

How was it that the UK-based firm Excalibur Health Care Services, led by Professor Sir Christopher Evans, a leading bioscience, medical and healthcare entrepreneur, was overlooked by the government in favor of Innova, an obscure start-up?

Nevertheless, armed with the Innova kit, the mass testing rollout planned by the government to coincide with the return to school and college[410] on March 8 this year, went ahead. Secondary school and college students were to take an initial three tests at school and then twice weekly at home, all to be administered by themselves, not by trained professionals. Further plans for expanding community testing were announced in April in which everyone was to be given access to two free tests a week.[411]

Today, the Government's contracts with Innova Medical Group total £3.2billion,[412] an astonishing sum to go to one single start-up company based in California for a test that has proved to be unreliable, on the basis only that it would quickly be able to supply the vast quantities of the test the Government assumed it needed. Daniel Elliott, IMG's chief executive, explained: 'There was a lot of discussion of course about the technology, but it also came down to our ability to supply. Nobody else was anywhere near our production capacity.'[413]

How did this fledgling California start-up get so far ahead of the game in being able to supply vast quantities of tests, not only to the UK but also delivering "over 500million Innova SARS-CoV-2 rapid antigen test kits to over 20 countries"?

Closer inspection suggests that the UK contracts were integral to this new company's success. IMG was set up only 15 months ago, in March 2020, in Nevada, the U.S. state that happens to have the most personal liability protection for directors over corporate wrongdoing and prevents creditors from pursuing companies' assets.

**Company Information**

| | |
|---|---|
| Company Name: | INNOVA MEDICAL GROUP, INC. |
| Entity Type: | FOREIGN CORPORATION |
| File Number: | C4576602 |
| Filing State: | California (CA) |
| Domestic State: | Nevada (NV) |
| Filing Status: | Active |
| Filing Date: | March 27, 2020 |
| Company Age: | 1 Year 2 Months |
| Registered Agent: | Shuning Luo<br>800 E. Colorado Blvd., Ste 288<br>Pasadena, CA 91101 |
| Mailing Address: | 800 E. Colorado Blvd., Ste 288<br>Pasadena, CA 91101 |
| Source: | California Secretary of State |

In a recent interview with the *Financial Times*[414] Elliott claimed they "were ahead of the competition in terms of developing these products but also scaling at mass." He said: "The UK is a key market to us . . . we've been a good partner to the government, the government's been a good partner to us." They were certainly ahead- in being given so much upfront UK taxpayer money.

The UK remains IMG's biggest market for its lateral flow devices. The company says it has spent more than £100million[415] transporting them from China. Now it says that it plans to start manufacturing in the UK. A factory in Wales is promised to begin producing a million tests a day from this summer. Perhaps someone in Government has begun to worry about the billions already spent not benefiting the UK manufacturing industry or its workers?

You would be forgiven for thinking that IMG, given its massive underwriting by the UK, was perhaps part owned by UK PLC but no, it is wholly owned by Pasaca Capital Inc, a private equity firm founded in 2017 by the Chinese-born billionaire Dr. Charles Huang (PhD in marketing) who was born and studied in Wuhan, the center of the pandemic.

IMG and Pasaca Capital are the same. The head office address for IMG is the same as Pasaca Capital's. The board of Pasaca Capital is the same as that of Innova. Prior to COVID-19, there was no history for IMG; their website domain "innovamedgroup.com" was registered only on 15 May 2020. (The website is no longer available online.)

The following extract from Pasaca's website shows how closely intertwined IMG's start-up was with the UK's LFT order: "In October 2020, as the world started to get a better understanding of the virus, the stellar team at Innova secured a significant order from the United Kingdom as it launched Project Moonshot – the British government's ambitious mass testing program. In a highly competitive and heavily scrutinized process led by scientific analysis conducted by the renowned experts at Porton Down and Public Health England, Innova won the contract due to the superior performance of its antigen tests and Innova's unparalleled capacity to supply."

The facts appear to be otherwise: Innova won a significant tranche of the contracts well before the "highly competitive and heavily scrutinized process" was completed. It is hardly surprising then that, as the website says, "In 12 months, Pasaca had transformed Innova from a small start-up to a multi-billion-dollar company, becoming the world's leading manufacturer and distributor of COVID-19 rapid antigen test kits."

But it wasn't Pasaca Capital that has catapulted IMG from an obscure start-up to a major player in COVID-19 testing kits. It was the £ 2.8 billion of UK taxpayers' money[416] handed to the company as of April 2021, making IMG the largest single recipient of payments from UK government contracts during the pandemic.

CEO Daniel Elliott told the Financial Times that "Pasaca Capital invested tens of millions in the early months of the pandemic." That evidence would be welcome. It certainly made a good return on whatever it did invest.

All that Pasaca's webpage[417] tells us is that: "In early 2020, as Covid hit the U.S. and the world, Pasaca's founder, Dr. Charles Huang, and the team of seasoned scientists, top analysts, and sales and marketing experts foresaw that the fight in stemming the spread of the virus necessarily must revolve around repeated mass testing."

IMG's website states that after Huang set up IMG in March 2020, "the Innova team, together with its primary contract manufacturer, Xiamen Biotime Biotechnology Co Ltd, based in Fujian, China, spent several months designing a highly accurate rapid antigen test for COVID-19."

Thanks to its exclusive global rights to the mass-produced rapid antigen tests made by its partner Xiamen Biotime Biotechnology in China, IMG has made itself the UK's sole supplier.

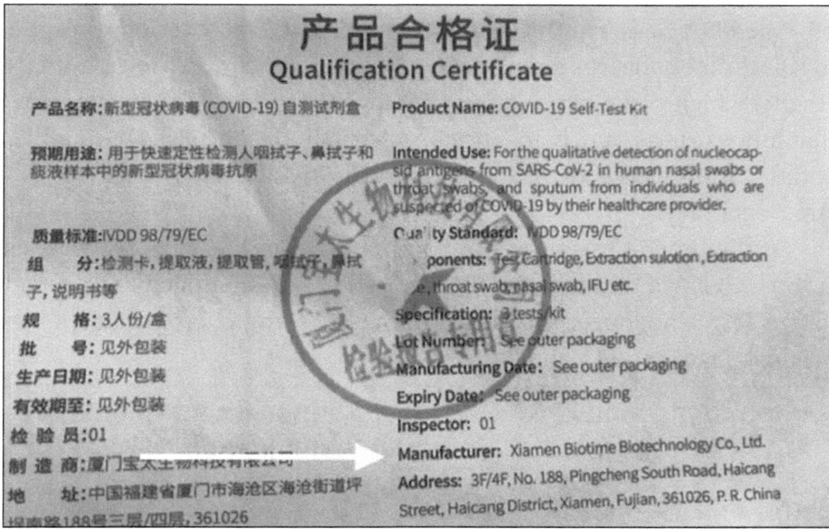

产品合格证
Qualification Certificate

产品名称：新型冠状病毒(COVID-19)自测试剂盒
Product Name: COVID-19 Self-Test Kit

预期用途：用于快速定性检测人咽拭子、鼻拭子和痰液样本中的新型冠状病毒抗原
Intended Use: For the qualitative detection of nucleocapsid antigens from SARS-CoV-2 in human nasal swabs or throat swabs, and sputum from individuals who are suspected of COVID-19 by their healthcare provider.

质量标准：IVDD 98/79/EC
Quality Standard: IVDD 98/79/EC

组　分：检测卡，提取液，提取管，咽拭子，鼻拭子，说明书等
Components: Test Cartridge, Extraction sulotion, Extraction tube, throat swab, nasal swab, IFU etc.

规　格：3人份/盒
Specification: 3 tests/kit

批　号：见外包装
Lot Number: See outer packaging

生产日期：见外包装
Manufacturing Date: See outer packaging

有效期至：见外包装
Expiry Date: See outer packaging

检 验 员：01
Inspector: 01

制 造 商：厦门宝太生物科技有限公司
Manufacturer: Xiamen Biotime Biotechnology Co., Ltd.

地　址：中国福建省厦门市海沧区海沧街道坪埕南路188号三层/四层，361026
Address: 3F/4F, No. 188, Pingcheng South Road, Haicang Street, Haicang District, Xiamen, Fujian, 361026, P. R. China

Qualification Certificate found inside the NHS Test and Trace COVID-19 self-test kits.

In April this year the *Guardian*[418] once again questioned the lack of transparency of the government's Covid contracts, saying that a fifth of them raise red flags for corruption thanks to Johnson's VIP lane set up by the Cabinet Office and the Department of Health and Social Care in the early days of the pandemic.

Innova's brief history raises other equally worrying questions. First, how did Huang of Pasaca Capital know in early 2020 that the world was going to need hundreds of millions of rapid COVID-19 testing devices when in early March[419] there were only 35 reported cases in the UK and 89 cases in the U.S.? When mass testing for a virus had never been conducted before?

How was his Chinese manufacturing partner, Xiamen Biotime able so quickly to provide a solution to the problem? Did they have some information that gave them a significant head start in forming a company with an unparalleled capacity to supply?

• • •

On June 10, 2021, the same day the second part of my investigation was published in *TCW*, the FDA urged the U.S. public to stop using Innova Medical Group's SARS-CoV-2 Antigen Rapid Qualitative Test and "to throw them in the trash."

The FDA classified this as a Class I recall, the most serious type, due to significant concerns about the test's performance and the risk of false results, which could pose serious public health risks. The agency noted that Innova's tests were being illegally distributed in the U.S. without FDA authorization, clearance, or approval, and lacked adequate data to demonstrate accuracy.

At the time of this book's publication, the specific FDA webpage issuing the Class I recall for the Innova SARS-CoV-2 Antigen Rapid Qualitative Test is no longer available, but the following is a screenshot of the original page.

**Stop Using Innova SARS-CoV-2 Antigen Rapid Qualitative Test: FDA Safety Communication**

**Date Issued: June 10, 2021**

The U.S. Food and Drug Administration (FDA) is warning the public to stop using the Innova SARS-CoV-2 Antigen Rapid Qualitative Test for diagnostic use. The FDA has significant concerns that the performance of the test has not been adequately established, presenting a risk to health. In addition, labeling distributed with certain configurations of the test includes performance claims that did not accurately reflect the performance estimates observed during the clinical studies of the tests. Finally, the test has not been authorized, cleared, or approved by the FDA for commercial distribution or use in the United States, as required by law.

Part 3 asks why did the UK discount the U.S. FDA's scathing critique and continue pouring taxpayer money into a test experts deemed unfit? How did a little-known California start-up secure such massive funding ahead of better-established competitors? And who benefited from this extraordinary expenditure of public money?

The following is the third installment[420] of my investigative series, published on June 14, 2021.

## The Innova Scandal: Part 3

In an unanticipated announcement at the end of last week, the U.S. Food and Drug Administration (FDA) warned the public to stop using the Innova lateral flow test. In the most stringent of terms, it stated: "The FDA has significant concerns that the performance of the test has not been adequately established, presenting a risk to health."

The Innova SARS-CoV-2 Antigen Rapid Qualitative Test is the very same test that was correctly described that night in BBC Newsnight's June

11, 2021, report of this news as the "cornerstone" of the British Government's anti-Covid strategy. The FDA's press release, they said, was "scathing and damning" about the Innova test while Allyson Pollock, a public health doctor appearing on the program, declared it unfit for purpose, adding for good measure that there is no evidence that mass-testing and 'Test and Trace' reduces transmission.

As I reported in Part 2 of my investigation, this is the test that was favored by the UK above 120-plus other contenders for its Covid mass screening program (initially called Moonshot but renamed NHS Test and Trace) after the operation had to shift from sole reliance on the flawed PCR test. It is the test to which both Sir John Bell, Regius Professor of Medicine at Oxford, and Susan Hopkins from Public Health England (PHE) gave their imprimatur.

It is the test for which the Department of Health (DHSC) committed hundreds of millions of UK taxpayer pounds to a Californian start-up company some six/seven weeks before the clinical evaluation overseen by Sir John Bell was published or the piloting of the finally chosen Innova test completed.

It is also the test that made one new California start-up, the largest single financial beneficiary of UK Covid contracts, for which the Government has committed £3.2billion to date.

The FDA's press release reported that some weeks earlier, on April 23, 2021, Innova Medical Group (IMG) had sent a medical recall letter to all those using the Innova test manufactured between September 1, 2020 and March 3, 2021 as a result of which at least 77,339 of the Innova SARS-CoV-2 Antigen Rapid Qualitative Test in the U.S. were recalled. The FDA identified this recall as a Class I recall, the most serious type of recall.

Curiously, the same type of test used in the UK, not in the thousands but in the hundreds of millions, has not been recalled. Millions have been purchased by our government since the April 23 recall. Is the UK test any way different? There is nothing to suggest whether it is or that the same basis for recall does not exist in Britain.

The FDA criticized: "Labelling distributed with certain configurations of the test includes performance claims that did not accurately reflect the performance estimates observed during the clinical studies of the tests." It also stated that "the performance characteristics of the test have not been adequately established, presenting a risk to health."

This was the conclusion (and the concern) articulated by other experts in the UK about the test within days of the PHE Porton Down evaluation publication early last November – expert criticism that the DHSC ignored.

In fact key limitations of the test were acknowledged by the manufacturer and are to be found in the original instructions for use of the Innova SARS-CoV-2 Antigen Rapid Qualitative Test. Namely that it was only ever intended for use in patients with COVID-19 symptoms (i.e. symptomatic patients) meaning that the Innova SARS-CoV-2 rapid antigen test was never designed to screen the asymptomatic but only to detect active infections (when symptoms are present).

The instructions say: "The SARS-CoV-2 Antigen Rapid Qualitative Test is . . . intended for the qualitative detection of nucleocapsid antigens from SARS-CoV-2 in human nasal swabs or throat swabs from individuals who are suspected of COVID-19 by their healthcare provider. within the first five days of the onset of symptoms." [Punctuation as in the leaflet.]

This of course makes a complete mockery of the UK government's Test and Trace mass screening intention, and of their fundamental justification for buying 20million of these tests in October 2020 (prior to the test's evaluation) and subsequent purchase of millions more, all with the main intention to catch infections in asymptomatic people (those showing no symptoms)!

The Innova tests, however, were repackaged for the NHS with a different version of the instructions, which stated (in the November 24, 2020, NHS version): "You can use this self-test kit if you have symptoms or if you are asymptomatic (you do not have symptoms)."

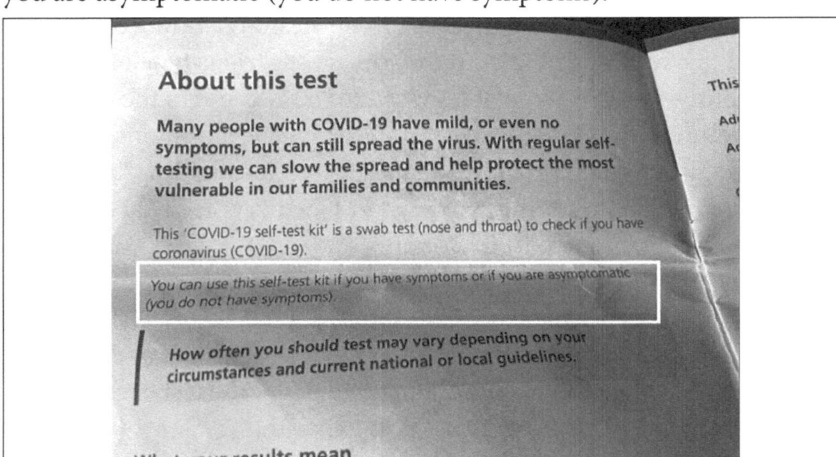

Source: NHS COVID-19 Self-Test Kit

Alarmingly, the NHS instructions have been updated[421] since then, with the removal of the referenced sentence above in the January 16, 2021 version.

The original Innova instructions also state that the test 'is intended for use by trained clinical laboratory personnel . . . and individuals similarly trained in point of care settings.'

In the NHS Test and Trace version, the test is intended for use by any member of the public aged 12-plus. Included in the original Innova instructions are the limitations of the procedure. These are omitted in the NHS version.

The Innova instructions say:

1. Clinical performance was evaluated with frozen samples, and test performance may be different with fresh samples.
2. Users should test specimens as quickly as possible after specimen collection.
3. Positive test results do not rule out co-infections with other pathogens.
4. Results from SARS-CoV-2 Antigen Rapid Qualitative Test should be correlated with the clinical history, epidemiological data, and other data available to the clinician evaluating the patient.
5. A false-negative test result may occur if the level of viral antigen in a sample is below the detection limit of the test or if the sample was collected or transported improperly; therefore, a negative test result does not eliminate the possibility of SARS-CoV-2 infection.

This disparity was picked up by the *Daily Mail*[422] in January 2021, which headlined its article: "Department of Health puts NHS branding on rapid Covid tests so it can get around manufacturer's instructions that people should NOT swab themselves."

Scandalously the government appears to have ignored this, spending further millions with Innova for school and home testing.

*The Telegraph*[423]also noted a "confusion" with the conflicting instructions for use, reporting that the "Chinese-made lateral flow tests handed to millions of schoolchildren" included the original manufacturer's instructions inside the box. The paper said the "out of date" instructions "erroneously" stated that the tests were for use by people "suspected of COVID-19 by their healthcare provider."

Had *The Telegraph* pursued their investigations, they would have found that the original manufacturer (Xiamen Biotime Biotechnology sold through Innova) did not make a mistake. The instructions were not out of date. The only factor that had changed was the Government's repurposing of the test to catch virus infections in asymptomatic individuals.

*The Telegraph* article went on to state that the official guidelines are that "people with symptoms are supposed to get a PCR laboratory test, the results of which are reported automatically, triggering the contact tracing process." This still contradicts the NHS instructions which are that Innova test is to be used in both the asymptomatic and symptomatic. *The Telegraph* quoted a Downing Street spokesman as saying that lateral flow tests had been "rigorously evaluated and we believe they are both accurate and incredibly useful in terms of being able to spot asymptomatic cases of the virus."

The truth is as Professor Allyson Pollock of Newcastle University told the paper: "The whole mass testing program is confusing, chaotic and the antithesis of good public health practice. If you do mass testing you need to do proper evaluation beforehand, which would identify problems like this. Lateral flow testing should have gone through the UK National Screening Committee for proper evaluation."

So, who is responsible for these major errors and this £3billion+ fiasco?

The joint PHE Porton Down and Oxford University's evaluation led by Sir John Bell, rapidly validated the Innova Test, leading the UK government to spend billions that would later be shown to have significant limitations. The Department of Health and Social Care who then changed the manufacturer's original instructions for intended use, rebranding it as an NHS COVID-19 self-test kit with a modified protocol, while publicly blaming the manufacturer for including "out of date" and "erroneous" instructions.

• • •

What started as a reckless, pre-evaluation procurement through the infamous VIP lane would soon unravel into a web of fraud allegations detailed in civil lawsuits, disputed fortunes, luxury estates, and executive excesses against the very individuals who profited most. The next chapter uncovers the fallout.

CHAPTER EIGHT

# INNOVA: THE FALLOUT

*"Corruption is like a ball of snow, once it's set a rolling it must increase."*

~Charles Caleb Colton, Lacon, vol. 1 (1820)

As the UK government doubled down on its exclusive partnership with Innova Medical Group, pouring nearly £4 billion into a product plagued by accuracy doubts and VIP favoritism. The United States issued stark warnings, deeming the tests unfit and urging their disposal. Yet, across the Atlantic, the contracts rolled on, fueling private jets, luxury estates, and executive excesses at taxpayer expense. This chapter looks at the fallout: from probing the dubious backgrounds of Innova's key players and their "get ahead of the science" maneuvers, to the explosive legal battles that ensued, including fraud allegations and misappropriated fortunes. Drawing on fresh FOI disclosures, court filings, and investigative updates, it poses the questions the establishment has evaded: How deep did the corruption run, and who will hold the government accountable? The following is the fourth installment[424] of my Innova series, first published by *TCW* on June 21, 2021.

## The Innova Scandal: Part 4

The owner of Innova Medical Group, suppliers of the flawed lateral flow tests on which British taxpayers have spent billions of pounds, is Chinese-born American businessman Dr. Charles Huang, (who holds a PhD in marketing from Strathclyde University). Despite the U.S. FDA later declaring the tests unsafe and urging Americans to throw them in the trash, the UK government has continued its exclusive partnership with Innova.

Huang has been associated with scandal in the past. As the financial director of a Chinese automotive manufacturer, Brilliance Group, he "played a key role in the strategic alliance between China's Brilliance Group and MG Rover Group in the UK in 2002." This is what his biography page[425] on Pasaca Capital, the company that wholly owns Innova Medical Group (IMG), at the heart of my investigation, proudly tells us.

In fact, it is nothing to boast about. It was an ill-fated joint venture which was embroiled in scandal. MG Rover, the last of the domestically owned mass-production UK car manufacturers, went into administration in 2005 and inspectors were appointed by the Department for Trade and Industry to investigate the affairs of its parent company, Phoenix Venture Holdings (PVH). Written evidence[426] submitted by PVH to the Parliamentary Select Committee on Trade and Industry in 2004 reveals that MG Rover Group had been working in partnership with China Brilliance and that "unfortunately, a major dispute between the owner and the Provincial Government (had) resulted in China Brilliance's inability to complete the project."

The "major dispute" refers to the sudden departure[427] to the U.S. of Brilliance's chairman Yang Rong, who was wanted in China for alleged involvement in "economic crimes." The head of Brilliance, Dr Brian X Sun, was also being investigated by the Chinese authorities and an arrest warrant had been issued for him too. The reason for the termination of their joint venture with MG Rover was stated to be the "result of the non-receipt of payments due to MG Rover from the China Partner."

In the 838-page report into the affairs of PVH,[428] (compiled at a cost to the taxpayer of £14.8million) MG Rover Group's joint venture with Brilliance Group, also referred to as "Project Sunrise," Charles Huang's name is mentioned: "Mr. Howe [MG Rover's managing director] reported that during the course of the Board meeting he had taken a telephone conversation from Charles Haswell of the British Embassy in Beijing. He confirmed that he had requested the British Embassy to make enquiries on the

Company's behalf as to the identity and whereabouts of Yang Rong, Brian Sun and Charles Huang and the position in respect of the Brilliance Group of companies. Mr. Haswell reported back that Mr. Yang appeared to have fled to the United States of America where he was expected to stay. He further reported that Brilliance as a group of companies had never had any intention of building motor vehicles with the Company." The whereabouts of Dr. Huang were not detailed. The report also included an extract from an article in the Financial Times: "Several senior executives at Brilliance China Automotive Holdings Ltd . . . are under investigation over suspected asset stripping among the group's sprawling network of subsidiaries."

If so, it was certainly ignored when it came to the Department of Health (DHSC) awarding its premature IMG contracts – the first one of which, as I revealed in Part 3, was for £103million and was agreed nearly two months before the clinical trial evaluation was completed and published, or the pilot using IMG LFTs started. Nor did Dr. Huang's history stop the UK government from continuing to pay out close to £3billion to the Huang-owned IMG over successive months from 2020 to 2021 for more of its highly inaccurate Innova lateral flow tests which distinguished UK scientist John Deeks, in January 2021, again warned[429] the government about before their planned mass roll-out, and which the U.S. Food and Drug Administration (FDA) has now abandoned.

How did Innova Medical Group come to get these lucrative UK government contracts in the first place? Who made the introduction? How was this one company chosen? Why was Innova given such preferential treatment by the joint PHE and Oxford University evaluation program run by the DHSC, chaired by Matt Hancock and overseen by Sir John Bell of Oxford University?

Some of this I touched on in Part 2. A *Guardian* report on the millions spent by the Government "on controversial covid tests for Dominic Cummings's scheme," last January confirmed that the context was the imminent collapse of Operation Moonshot, Cummings's mass testing idea that preceded the LFT invention.

According to Professor Tim Peto, the chief investigator for the lateral flow tests under Sir John Bell, fellow Oxford academic and overseer of LFTs for the government, "LFT was the knight in shining armor to save the day." How long before the clinical trials were published that they decided that "Innova was top of the pile," he does not reveal. But by last summer a Cabinet Office Covid taskforce, including the Prime Minister's chief strategist Sir Edward Lister, was pressing "cities around the country with rising caseloads" to pilot the new tests, well before their clinical evaluation.

A senior public health source indicated the pressure they were put under: "Ed [Lister] and his team came to visit areas with high rates of Covid and kept mentioning LFTs and that the PM was very keen . . . When we raised questions, we were told . . . it was in Moonshot and was a proposal with endless amounts of money. The phrase they constantly used to us was 'No regrets' and that Dominic Cummings's phrase was: 'We want to get ahead of the science'..."

"Get ahead of the science," Cummings did. He also appears to have "got ahead" of the Government's normal protocols for clinical evaluation and procurement, detailed in Part 2. An irregularity, which opened the way to an unknown start-up becoming the Government's highest-paid single Covid contractor and turning over a multi-billion-pound operation.

According to the *Guardian* the Oxford (LFT Clinical Evaluation) team presented the results of their evaluation of Innova's tests to Cummings in late October, with the health secretary, Matt Hancock. The decision to roll the tests out in a large field pilot as soon as possible was then pushed by Cummings, a couple of weeks before he resigned, with Innova being the lucky winner of this opportunity. MHRA (Medicines and Health products Regulatory Agency) approval quickly followed. Mr. Cummings resigned on November 13, 2020. Why did he and Hancock discount the other LFTs that made it through the screening process?

In a joint webinar from the joint Royal College of Pathologists and British Infection Association (BIA), published on November 10, 2020, test investigator Professor Tim Peto of Oxford University is recorded saying "Four or five got through the screening process and one, Innova, was done first and we've got more data on that because of time – I'm not saying that the others aren't as good – and I'm going to present to you the Innova data because I think that is going to be distributed widely in the short term." (At the time of this book's publication, the BIA has removed the content.)

This admission from Peto that other tests were potentially as good, but that Innova was "done first" and its data was presented because he believed that it was going to be "distributed widely" appears to be a nod to the first contract with IMG before the clinical evaluation was completed. It was also Professor Peto who, in reference to the early procurement of the Innova test, admitted: "We had to buy before we knew they worked."

Questioned earlier this year on how IMG came to secure its huge UK government contracts in the first place, its CEO, Daniel Elliott mentioned[430] one company as "key in helping them beat more established industry giants to secure the first lucrative deal last Summer"- the Northamptonshire-based, Disruptive Nanotechnology Ltd. It agreed, he said, to help IMG negotiate the bureaucracy and the trials the test had to go through to win this Government deal.

The man once in charge of that company, a Northamptonshire-based businessman called Kim Thonger, today is in charge of marketing and operations at Tried & Tested,[431] the company that later won its way to being the sole UK distributor of Innova's tests. However, this sole distributor of the Innova LFT was not always called Tried & Tested. It originally traded under the name of Disruptive Nanotechnology Ltd, the company that helped Elliot secure the IMG contract, a small company which until recently showed debts exceeding assets by a couple of thousand pounds.

Described by the *Daily Mail*[432] "as a man with no previous healthcare background who once worked for DKNY shoes and Dr Marten's." Mr. Thonger managed to help Mr. Elliott (and Dr. Huang presumably) negotiate the biggest value Covid contract between the UK government and a single company. He has been aided latterly by his new partner Charles Palmer, who runs the company under its new name.

A spokesperson for Tried & Tested told the *Mail*[433] that "the company is the sole distributor of Innova lateral flow devices to the UK commercial market and is not involved with Innova's UK government contract."

A single box of 25 Innova rapid antigen tests costs £207.50. Thonger and Palmer are reported to get "a few pence" for every test sold. With hundreds of millions of Innova tests purchased, a few pence for each, is not insignificant.

It would be interesting to know how a former shoe salesman came to be pivotal in securing Innova's early contracts and how this same man, working under a new company name, came to be, according to his LinkedIn page, the "exclusive UK and EU distributor" for the Innova Medical Group rapid antigen test in the commercial market.

The Private Eye issue of December 4-17, 2020, questioning the highly lucrative Innova deal with the UK Government and Disruptive Nanotechnology's involvement, which "looked to be among the most questionable of the many previously unheard-of recipients of pandemic deals," throws further light on Mr. Thonger's rebranded company: "What little activity can be seen since it set up in 2015 is an unsuccessful attempt to sell Light-Cleanse, a technology coating surfaces in titanium dioxide that reacts with light to produce oxidants to clean the surface. Health concerns allegedly scuppered it. On latest figures (to December 2018) the firm was technically insolvent, with debts exceeding assets by a couple of thousand pounds. It is run by directors Kim Thonger and Charles Palmer, whose careers have taken in shoe retail and property respectively."

The significance of this nanotechnology connection, also highlighted by the *Daily Mail*, between Thonger and Elliott remains obscure.

What we do know is that both men secured lucrative Innova LFT deals, thanks to the UK Government and at the taxpayer's expense. This is more than an "Operation Shambles,"[434] as the *Daily Mail* has called the LFT and Moonshot/NHS Test and Trace saga. Despite a litany of warnings from some of Britain's top scientists about the deeply flawed nature of the test, the government not only determined to go ahead with this hubristic and ill-conceived program but proceeded with a deeply questionable tendering and procurement process.

Nor has the FDA's thumbs-down to the Innova lateral flow device and IMG's own product recall in the U.S. some months earlier, discussed in Part 3, made any difference to the intransigent UK government. Disregarding the FDA's safety concerns, the MHRA announcement[435] on June 17 extended the UK's emergency use authorization (EUA) of the (Innova) lateral flow devices used in the NHS Test and Trace program through to August 28, 2021. Graeme Tunbridge, MHRA Director of Devices, said: "A full risk assessment was undertaken by DHSC as legal manufacturer of the LFDs in the UK and the MHRA has undertaken a thorough review to ensure that we were satisfied with the assessment and any action proposed."

Yet this investigation has shown that the Chinese Xiamen Biotime Biotechnology is the actual manufacturer of the Innova test, not the DHSC, and if the latter were the legal manufacturer a wholly independent risk assessment should have been done, not by the DHSC themselves. The UK public deserve to be shown the evidence of the "thorough review" undertaken by the MHRA.

For the fortunate folks at IMG, Pasaca Capital, the Chinese manufacturer of the tests Xiamen Biotime and Tried & Tested, the gravy train rolls on. Not so for the UK public: so far, £3.2billion of their money has been spent on the Government's relentless testing of the asymptomatic using this unreliable product, greatly inflating the number of Covid cases (while putting others at risk) to justify the draconian restrictions imposed on them.

• • •

Since the fourth installment of my original series in *TCW*, further revelations have emerged via Freedom of Information requests and legal action. Emails[436] secured by the Good Law Project, between Kim Thonger and Dominic Cummings (then Chief Adviser to Prime Minister Boris Johnson).

These emails, dated from July 29- August 4, 2020, which precede Innova's first £103 million contract (September 2020), highlight the unusually fast escalation from an unsolicited pitch to senior government engagement. The fact that Cummings' email address was accessible to Thonger, the unusually familiar tone, and the immediate involvement of William Warr (Special Adviser at Number 10), strongly suggests pre-existing connections.

**From:** Kim Thonger <*Redacted*>
**Date:** Wednesday, 29 July 2020 at 10:39
**To:** Dominic Cummings <*Redacted*>
**Cc:** Charles Palmer <*Redacted*>; *Redacted* <*Redacted*>
**Subject:** 15 minute accurate effective saliva antigen Covid-19 test

Good morning Dominic,

I attach a letter to you about our new antigen test.

**Features**

1. 15 minute result
2. No machine
3. No lab
4. Saliva based
5. Low cost compared to PCR
6. 100% specificity

We are selling it combined with our antibody test. We call it DoubleTest™, see this pdf.

Best regards
Kim

Kim Thonger
Director
<*Redacted*>
<*Redacted*>
www.triedandtested.tech

Within less than an hour, William War, a senior Special Adviser, responds in a familiar tone, expressing "very keen" interest in supporting rapid antigen tests.

> On 29 Jul 2020, at 11:35, William Warr <*Redacted*> wrote:
> Dear Kim,
>
> Thanks for this note to Dom. We are very keen to support rapid antigen tests. Please can you provide some further details about your test and some data to Emma cc'd who leads testing innovations in the testing programme.
>
> Many thanks,
>
> Will

The email exchanges contain no indication of initial scrutiny regarding the credentials of Innova or Disruptive Nanotechnologies. Thonger's assertion of the test achieving "100% specificity" is made without accompanying data to substantiate the claim, yet it still triggers government response. These communications further bolster criticisms surrounding the highly contentious VIP lane process, through which the UK government awarded contracts post 3/11, with little to no competitive tendering.

Notably in January 2022, the UK High Court ruled[437] that the Covid PPE VIP lane was "unlawful," finding it breached equal treatment obligations under procurement laws. Mrs. Justice O'Farrell noted a lack of objective justification for prioritizing certain offers, a decision stemming from a case brought by the Good Law Project (GLP) and EveryDoctor.

This sets the stage for the fifth instalment of my investigative series, "How The Test Firm Flashed the UK Taxpayer's Cash,"[438] published in *TCW* on September 15, 2021.

## The Innova Scandal: Part 5

The golden child of lateral tests was fast-tracked through Public Health England's Porton Down laboratory and Oxford University's allegedly rigorous evaluation program. It was given special VIP status, by being placed "on top of the pile."

In December 2020, it was granted Exceptional Use Authorization (EUA) by the Medicines and Healthcare Products Regulatory Agency (MHRA), without the standard regulatory approval process because of "exceptional circumstances." Professor Tim Peto, chief investigator of the joint evaluation program (overseen by Sir John Bell, Regius Professor at Oxford University and Susan Hopkins from PHE) admitted in relation to the Innova LFTs, "we had to buy before we knew they worked."

This fully explains why the first round of multi-million-pound contracts with Innova Medical Group were already greenlit by the Department of Health and Social Care (DHSC), chaired by the former Health Secretary Matthew Hancock, weeks before the evaluation report was even published. Considerable evidence points to the fact that the tests were also inaccurate, unreliable[439] and still are "not fit for purpose." The Chinese-made, and US-supplied Innova test was the sole brand of LFT used, as part of the Government's discredited NHS Test and Trace scheme, with an allocated budget of £37 billion with no evidence that it made a measurable difference.[440]

An article[441] posted on the Good Law Project's website provides yet another dimension to this saga of ineptitude and possible corruption. Quoting the Public Accounts Committee[442] report on Test and Trace, which stated that, despite "unimaginable resources," the program "cannot point to a measurable difference to the progress of the pandemic." The article though goes on to find the one measurable difference, which was "for the owners of the biggest of the pandemic contract winners, Innova."

The GLP adds a Los Angeles Times report[443] on how the Innova owners flashed a bank statement "with a $175million balance as proof of funds" and also went on "a corporate and personal luxury buying spree, including several Gulfstream jets and luxury houses."

The welcome news is that the GLP has been granted court permission to bring a judicial review, questioning the decision to make Tory life peer Dido Harding head of NHS Test and Trace from May 2020 to May 2021. This was the period when she was "in charge of the program that delivered unimaginable wealth to Innova's owners yet made no measurable difference to the progress of the pandemic."

Up until now, roughly £4billion of taxpayers' money has been handed over to Innova Medical Group, (the last contract awarded in July 2023 was worth a hefty £144million) an unknown California start-up, formed coincidentally around the start of the pandemic by the US-Chinese billionaire Charles Huang, founder of Pasaca Capital, a private equity firm.

Revealed in the article is the critical fact that John Penrose MP[444] the Government's anti-corruption champion, who "rather than chasing corruption ... seems to spend his time besmirching those who do" is the husband of Harding. This fact was found "laughable" by Jolyon Maugham, chairman of GLP and I concur.

How can an independent inquiry ever be launched if it is your own spouse you are supposed to be investigating? This glaring conflict of interest has been shockingly ignored by the mainstream media.

The Penrose-Harding connection was raised in Parliament by Tonio Antoniazzi, Labour MP for Gower, in the Government Contracts: Covid-19[445] debate on June 21, 2021. Antoniazzi said: "Some people might want to raise the issue of apparently cozy contracts, the lack of a tendering process and the inability to declare contracts, but who would they turn to? Perhaps they could approach the Government's own anti-corruption champion, the Hon Member for Weston-super-Mare (John Penrose), although he might not be open to receiving complaints as he is married to Baroness Harding."

I welcome the GLP's pursuit of the rampant Test and Trace corruption and for drawing the public's attention to the lucrative contracts made to the owners of Innova.

According to the Los Angeles Times, when a real estate agent asked for proof of payment from one of the Innova executives, he waved the company's bank statement showing a deposit of $128million from the UK government.

Maugham, however, reveals only a fraction of the scandals surrounding the Innova lateral flow test. I believe the lateral flow test program stands out as one of the most flawed and over-hyped aspects of the COVID era, riddled with issues around accuracy and misuse, at a catastrophic cost to the UK public. In my investigative report, I revealed the many Innova anomalies, such as the drastic changes the DHSC made to the instructions for use of the test. Essentially, this involved repurposing the test from being intended only for use by laboratory-trained professionals on symptomatic patients (those showing symptoms), as laid out in the original manufacturer's instructions (these instructions are no longer available online) to being used by anyone over the age of 12 with no symptoms (asymptomatic).

The false justification given for using Innova as the sole supplier without a call for competition (bypassing the standard tendering process) was that it was in accordance with Article 32 of the contract conditions: "Innova are the only available supplier of home use lateral flow tests for COVID-19 as there is currently no other supplier whose COVID-19 tests are authorized by the relevant regulator, the Medicines and Healthcare products Regulatory Agency, for self-test use in the UK."

The existing link I had used as my source in Part 2 of my original report now gives this message: "This content has been deleted, doesn't exist, or can't be previewed." There could be a legitimate technical reason for this, of course, or perhaps it might be the case of covering up the evidence.

Article 32 is not true, because there were other LFTs, some even UK-made, that passed the evaluation process at the same time as Innova and were granted MHRA approval very soon after.

Thanks to an anonymous source, there is yet another scandal that has been drawn to my attention in connection with the executives at Innova Medical Group. Daniel Elliott, the CEO of Innova and President/Partner of Pasaca Capital, was the former CEO of EnerBlu, the now-bankrupt battery manufacturer.

In late 2017, Enerblu announced plans to invest $400million for a new battery manufacturing plant in Pikeville, Kentucky, creating 875 jobs. Kentucky officials approved $30million in tax incentives and pledged millions in grants.

However, the only thing to materialize from the new plant proposal were lawsuits launched against the executives at EnerBlu, many of whom happen to sit on the board at Innova and Pasaca Capital, including Daniel Elliott and Darin Marino.

The Florida investor group Dapco invested $3million into the development of the proposed EnerBlu plant. But, according to its representative, all it got in return was "a bogus Eastern Kentucky battery plant[446] that was never more than drawings on a piece of paper."

The investors filed a lawsuit against EnerBlu's executives, accusing them of fraudulent misrepresentation, fraud by omission and unjust enrichment. They accused EnerBlu of using "little to none" of the $9.6million it raised for developing products or technology. Instead, Elliott and the other defendants "were travelling around the world at great expense, purporting to be closing in on investments from some of the wealthiest people and entities on the planet."

Elliott was reportedly fired from EnerBlu in January 2019 and shortly afterwards moved to California, where he joined forces with the elusive Charles Huang. Huang, like Elliott, is no stranger to controversy, as detailed earlier in part 4.

• • •

In June 2022, the multi-million pound COVID-19 inquiry, chaired by Baroness Heather Hallett, was launched to "examine the UK's response to and impact of the COVID-19 pandemic, and learn lessons for the future."

The glaring irony of the UK's COVID-19 response can be epitomized by a question that the inquiry committee will likely never dare ask: Why did the UK Government blow nearly £4 billion on the infamous Innova lateral flow tests?

Adding to the absurdity, according to *The Telegraph*,[447] "the COVID-19 inquiry is demanding that the attendees test for the virus more than a year after the Government scrapped lateral flow tests."

Notably, in April 2023, the UK public sector contract site, BidStats, published a jaw-dropping contract from 2021. The Department of Health and Social Care signed off on a staggering £1.2 billion deal for Innova's rapid antigen tests in just a brief 1.5-month contract period.

**SARS-CoV-2 Antigen Rapid Qualitative View Notice elf-Tests)**

*Source:* Contracts Finder
*Published:* Thu 13 Apr 2023
*Closed:* Fri 12 Mar 2021

The contract is to purchase Innova SARS-CoV-2 Antigen Rapid Qualitative test kits for self-test use.

*sars; diagnostic kits; rapid qualitative tests; procurement of sars-cov-2 antigen; self-tests; self-test use; innova sars-cov-2 antigen; rapid qualitative test kits; covid-19 self-test kit; self-test;*

1.5 month contract, ended Apr 2021

award: Innova Medical Group £1.2B

And what happened to the key players at Innova? They became heavily embroiled in a web of legal disputes. The following is based on public court records and filings in ongoing litigation. All allegations are disputed by the defendants, and no court has yet determined their validity.

Robert Kasprzak (Innova's former chief legal officer) filed a lawsuit[448] in Los Angeles County Superior Courts against Charles Huang (founder of Innova and Pasaca Capital). Kasprzak alleges Huang misappropriated over $1 billion of Innova's profits, including $200 million transferred to Hong Kong and Singapore, and spent on personal luxuries.

According to the plaintiff's filings, "Huang deceived Kasprzak for years, and when Kasprzak finally realized the true extent of Huang's self- dealing, lies, and ineptness and sought to exit their business relationship, Huang reneged on the promises he made to induce Kasprzak to remain at their company, and instead terminated Kasprzak, falsely accused him of stealing from the company, and defamed him with salacious and false statements."

Kasprzak alleges that, "Huang is a high-end con artist who claims he can 'see the future.' He hoodwinked his purported business partners, including Kasprzak, by falsely holding himself out as a wealthy, successful, and respected businessman and investment banker. When the company became successful, Huang plundered hundreds of millions of dollars of company resources. Without due diligence or board approval, he invested and lost more than $200 million on flailing businesses owned by friends and colleagues."

According to the complaint: "Huang used billions of dollars generated by Kasprzak and a handful of others to enrich himself, his family, and his friends, while claiming sole credit for the company's success. Huang's astonishing megalomania is demonstrable-he is literally attempting to produce a self- aggrandizing movie telling his (fictionalized) life story, entitled 'Overnight Billionaire,' and has been trying (unsuccessfully) to get himself knighted in the United Kingdom."

Huang has denied the claims and accused others (including Kasprzak) of misconduct in separate filings.

Legal action did not stop at the doorstep of Innova, Disruptive Nanotechnology Ltd. (also known as Tried and Tested, a UK-based company acting as Innova Medical Group's UK agent) filed a lawsuit against Daniel Elliott (former CEO of Innova), Robert Kasprzak, and Charles Huang. Disruptive Nanotechnology alleged it was defrauded out of approximately $500 million in commissions (10% of UK contract sales) due to a reduction or diversion of payments by the defendants.

According to a *Los Angeles Times*[449] article published in July 2024, Daniel Elliott is reported as saying "Charles [Huang] called me in January [2020], and said, 'Hey, do you want to get into the COVID-testing business?' and I was like, 'What the hell do I know about COVID testing?'

This confirms the questions I raised earlier in my 2021 investigation. In January, months before 3/11, how would Huang have known to "get into the COVID- testing business"? Perhaps, he did have the ability to "see the future" as he self-claimed, according to Kasprak's filings, or maybe he simply had insider knowledge.

CHAPTER NINE

# THE LONG SHOT

*"What if we have a global pandemic and it's a novel pathogen? That will be catastrophic. We can't wait the normal 3 to 10 years for a vaccine. And what if instead we could use mRNA to create a vaccine in days and weeks instead of the normal year-long timelines, 3 to 10 years?"*

~Dan Wattendorf,
DARPA Program Manager, 2010

This chapter unravels the improbable ascent of messenger RNA (mRNA). From a fragile "missing link" in 1961's molecular biology to the cornerstone of COVID-19 "vaccines," propelled by serendipity, secrecy, and strategic funding. It chronicles a half-century odyssey, shadowed by toxicity woes and patent skirmishes, culminating in a "Hail Mary" windfall, post 3/11. Overnight, mRNA leaped from lab curiosity to global salvation, birthing Spikevax and Comirnaty in record time, turning the industry's long shot into billion-dollar COVID shots.

## The mRNA Story

The discovery of mRNA in 1961 was a pivotal moment in molecular biology. It revolutionized the understanding of genetic information transfer by providing the missing link between the genetic code found in DNA and the production of proteins. The "messenger" is the "m" in mRNA that transmits the genetic information found in a cell's nucleus to the body's protein-making factory. The key researchers involved in its discovery were François Jacob, Jacques Monod, and Sydney Brenner, who were working at the Pasteur Institute in Paris at the time. Matthew Meselson and Franklin Stahl from the California Institute of Technology also played a significant role in confirming the existence of mRNA. Brenner, Jacob and Meselson went on to work on a series of experiments, the results of which were published in *Nature* in a landmark paper[450] entitled, "An unstable intermediate carrying information from genes to ribosomes for protein synthesis." As noted in the paper the mRNA molecule is highly unstable. It degrades quickly because of ribonucleases (RNases), which are enzymes that break down RNA molecules into smaller components.

In 1978, the Greek researcher Giorgos Dimitriadis[451] conducted a series of experiments encasing different types of RNA into liposomes (tiny globules of fat). He showed that when rabbit globin mRNA was introduced into mouse spleen cells it directed the synthesis of globin protein. The liposomes protected the mRNA from being degraded by RNases. This was the discovery of the first mRNA-liposomes formulation.

Later in 1984, Paul A. Krieg, Ph.D., Douglas A. Melton, Ph.D., Tom Maniatis, Ph.D., Michael Green, Ph.D. and colleagues at Harvard University conducted significant experiments that played a critical role in understanding RNA synthesis and its applications. In a pioneering study,[452] molecular biologists synthesized RNA enzymes to make biologically active messenger RNA (mRNA) in a lab for the very first time.

In the late 1980s, while working at the Salk Institute for Biological Studies, the physician and biochemist, Dr. Robert Malone, conducted a series of experiments that demonstrated the potential for mRNA to be used as a therapeutic tool. In *Nature's*, "The tangled history of mRNA vaccines"[453] Elie Dolgin writes: "In 1987, Malone performed a landmark experiment. He mixed strands of mRNA with droplets of fat, to create a kind of molecular stew. Human cells bathed in this genetic gumbo absorbed the mRNA, and began producing proteins from it." Following on from those experiments, a landmark paper by Malone et al.[454] showed the very first in-vivo RNA transfection data. It marked the first time a scientist had used droplets of fat to introduce mRNA into a living organism. The researchers wrote: "We report the use of RNA transfection mediated by lipofectin (a liposome containing a cationic lipid) for efficient and reproducible RNA introduction and expression in tissue culture cells." They went on to state: "The RNA/lipofectin method can be used to directly introduce RNA into whole tissues and embryos raising the possibility that liposome-mediated mRNA transfection might offer yet another option in the growing technology of eukaryotic gene delivery, one based on the concept of using RNA as a drug."

A pioneering study in 1990 by Wolff et al.[455] (with Malone credited as one of the researchers) proved that direct injection of DNA into muscle tissue of mice could lead to the expression of a foreign gene.

My first interview[456] with Dr. Robert Malone took place in June 2021. It was abruptly removed "for violating YouTube's community guidelines" but resurfaced on the platform in May 2024. Malone shared some critical information in relation to his early discoveries on mRNA: "I was right at the center in a series of discoveries that happened in the late 1980s at the Salk Institute. It was when I was a graduate student. I was only 28/29 during that period. It resulted in a large number of patents. Those patents were filed by both the Salk Institute and by a company that I left the Salk for and joined shortly thereafter and brought all my technology reagents and protocols.

We had other discoveries, follow-on discoveries there and it was at that company Vical that the use of RNA and DNA for vaccination purposes was first reduced to practice, resulted in a large number of domestic U.S. and worldwide patents and those patents were used quite aggressively by Vical and then by Merck, which licensed that whole patent estate to prevent others from entering the field for the 20-year life of the patents.

So, often the question comes up: 'How come there was this big gap in commercial development between when you had your discoveries in the late 80s and the current situation?' And the truth is that Vical and Merck, although they were not able to actually make a product themselves, and I was long gone at that time. I was an academic by that point but they were never able to develop anything commercially after spending literally over a billion dollars but they kept everybody else from doing anything. And then when those patents expired suddenly, the field opened up. So, that was a little over 10 years ago, so that's the story. I was an industrial scientist at the time when those patents were filed, I got a total of $1 for compensation but the people that held the patents used them to prevent others from commercializing the tech and that's the core story."

Another scientist who played a prominent part in the mRNA technology story is the biochemist, Katalin Karikó, who first started working on RNA molecules in the 1980s at the Szeged Biological Research Centre in her native Hungary. In an interview, Karikó admitted that she was an asset for the security services during Hungary's Communist era. After coming to the U.S., Karikó was hired by the University of Pennsylvania (UPenn) in 1989 to work with cardiologist Elliot Barnathan on mRNA.

She continued to doggedly pursue transforming mRNA into a drug platform and build on Robert Malone's protocols.

However, during the next decade much of the early excitement surrounding mRNA began to quickly fade as scientists discovered that once injected into animals, foreign mRNA induced such a severe inflammatory response that the animals in the experiments died. It was also at this time, when mRNA research had fallen out of favor, that Karikó met Drew Weissman, an immunologist who joined UPenn in 1997 from the National Institute of Allergy and Infectious Diseases (NIAID). Notably, Weissman had trained as a fellow under the supervision of Dr. Anthony Fauci, who would become the self-referred "Science" on the control of Covid in the United States.

Karikó eventually joined Weissman's lab at the Perelman School of Medicine at UPenn, which was working on an HIV vaccine funded by the NIH. They collaborated on how to overcome major challenges of mRNA technology as "RNA had failed in clinical trials, and pretty much everybody had given up on it," Weissman later told *Time*.[457] Both were extremely interested in the delivery of synthetic mRNA to generate highly targeted therapeutic proteins.

In 2005, they worked on a series of landmark studies funded by the NIH, where they discovered that when uridine (one of the nucleosides or "building blocks" of mRNA) was replaced with a modified version, pseudouridine, it led to a reduced immune response. In other words, the modified nucleosides could "camouflage" the synthetic RNA from the innate immune system. Karikó and Weissman's pivotal paper was published in Cell, entitled "Suppression of RNA Recognition by Toll-like Receptors: The Impact of Nucleoside Modification and the Evolutionary Origin of RNA."[458]

In their discussion, the scientists pointed out that: "Insights gained from this study could advance our understanding of autoimmune diseases where nucleic acids play a prominent role in the pathogenesis, determine a role for nucleoside modifications in viral RNA, and give future directions into the design of therapeutic RNAs."

In 2006, UPenn went on to file two patents on behalf of the scientists' discoveries, which went largely unnoticed in the scientific community. The following year, Karikó and Weissman founded the company RNARx while both at UPenn. They received $97,396 in small-business grant funding from the U.S. government.

The German company BioNTech (founded in 2008 by husband-and-wife team, Uğur Şahin and Özlem Türeci, along with Christoph Huber) took notice of Karikó and Weissman's discoveries. In 2009, they first licensed the mRNA technology for their development of cancer treatments, which later proved crucial for their eventual COVID-19 vaccine, produced in collaboration with Pfizer. Karikó later joined BioNTech in 2013, where she became senior vice president.

Notably, for over a decade, BioNTech failed to secure a single regulatory approval from their expansive pipeline of mRNA therapeutics. However, following 3/11, their fortunes changed dramatically. BNT162b2, later marketed as Comirnaty would become BioNTech's first and most successful product ever, mirroring Moderna's trajectory, later detailed in this chapter.

In October 2023, Karikó and Weissman were jointly awarded the Nobel Prize in Physiology or Medicine[459] "for their discoveries concerning nucleoside base modifications that enabled the development of effective mRNA vaccines against COVID-19."

However, just a mere two months after this prestigious award, a study published in Nature by Mulroney et al.[460] cast a shadow over this achievement. The research unveiled a critical flaw: the mRNA technology, specifically when using N1-methylpseudouridine (m1Ψ), was susceptible to ribosomal frameshifting. This meant that instead of producing the intended spike proteins to train the immune system, the body was potentially manufacturing unintended, rogue proteins with unknown consequences. This revelation pointed to a "bug" in what was heralded as "revolutionary" medical technology, raising serious questions about the safety and efficacy of these globally distributed experimental mRNA vaccines, which are further investigated in chapter 12.

## Moderna's Meteoric Rise

Another scientist who took notice of Karikó and Weissman's landmark paper, was stem-cell biologist Derek Rossi, a faculty member at Harvard Medical School. He told the *Financial Times*:[461] "We saw that paper and thought maybe we can take these damn mRNAs and get them to flip into the cell and not be recognized."

Building on Karikó and Weissman's protocols, Rossi secured success with his own work on synthetic modified mRNAs.[462] *Time*[463] even did a feature, where he was one of 2010's "people who mattered." Around that time, Rossi reached out to chemical engineer Robert (Bob) S. Langer, an expert in nanotech drug delivery systems and tissue engineering, with a slew of patents to his name and eighth most-cited researcher in the world. Langer, an Institute Professor at Massachusetts Institute of Technology (MIT), which has often been involved with DARPA-funded projects, is a close associate with Bill Gates and is no stranger to controversy. For instance, the concept for a remote controlled contraceptive implant[464] originated when Gates visited Langer's lab at MIT. His creation of an invisible quantum dot "tattoo"[465] only visible by a special smartphone camera app and filter, intended to be used as a vaccination ID for children in Africa, was funded by the Bill and Melinda Gates Foundation.

Langer introduced Rossi to Noubar Afeyan (CEO of biotech investment firm, Flagship Ventures, now known as Flagship Pioneering) a biochemical engineering doctoral graduate of MIT and recipient of the Technology Pioneer award from the World Economic Forum. The three went on to establish the Cambridge, Massachusetts-based biotech company, Moderna (known formerly as ModeRNA Therapeutics) with its premise to develop mRNA therapeutics: "turning the body's cells into ad hoc drug factories." Cardiovascular biologist, Kenneth Chien of Harvard Medical School, also came onboard as cofounder.

The following year, Noubar Afeyan hired the slick salesman, Stéphane Bancel to head up Moderna, even though he had no scientific background. Bancel was the former CEO of the French diagnostic testing company, bioMérieux, with significant ties to China. It assisted in the design and oversaw the construction of the first ever level 4 bio facility (BSL-4) for the People's Republic of China's infamous Wuhan Institute of Virology, previously mentioned in chapter 1.

In 2013, the Pentagon's military tech arm, DARPA, awarded Moderna Therapeutics, a grant for up to $25 million[466] to develop Messenger RNA Therapeutics™ "to protect against a wide range of known and unknown emerging infectious diseases and engineered biological threats." It was seen as an unusual move at the time, given Moderna was not specializing in vaccines for infectious diseases but therapeutics for very rare diseases, as well as cancer.

DARPA's grant proved pivotal as it paved the way for Moderna to sign a five-year agreement with AstraZeneca for $240 million[467] the following year, to develop mRNA-based therapies for cardiometabolic diseases and cancer, despite the start-up failing to bring a single product to market.

In late 2013, Moderna was added as a member of the World Economic Forum's ("committed to improving the state of the world") community of the fastest-growing "Global Growth Companies."[468] Two years later, Moderna was catapulted to "unicorn" status with a market valuation of $1 billion. (A company is described as a unicorn by the venture capital industry when a privately held start-up has achieved a valuation of over $1 billion.) This immense feat was achieved without a single Phase 1 clinical trial underway from its 92 drugs in the pipeline.

A year later, Moderna partnered with Merck in a $100 million deal[469] to launch a venture company, Valera, focused exclusively on using Moderna's mRNA platform to develop five product candidates "against four undisclosed viruses."

2016 proved to be a busy year for Moderna. In January (six years after the company was founded) Moderna announced that their first ever Phase 1 studies were under way for two mRNA vaccines that "target influenza strains with pandemic potential: mRNA-1440 for influenza A subtype H10N8 and mRNA-1851 for influenza A subtype H7N9."

Concurrently, the Gates Foundation pledged up to $100 million to Moderna, including an initial grant of $20 million[470] "to develop a new affordable combination of messenger RNA–based antibody therapeutics geared toward preventing HIV infection" led by Moderna's infectious disease-focused venture company, Valera.

Notably, in early 2016 Moderna filed their infamous patent for modified nucleotides (with Stéphane Bancel listed as one of the inventors) as part of their cancer research. Moderna's patent happened to encompass a perfect match for a nucleotide sequence that codes for the Furin Cleavage Site (a critical component of the SARS-CoV-2 spike protein enabling the virus to latch onto human lung epithelial cells and replicate) previously mentioned in chapter 1.

Moderna Therapeutics received up to $125 million[471] from the Biomedical Advanced Research and Development Authority (BARDA) toward developing a Zika virus vaccine (mRNA-1325) the same year. Interestingly, Moderna said at the time it had already carried out preclinical work for the Zika mRNA vaccine, funded through a grant from DARPA.

2016 was also the year that NIAID's Vaccine Research Center scientists: Barney Graham (director of the VRC's Viral Pathogenesis Laboratory), Jason McLellan, Kizzmekia Corbett and others stabilized[472] the coronavirus "spike protein" that enables HKU1, a form of the common cold, invade cells. This was the first time NIH scientists and Moderna began to collaborate on a general vaccine design using viral mRNA that could be quickly adapted to protect people from emerging viruses such as Nipah virus and Middle East respiratory syndrome (MERS) coronavirus.

By December 2018, Moderna had completed the biggest initial public offering (IPO)[473] for a biotech on record, securing a valuation of $7.5bn. However, Moderna's feat was muddied by STAT News reporting that "safety issues forced the company to abandon its most advanced drug candidate, a treatment for a rare disease, and instead prioritize the less lucrative field of vaccines. And over the past 12 months, the company has consistently lost top executives, including the heads of its vaccines, cardiovascular, and rare disease divisions."

Moreover, Moderna's SEC filing[474] for that year revealed: "No mRNA drug has been approved in this new potential category of medicines, and may never be approved as a result of efforts by others or us. mRNA drug development has substantial clinical development and regulatory risks due to the novel and unprecedented nature of this new category of medicines." These pressing problems for Moderna are discussed in further detail later in this chapter.

After 3/11, Moderna "struck gold" with Spikevax (mRNA-1273), which was granted emergency use authorization on December 18, 2020. From April 2020 to July 2022, DoD and HHS contracts worth just over US$10 billion in total were lavishly awarded to Moderna for its mRNA 1273 vaccine, which it developed in partnership with the NIH and funding from Coalition for Epidemic Preparedness Innovations (CEPI), a global partnership established to accelerate the development of vaccines against epidemic/pandemic threats.

CEPI was the brainchild of Sir Jeremy Farrar, then head of the Wellcome Trust, Dr Stanley A. Plotkin (known as the "godfather of vaccines") and Adel Mahmoud, developer of the HPV and rotavirus vaccines. The idea was first proposed in their July 2015 co-authored paper in the *New England of Journal of Medicine*, titled "Establishing a Global Vaccine-Development Fund"[475] and was launched at the World Economic Forum in Davos, Switzerland, in January 2017. The organization was established with the financial backing of US$460 million from the Bill & Melinda Gates Foundation, the Wellcome Trust and the governments of India and Norway.

Turning back to the DoD and HHS contracts worth billions, which encompassed the research, development, testing and procurement of mRNA-1273, where $2 billion alone was given to support Moderna's clinical trials. It was BARDA which awarded the initial grant of $483 million to the biotech in April 2020, to accelerate the development and manufacturing of Moderna's Covid vaccine.

BARDA also collaborated with "DoD Joint Program Executive Office for Chemical, Biological, Radiological and Nuclear Defense and Army Contracting Command" by providing a heftier contract worth $1.5 billion[476] to Moderna to manufacture and deliver the vaccine to government-designated locations across the United States, astonishingly regardless of whether their mRNA-1273 vaccine would even obtain FDA approval. Moreover, any liability for patent infringement was transferred to the U.S. government and thus, the U.S. taxpayer.

In response to Harvard Medical School's assistant professor, Ameet Sarpatwari's testimony[477] (before the United States Senate Committee on Health, Education, Labor, and Pensions) on Moderna's intention of a four-fold price hike (which it went ahead and implemented) on its COVID-19 vaccine, legal scholar, Christopher J. Morten wrote:[478] "The U.S. government's August 2020 procurement contract with Moderna- worth $1.5 billion, in exchange for 100 million doses of the NIH-Moderna vaccine- was apparently executed at risk. This means the contract seemingly committed the government to pay Moderna even if the vaccine never obtained FDA authorization or approval." Morten went on to state:

"As such, this first procurement contract 'derisked' Moderna's development process enormously. Second, Sarpatwari observes that, with the same contract, the U.S. government attempted to shield Moderna from any liability it might face for infringing other companies' patents in the course of manufacturing and distributing the vaccine. In February 2023, the Department of Justice confirmed[479] the government's intent to provide this additional subsidy to Moderna: 'the effect of the Government's 'authorization and consent' is to relieve Moderna of any liability for patent infringement resulting in performance of the [August 2020 procurement contract] and to transfer to the United States any liability for the manufacture or use of the inventions claimed in [patents asserted against Moderna] resulting from the authorized and consented acts.' This liability shield may be worth tens or even hundreds of millions of dollars, as Moderna defends itself from claims of patent infringement brought by Alnylam, Arbutus, and Genevant, all of which hold patents on lipid nanoparticle technology used in mRNA delivery."

These ongoing patent disputes are discussed later in this chapter. By September 2021, Moderna was valued at a staggering $180 billion, surpassing biopharma behemoths, such as Sanofi and Bristol Myers Squibb, with its shares up nearly 2,140 percent since going public.

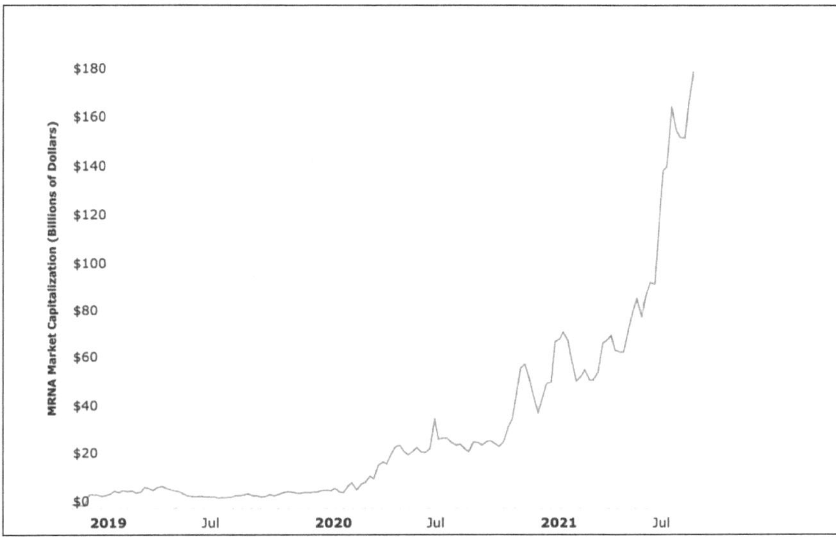


Source: Macrotrends[480]

The company amassed an astonishing $18.5 billion[481] in revenue for 2021, compared to just $803 million the year before. Moreover, as per the *Wall Street Journal*,[482] "in the two main COVID-19 vaccination years—2021 and 2022—the company made in excess of $20 billion in profits on more than $37 billion in revenue."

Dr. Stephen Hoge, Moderna's president and Bancel's right-hand man, told the *Financial Times*[483] that the success of the jabs gave the industry the "home run" that it had always craved. "What happens with the pandemic is that all of a sudden, a year forward, everyone believes in [mRNA] for all the right reasons."

Moderna's "home run" was achieved with the help from its "strategic collaborators." The U.S. government's lavish expenditure of taxpayers' money increased the personal wealth of the company's CEO, Stéphane Bancel, to $4.7 billion[484] at its peak in 2021-2022, while co-founders Robert Langer and Noubar Afeyan saw their net worth rise to around $1.7 billion and $1.8 billion, respectively, during the same period. It is noteworthy that Hoge failed to mention that the industry's "home run" was not just "craved" but desperately needed for Moderna to stay afloat. The company's troubles are investigated later in this chapter.

On the day Moderna's Covid vaccine received emergency use authorization from the FDA, CEO Stéphane Bancel shared in an interview:[485] "When I resigned from my last company, bioMerieux, to start on this journey at Moderna, I told my wife there was only a 5% chance it would work out."

It is puzzling why the French national decided to leave his lucrative position as CEO of an established company for an obscure start-up, with a success rate, according to Bancel, of just 5 percent? Perhaps he had good reason to believe that Moderna would benefit from strong U.S. government support. The type of support that was willing to provide funding, guarantees, or even bailout measures to mitigate any risks, greatly magnifying the company's odds of success: from unknown start-up to biotech behemoth.

Moncef Slaoui, the former head of vaccines at GlaxoSmithKline (GSK), while serving as the head of "Operation Warp Speed,"(a collaboration between the HHS and the DoD aimed at speeding up the development of COVID-19 medical countermeasures), openly acknowledged the immense support provided to Moderna, a company where he previously held a position on the Board of Directors right up until May 15, 2020. Slaoui candidly admitted: "We held Moderna by the hand on a daily basis."

## DARPA's Helping Hand

Notably, from its inception, Moderna was also held by another hand, that of the Pentagon's enigmatic research arm, DARPA. In a December 2020 revelatory interview[486] with Yahoo Finance's Anjalee Khemlani, former director of the Defense Advanced Research Projects Agency, Regina Dugan, discussed how the secretive agency played a key role in the development of mRNA technology. The following is an extract from that interview.

Regina Dugan: Well, you should know that DARPA was formed after Sputnik in 1958 with the goal of preventing and creating strategic surprise. So big questions about risks and vulnerabilities and new capabilities that we might create were routine at DARPA. And what I remember was a pivotal moment in 2010. So we were contemplating new programs, and a program manager by the name of Dan Wattendorf asked two big what ifs. He said, "What if we have a global pandemic and it's a novel pathogen? That will be catastrophic. We can't wait the normal 3 to 10 years for a vaccine. And what if instead we could use mRNA to create a vaccine in days and weeks instead of the normal year-long timelines, 3 to 10 years? So what's important is that at that time DNA vaccines had been tried. They made protein, but they didn't produce enough. They lacked potency, so there wasn't a strong immune response. And Dan argued that mRNA could be different. And there were a lot of critics at the time. They argued that there was no evidence it would work, and Dan argued there was no evidence that it wouldn't work. And if it did, someday it would matter, and that day has come.

Anjalee Khemlani: Regina, I know that one of the things that's really interesting about this is that the mRNA technology is getting its time in the limelight right now. We have seen the Pfizer rollout. We've also seen some of the concerns about, you know, whether or not-- the myth about whether or not it can alter your DNA, but then also some of the side effects. And so I wonder, you know, based on what you're seeing and based on your understanding of the technology, you know, is this something we can expect? Is it normal to kind of go through this process of side effects, et cetera, with the vaccine?

Regina Dugan: I think that's a normal progression in the investigation of safety for vaccines. Now remember, our charge was to create the possibility, and I think we need to understand how remarkable an achievement this is. We went from virus sequence to first dosing in humans in 63 days. It's unprecedented. Now, we still have the hard work to do to determine efficacy and to understand distribution and all of those things, but the first step is to have a vaccine candidate that creates an immune response and offers protection. Now, my sense is that this will be one of the most important scientific achievements of our generation and certainly in the top-five contributions for DARPA, which was also responsible for the early investments in the internet and GPS.

Anjalee Khemlani: Absolutely. Regina, when we're talking about, you know, health care right now and the speed at which this was done, we know that this administration specifically focused a lot on public-private partnerships dealing with not just the health-care companies but also the tech companies for the rollout of software that will track some of these adverse events and the safety monitoring. You have been part of that world before, and I just wonder what is your sense of the ability for big tech to really, you know, walk into this health-care space that has been kind of technologically slow but also is so complex?

Regina Dugan: Well, look, I firmly believe in public-private partnerships. And, in fact, when we made the investment in Moderna at DARPA, there were three people. And these early investments are important, and now we see what's happened with the investment of private capital. We now also have to consider what other established tech companies might bring to the table in terms of their reach, in terms of their scale. These are very important considerations. But I think central to the question is also what do we need by way of new breakthroughs? How do we ask the new "what if?" questions for public health and human health. And, in fact, it's the reason I accepted the CEO role at Welcome Leap, which was formed by the Wellcome Trust with an initial funding of $300 million and a specific mandate. And that is to ask the next "what if?" questions, to create the next round of breakthroughs for human health. We need to do those things at scale, and we need to do them in partnership.…It's an amazing organization [DARPA] with respect to the leverage it offers- small investment but right at these pivotal places where we need the kind of risk-tolerant investments. But in health we also see private organizations like Wellcome Trust, like the Gates Foundation, others stepping up and beginning to ask those kinds of "what if?" questions as well. We definitely need to do that at scale. And I think it's clear human health, global health is going to require that of us. It is not only a moral investment. It is also an economic investment, as we're seeing in this current pandemic.

Several key points emerge from Dugan's candid interview. Firstly, the Pentagon's clandestine agency oversaw the development of mRNA technology by being "an early investor" in Moderna (and later investing in Pfizer). On the back of Wattendorf's lobbying, it was Dugan herself who signed off on strategic grants that were awarded to both pharmaceutical companies.

When questioned on the safety of the experimental mRNA vaccines, the former DARPA director shifted the conversation, focusing instead on DARPA's success in making such technology feasible. "Our charge was to create the possibility and I think we need to understand how remarkable an achievement this is," she remarked. This strategic deflection suggests that DARPA's priority was not on making the new mRNA technology safe for human use, but to simply make it possible.

"Public-private partnerships," which are collaborative agreements between government entities and private sector companies, designed to allegedly serve the public interest, was also emphasized by Dugan. Notably, in the prescient October 2019 training tabletop exercise, known as "Event

201," (organized by the Bill and Melinda Gates Foundation, in partnership with The John Hopkins Center for Health Security and the World Economic Forum), which practiced the steps that would be taken during a fictional coronavirus pandemic, one of their primary recommendations was the call for "public-private cooperation for pandemic preparedness and response."[487] This simulation exercise is discussed in greater detail in chapter 16.

Perhaps, one of the most notable outcomes of a public-private partnership, is the development of the mRNA Covid vaccines. A *BMJ* study[488] revealed: "The U.S. government invested at least $31.9bn to develop, produce, and purchase mRNA COVID-19 vaccines, including sizable investments in the three decades before the pandemic through March 2022." A total of 34 NIH funded research grants directly related to mRNA COVID-19 vaccines, were identified. A further breakdown of the results from the study showed: "Pre-pandemic, the NIH invested $116m (35%) in basic and translational science related to mRNA vaccine technology, and the Biomedical Advanced Research and Development Authority (BARDA) ($148m; 44%) and the Department of Defense ($72m; 21%) invested in vaccine development."

As per *Britannica*,[489] "DARPA is renowned for funding 'revolutionary' ideas, in line with DARPA's overall strategy of making high-risk, high-return investments." It appears the DoD's secretive branch was betting big on the "unproven bet" of mRNA-based therapeutics in the years before 3/11 and expecting a sizable return from its investment. These "sizeable investments" amassed to a total of $337 million being spent by the U.S. government on mRNA vaccine technology in the years prior to the pandemic being declared. Post 3/11, a staggering $29.2 billion of U.S. public funds was spent on purchasing Covid mRNA-based vaccines and $2 billion on supporting clinical trials, mentioned earlier in this chapter.

Around 2012/2013, significant funds began to flow into the mRNA tech industry thanks to DARPA's helping hand. As mentioned earlier, DARPA awarded Moderna Therapeutics a grant for up to $25 million to develop Messenger RNA Therapeutics™ to protect against pathogens. This grant came under DARPA's program ADEPT: PROTECT[490] (Autonomous Diagnostics to Enable Prevention and Therapeutics: Prophylactic Options to Environmental and Contagious Threats) which started in 2012, with the goal to "develop platform technologies that can be deployed safely and rapidly to provide the U.S. population with near-immediate protection against emerging infectious diseases and engineered biological weapons." Moderna's grant was specifically for the research and development of a mRNA vaccine to combat Chikungunya, a virus spread by mosquitoes. The outcome of which is discussed later in this chapter.

In 2013, DARPA awarded a further contract to Pfizer worth $7.7 million,[491] for the New York-based pharmaceutical company to "perform a research and development program designed to develop a technology platform to identify and subsequently induce the production of protective antibodies to an emerging pathogen directly in an infected or exposed individual."

Saliently, Regina Dugan told the *Financial Times*:[492] "It's not even clear that, without some pretty heavy pressuring, this activity — even at Moderna — would have been pursued versus other potential applications for mRNA that had a much clearer path to monetization, such as cancer treatment."

The "activity" Dugan refers to involves Moderna's shift in focus away from the development of mRNA therapeutics for cancer treatment (which was more appealing to investors) to creating vaccines for infectious diseases. It is interesting how she admits Moderna was subject to this "heavy pressure," leading one to infer that perhaps DARPA was responsible for exerting the pressure.

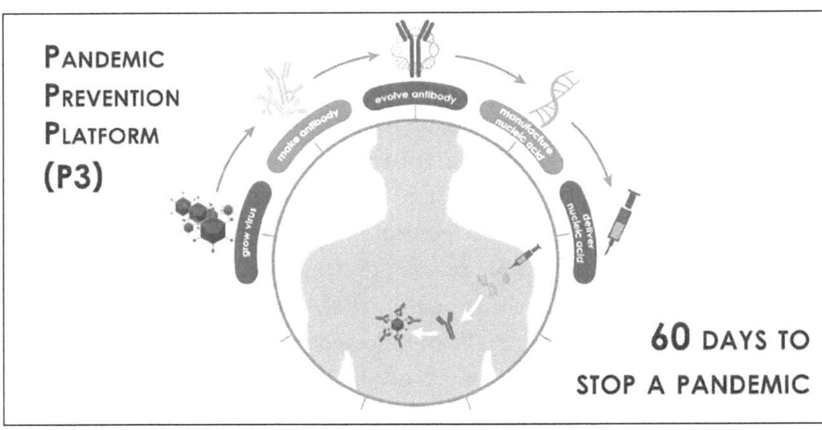


Source: DARPA: Pandemic Prevention Platform (P3) (ADEPT: PROTECT)[493]

In 2017, DARPA founded the Pandemic Prevention Platform (P3), a follow-on effort to its ADEPT: PROTECT program set up in 2012. According to the agency, P3 "aims to take pandemics off of the list of humanity's angsts with a range of technologies and practices marked by early detection of an outbreak and, within 60 days, development and widescale deployment of protective countermeasures."

Moderna's adoption of DARPA's mission to manufacture nucleic acids (mRNA) to rapidly combat emerging infectious diseases, is evidenced in their 2017 advertisement feature published in *Nature*:[494] "Vaccines to prevent infectious diseases have an enormous impact on public health, and currently protect people against more than 25 different diseases. However, traditional vaccine approaches involve long, complex, and costly development and production processes. As a result, the global health community remains woefully unprepared to address rapidly emerging infectious diseases, as evidenced by the recent epidemics of Zika, Ebola, and chikungunya virus, among others. In addition, many persistent pathogens for which there are no effective vaccines continue to cause widespread sickness worldwide. Moderna Therapeutics is addressing these challenges by pioneering a new class of vaccines made of mRNA, molecules that carry instructions copied from DNA for the assembly of proteins active in preventing or fighting disease."

By this point, it appears that the Pentagon's research agency was not just collaborating with Moderna as a "private partner" but using it as an extension of its own strategic objectives. DARPA's P3 mission: the development of protective countermeasures "within 60 days," was accomplished with Spikevax (give or take a few days). Dugan reflected on this achievement by saying: "We went from virus sequence to first dosing in humans in 63 days." The "we" underscores how DARPA was pivotal in this accomplishment.

Dan Wattendorf, the clinical geneticist and former DARPA program manager, who back in 2010 envisioned the dire scenario of a global outbreak from a new pathogen, while swiftly providing the solution: experimental mRNA vaccines, went on to become director of the Bill & Melinda Gates Foundation's Accelerator program,[495] the foundation's technology innovation team.

Regina Dugan, former DARPA director whose tenure was shadowed by controversy over her close ties to RedXDefense (the defense contractor she founded) has since carved out an extraordinary career in Silicon Valley. She led Google's secretive "Building 8" unit, focused on moonshot technologies, then moved to Meta to head its equivalent advanced research division. Today, Dugan serves as CEO of Wellcome Leap,[496] an initiative launched by Sir Jeremy Farrar with an initial $300 million from the Wellcome Trust. As Dugan herself described it: "We were formed... with a specific mandate. And that is to ask the next 'what if?' questions, to create the next round of breakthroughs for human health." In essence, Wellcome Leap is positioning itself as a global DARPA for health

## How The Secretive Unicorn Lost Its Sparkle

3/11 was the catalyst that propelled Moderna's Spikevax vaccine to score its monumental "home run." Moreover, it served as a critical lifeboat to Moderna in its deep sea of financial and legal troubles. Around 2016 onwards, the biotech unicorn was significantly losing key executives and major investors. An in-depth STAT investigation[497] "found that the company's caustic work environment has for years driven away top talent and that behind its obsession with secrecy, there are signs Moderna has run into roadblocks with its most ambitious projects."

According to STAT: "Bancel [Modern's CEO] had driven away top talent from Moderna with a culture of recrimination and a caustic work environment, including on-the-spot firings for failed experiments...At least a dozen highly placed executives have quit in the past four years, including heads of finance, technology, manufacturing, and science. In just the past 12 months, respected leaders of Moderna's cancer and rare disease programs both resigned, even though the company's remarkable fundraising had put ample resources at their disposal. Each had been at the company less than 18 months, and the positions have yet to be filled."

Joseph Bolen, a distinguished chief scientific officer who led Millennium Pharmaceuticals to FDA approval for a blockbuster cancer drug, abruptly resigned as Moderna's head of research and development, where he served for a mere two years- signaling serious concerns. A company insider told STAT that "no scientist in his right mind would leave that job unless there was something wrong with the science or the personnel." At the time of Bolen's resignation, Moderna was under scrutiny for its preference of "stealth over disclosure" of any published data indicating whether or not its mRNA technology worked.

A plausible reason for Moderna to shroud its data in secrecy, along with sudden departures from key staff, could be the fact that the unicorn's drug results were far from "revolutionary." Moderna's former director of chemistry, Dr. Suhaib Siddiqi, said Bancel punished technicians for failed experiments. "Ninety percent of the things in science fail – that's the way the inventions are made," Siddiqi told CNN.[498] "When it failed (at Moderna), he just shifted the blame to the technicians and fired them."

A former BARDA official, who worked with Moderna commented: "They've been a little tight-fisted about their data, and I interpret that to mean the results so far have been disappointing."

Following on from Bancel's presentation at the 2016 J.P Morgan Healthcare Conference about the "unbelievable future" of his company, the editors of *Nature*[499] criticized the biotech for its secrecy: "Moderna's coming-out party was highly anticipated and breathlessly reported. But something was missing: Moderna's scientists have yet to publish a single paper describing its therapeutic platform. That makes it difficult for outsiders to get a read on the company. And the Boston-based firm isn't alone in deprioritizing journal publication. Other prominent biotechs like Theranos and Kadmon have also chosen stealth over disclosure of data."

The infamous Theranos, founded by Elizabeth Holmes in 2003, was another secretive unicorn biotech, which claimed to have revolutionary blood testing technology. Its dramatic fall from grace was triggered by a series of articles[500] in The Wall Street Journal from investigative journalist John Carreyrou, questioning the validity of Theranos' technology and the accuracy of its tests.

In 2018, former Theranos presidents, Ramesh Balwani and Elizabeth Holmes, were charged with "massive fraud" by the SEC for making false statements about the company's technology and financial performance. In 2022, Holmes was sentenced to over 11 years in prison and ordered to pay a restitution of $452 million, while her former business partner and then-boyfriend, Ramesh "Sunny" Balwani, was sentenced to nearly 13 years in prison. Notably, former U.S. Secretary of State, the late Henry Kissinger, was also on the Theranos board. However, no public records indicate he was ever legally prosecuted or fined for his part in the disgraced company.

One could argue that Moderna and Theranos share certain similarities extending beyond their mutual attainment of their coveted unicorn status. Perhaps, there was "something wrong with the science" behind Moderna's mRNA technology.

Moderna's CEO has repeatedly asserted: "mRNA is like software: You can just turn the crank and get a lot of products going into development." However, from the beginning, safety problems or "bugs in the software" have arisen challenging Bancel's reductive view. According to a *STAT*[501] report by Damian Garde: "mRNA is a tricky technology. Several major pharmaceutical companies have tried and abandoned the idea, struggling to get mRNA into cells without triggering nasty side effects."

In 2014, Alexion Pharmaceuticals entered into a significant $100 million agreement with Moderna, focusing on developing treatments for rare and severe diseases, including Crigler-Najjar syndrome. However, the Crigler-Najjar treatment that harnessed Moderna's mRNA technology was "indefinitely delayed." An Alexion spokeswoman told STAT. "It never proved safe enough to test in humans, according to several former Moderna employees and collaborators who worked closely on the project." It was after the troubles with the Crigler-Najjar treatment, where Alexion severed ties[502] with Moderna, that Stephen Kesley, head of the unicorn's oncology division, parted ways with the company. The timing of his departure points to the plausibility that something was "wrong with the science."

Moreover, the STAT investigation emphasized how: "Moderna could not make its therapy work, former employees and collaborators said. The safe dose was too weak and repeat injections of a dose strong enough to be effective had troubling effects on the liver in animal studies."

The toxicity of the lipid nanoparticle (LNP) delivery system for the modified mRNA was explained as the problem: "For Moderna, that meant putting its Crigler-Najjar therapy in nanoparticles made of lipids. And for its chemists, those nanoparticles created a daunting challenge: Dose too little, and you don't get enough enzyme to affect the disease; dose too much, and the drug is too toxic for patients."

The report detailed how other pharmaceutical companies had abandoned their RNA projects because of the significant safety concerns with the LNPs: "those nanoparticles can lead to dangerous side effects, especially if a patient has to take repeated doses over months or years. Novartis abandoned the related realm of RNA interference over concerns about toxicity, as did Merck and Roche."

It went on to explain: "The indefinite delay on the Crigler-Najjar project signals persistent and troubling safety concerns for any mRNA treatment that needs to be delivered in multiple doses, covering almost everything that isn't a vaccine, former employees and collaborators said."

Despite the report's emphasis on the significant safety concerns with mRNA-LNP treatments requiring repeated doses, it simultaneously relied on the assumption made by "former employees and collaborators" that vaccines would not need multiple administrations. However, this assumption was turned on its head by the rollout of the experimental mRNA-based

COVID-19 vaccines. Both Moderna and the Pfizer/BioNTech's mRNA vaccines were launched as two-dose regimens, later supplemented with additional booster shots.

Ironically, the pivotal issue of toxicity caused by repeated doses of these products was highlighted even by Katalin Karikó, herself. She revealed to STAT[503]: "I would say that mRNA is better suited for diseases where treatment for short duration is sufficiently curative, so the toxicities caused by delivery materials are less likely to occur."

Yet, the Nobel laureate fell remarkably silent over the safety implications of repeated dosing required for the mRNA-LNP vaccines developed by Moderna, Pfizer, and BioNTech, where she was a senior vice president until 2022.

In September 2016, Moderna secured funding of up to $125 million from Biomedical Advanced Research and Development Authority (BARDA) towards developing a Zika virus vaccine (mRNA-1325). Notably, BARDA's substantial grant to Moderna was awarded during a period of transition within two highly significant public health roles. Firstly, the Assistant Secretary for Preparedness and Response (ASPR) at the HHS, which oversees BARDA, changed from Dr. Nicole Lurie to Dr. Robert Kadlec, although he was officially appointed the following year.

Robert Kadlec, a highly controversial figure in the field of biodefence and public health preparedness, was involved in "Dark Winter,"[504] the June 2001 bioterrorism simulation exercise depicting a smallpox outbreak in the U.S., eerily just months before the real anthrax letter attacks began. Then in 2019, Kadlec led "Crimson Contagion"[505] a pandemic simulation event, which ran from January to August, based on a novel influenza A (H7N9) virus that spread from China to the United States. These events are discussed in detail in chapter 16.

It is noteworthy that the same strain of influenza, H7N9, at the center of the simulation event, also happened to be one of the two strains of influenza "of pandemic potential" that Moderna had developed a mRNA vaccine against, which was noted earlier. Moderna's Phase 1 trial results for its mRNA vaccine against H7N9 was published in *Vaccines*[506] in May 2019, just when Crimson Contagion was in full swing.

The second significant public health position that underwent transition, around the time the Zika vaccine grant was awarded to Moderna, was BARDA's director role. Former vice president of global influenza programs at Novavax, Dr. Rick Bright, took over as director in November 2016 from Dr. Richard Hatchett. Prior to his plum position, Bright was Incident Commander of ASPR/BARDA's Zika Response from February through to November 2016. This meant that Bright would have been instrumental in green lighting BARDA's grant for the development of mRNA-1325 (Moderna's Zika virus vaccine candidate). Bright also served on the DoD's DARPA Scientific Advisory Board for Accelerated Manufacturing Program and for the Blue Angel Program for development of vaccines. From 2008-2010, he was a director at the non-profit PATH, where he developed, championed and managed scientific strategies of the global influenza vaccine program, funded by the Bill and Melinda Gates Foundation.

Notably, BARDA's hefty grant awarded to Moderna for developing its Zika virus mRNA vaccine, was issued when the World Health Organization (WHO) declared the Zika epidemic had ended.

Dr. Randall S. Bock's article for the *Washington Examiner*[507] based on his book entitled, "Overturning Zika, The Pandemic That Never Was" unveils another side of the Zika virus story. The following is an extract from his article. "In 2015, the Zika-microcephaly pandemic took hold in Recife, Brazil. Flavivirus Zika, for decades seen as harmless, was now suddenly deemed responsible for congenital microcephaly (small heads, diminished intellect). Massive panic predictably ensued." Bock went on to note: "In January 2016, the World Health Organization's Bruce Aylward acknowledged, 'In any unfolding crisis you're dealing with a lot of uncertainty (including the precise nature of any link between Zika and microcephaly).' By February 2016, the WHO had pivoted, declaring Zika a worldwide public health emergency…Federal funds of the National Institute of Allergy and Infectious Diseases were even 'borrowed' from other purposes to create such a vaccine, presuming that active infection would persist. It did not."

Why did BARDA spend $125 million of U.S. taxpayers' funds on the development of an experimental vaccine against a threat that no longer persisted? Was it because its primary objective was to launch a product using LNP-mRNA technology?

In March 2017, Moderna's first ever pre-clinical results for their BARDA-funded, mRNA-LNP Zika vaccine was published in the peer-reviewed journal, *Cell*, with much fanfare. Their scientists demonstrated that the mRNA vaccine candidate for Zika virus managed to protect mice against infection. The results were deemed to "bode well" for Moderna's planned clinical trial in humans. "I'm sure that five years from now we'll look at

2017 as the inflection point that Moderna went for a lift-off," Bancel declared during the 2017 J.P. Morgan conference presentation.

However, the year turned out to be the "lift-off" of Moderna's legal woes instead. Shortly after Moderna celebrated their disclosure of their first ever pre-clinical results (seven years after being in operation), legal disputes erupted over the LNP technology that Moderna had sublicensed from another company, Acuitas.

A *STAT*[508] article ran the provocative headline: "Moderna breaks its publishing silence, but can it sell its Zika vaccine?" The report revealed: "But while the disclosure may satisfy some of the company's skeptics, a messy legal dispute could imperil Moderna's ability to make money on its work." The truth of the matter was that the LNP technology, in fact, belonged to Arbutus. Legal proceedings revealed that Moderna's sublicense from Acuitas "violated the terms of the original deal, which doesn't cover vaccines." This meant that Moderna was "pressing toward the market with a technology it doesn't own." These ongoing patent wars are discussed in further detail later in this chapter.

Moderna's Zika vaccine pre-clinical (animal) trial did move on to Phase 1 of a clinical trial[509] on 90 healthy adults (aged 18-49 years) but it failed to progress further. Strikingly, it took roughly seven years from the trial start date for the results to be posted on ClinicalTrials.gov. Unlike the animal study, the clinical results on humans did not appear to "bode well" for Moderna. In the trial arm, where 25 participants were assigned a100mcg dosage (administered in two doses), disturbingly all suffered from some kind of adverse event. Moreover, there was a serious adverse event resulting in the death of a subject (from respiratory arrest) in the 25-participant group assigned the 10mcg dosage due to "toxicity to various agents."

The concerning trial safety data was heavily downplayed in the Moderna and BARDA funded study, which was published in *The Lancet*,[510] where researchers claimed: "All three dose levels of mRNA-1325 (10, 25, and 100 μg) were generally well tolerated, but the vaccine elicited poor Zika virus-specific nAb responses."

Turning to the DARPA-funded project aimed at developing a vaccine for the chikungunya virus. Moderna faced significant challenges there as well. As reported by *STAT*,[511] the trials of mRNA-1944 didn't go as planned either. Specifically, three out of the four participants who received the highest dose experienced significant reactions at the injection site. Additionally, one of these participants also reported symptoms of a rapid and irregular heartbeat.

Against the backdrop of toxicity issues concerning Moderna's pipeline of therapeutics, in a September 2017 closed-door presentation to one hundred of biotech's top investors, Moderna's president, Dr. Stephen Hoge, claimed "the company had solved the scientific issues that made its earlier mRNA treatments too toxic for clinical trials" according to *STAT*.[512] However, several of those who attended said they were not overly impressed as key questions remained unanswered, with one attendee saying, "None of the answers they have really seem like the 'a-ha' moment."

Over a year later, Hoge's claim was directly contradicted by a key section buried in Moderna's Securities and Exchange Commission (SEC) November 2018 filing:[513] "Most of our investigational medicines are formulated and administered in an LNP which may lead to systemic side effects related to the components of the LNP which may not have ever been tested in humans. While we have continued to optimize our LNPs, there can be no assurance that our LNPs will not have undesired effects. Our LNPs could contribute, in whole or in part, to one or more of the following: immune reactions, infusion reactions, complement reactions, opsonization reactions, antibody reactions including IgA, IgM, IgE or IgG or some combination thereof, or reactions to the PEG from some lipids or PEG otherwise associated with the LNP. Certain aspects of our investigational medicines may induce immune reactions from either the mRNA or the lipid as well as adverse reactions within liver pathways or degradation of the mRNA or the LNP, any of which could lead to significant adverse events in one or more of our clinical trials. Many of these types of side effects have been seen for legacy LNPs. There may be resulting uncertainty as to the underlying cause of any such adverse event, which would make it difficult to accurately predict side effects in future clinical trials and would result in significant delays in our programs."

By the end of that year, shortly after its $600 million IPO,[514] Moderna's stock price slumped 30 percent wiping out around $2 billion in market value. "A sign the company and its underwriters might have over-estimated demand for the richly valued company," STAT reported at the time. It was becoming apparent that the unicorn was losing its sparkle with investors, as it was clearly not living up to "the hype" but did that really matter, if its future was assured, regardless of the brewing storms?

Circling back to Bancel's December 2020 interview, the CEO candidly admitted: "The partnership we've had with the U.S. government has been important. Moderna isn't like a lot of pharma companies that have a strong balance sheet and cash flow coming from their drugs. We've never had a dollar of sales. And one of the reasons we've been able to grow so fast is that, due to government support, we've been able to take a lot of business risk so that we did not have to take any safety risk."

Indeed, Moderna's partnership with the U.S. government offered it protection against the "rainy days" of disappointing drug and vaccine trial outcomes, legal disputes, and its failure in bringing a single product to market. Here was a biopharmaceutical company, its sails yet to catch the wind of commercial success, seemingly buoyed by the lifeboat of taxpayer funds. But what was the rationale behind "Government support" for Moderna's unproven technology, considering the company's parade of disappointments? Could it be that the biotech industry's long shot, the "unproven bet" on mRNA technology, might just be the endgame?

## Patent Wars

Turning to Moderna's legal disputes, which sprang out from its early days as a fledgling biotech. Robert Langer informed[515] Stéphane Bancel that Moderna was too limited to create its own mRNA delivery system, so it needed to look to an external company to license the lipid nanoparticle (LNP) technology, an integral part of that system. LNP technology involves wrapping up the synthetic mRNA into tiny bubbles of fat that protect the mRNA from degradation and facilitate its entry into cells. The LNP compound consists of four components: ionizable cationic phospholipids, cholesterol, helper phospholipids, and PEG–modified phospholipids.

The biochemist, Prof. Pieter Cullis and his co-workers at his laboratory at the University of British Columbia (UBC) in Canada were the first to design LNP technology. Interestingly, SEC filings[516] show that patents relating to this technology were solely assigned to the University of British Columbia and then licensed back to the biotech company, Inex Pharmaceuticals, co-founded by the leading LNP scientists Drs. Pieter Cullis, Thomas Madden, and Michael Hope in 1992. The three went on to co-found Tekmira Pharmaceuticals (a wholly owned subsidiary of Inex Pharmaceuticals). However, in 2005 Cullis left Tekmira and by 2008, Tekmira was not interested in supporting the work that Drs. Madden and Hope were pursuing and terminated their employment.

The three united again to establish Acuitas Therapeutics in 2009 but not without filing a lawsuit which resulted in Madden being able to license the technology from Arbutus. Tekmira (later renamed Arbutus Biopharma) focused on the development lipid nanoparticles to deliver drugs based on small interfering RNA, "siRNA," (which are short pieces of RNA that interfere with the body's ability to make certain proteins that may cause disease). By 2012, Acuitas' focus was on the development of LNP technology for the delivery of mRNA. This was around the time that DARPA granted Moderna $25 million to develop mRNA technology.

Tekmira garnered the world's attention during the 2014 West African Ebola virus epidemic due to its experimental antiviral drug, TKM-Ebola. The Canadian biotech company was developing the drug under a $140 million[517] U.S. Department of Defense contract. During that time Tekmira's stock rose dramatically but it took a sharp hit when the development of TKM-Ebola was indefinitely suspended because the treatment was plagued by clinical setbacks[518] due to lack of efficacy. After the suspension, Tekmira changed its name to Arbutus Biopharma Corporation in 2015.

In Moderna's early days, it sub-licensed the rights to Arbutus' LNP technology through the small privately held company, Acuitas (where the world headquarters at the time was the CEO's house), instead of going direct to Arbutus. Why did Moderna do that? According to Bancel, it was because "Acuitas had the people and the capabilities."

However, problems quickly arose because Acuitas' deal with Arbutus never included Moderna. In 2016, Arbutus sued Acuitas claiming its sublicense to Moderna was illegal and won the case. This led to an injunction in 2017, which prevented Acuitas from further sublicensing the LNP technology to third parties. In 2018, a settlement[519] was reached before trial, which resulted in the termination of Acuitas' license to the technology. It also restricted Moderna's use of the LNP delivery system to only four vaccine candidates. The settlement stipulated "that the four non-exclusive viral vaccine sublicenses previously granted to Moderna are the only sublicenses to survive. These four sublicenses, previously granted by Acuitas to Moderna under the pre-April 15, 2010, Arbutus LNP patent families, are each limited to a specific viral target. Moderna has no other rights to Arbutus' broad suite of LNP intellectual property."

The intact 4 sublicenses did not extend to the viral target, SARS-CoV-2. This opened the door to further patent infringement lawsuits, when Moderna eventually brought its COVID-19 vaccine onto the market. However, Moderna's early contract with BARDA offered it protection from any patent infringement liability, which was unbelievably transferred to the U.S. government, as referenced earlier in the chapter.

Interestingly, Moderna took the trouble to try to invalidate the patent owned by Arbutus related to the lipid nanoparticle (LNP) technology crucial to the biopharmaceutical's mRNA medicines. However, in July 2020, the U.S. Patent Trial and Appeal Board rejected Moderna's challenge. After it lost, Moderna claimed[520] that its LNP technology had advanced well beyond the technology described in the Arbutus patent and it was "not aware of any significant intellectual property impediments for any products we intend to commercialize, including mRNA-1273."

In February 2022, Arbutus and its partner Genevant Sciences filed a lawsuit[521] against Moderna where it sought damages for the infringement of six of its patents related to Moderna's Covid vaccine, Spikevax. According to Reuters,[522] "Arbutus said it developed the so-called lipid nanoparticles that enclose the vaccine's mRNA payload, the patents related to which were licensed to Genevant Sciences, a joint venture between Arbutus and Roivant Sciences Ltd."

As part of Moderna's defense, it claimed to have created its own LNP technology, although the exact composition of the LNP delivery system used in Spikevax has never been disclosed. In April 2024, a U.S. judge issued an order that strengthened Arbutus' arguments in its patent infringement lawsuits against Moderna, resulting in a drop in its share price.

The following visualization shows the tangled web of Covid vaccine patents.

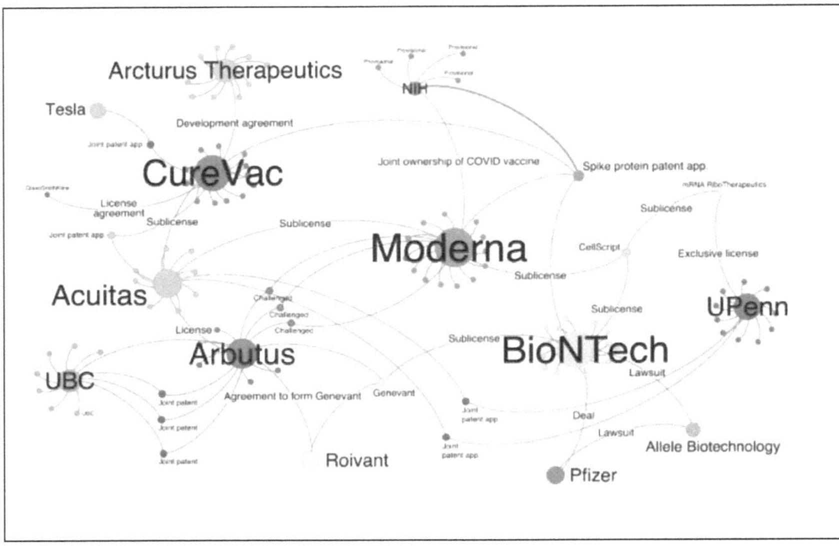


Source: A network analysis of COVID-19 mRNA vaccine patents[523]

It is an anomaly why Moderna, which had enough capital, did not fully investigate the licensing agreement between Acuitas and Arbutus at the time. Instead, they went ahead with using Acuitas' technology (that really belonged to Arbutus) for their pipeline of drugs and vaccines.

In a 2016 *Forbes* interview,[524] on the heels of the Acuitas/Arbutus lawsuit, Moderna's CEO, Stéphane Bancel, dismissed Acuitas' technology, stating, "We knew it was not very good. It was just okay." His statement was followed by an explanation that Moderna was in the process of producing its own nanoparticle lipids. As per Forbes reporting, "One such lipid, N1GEL (called "Nigel" internally), appears to cause less inflammation than Acuitas' version. Another is being licensed from Merck. Bancel says Moderna has stopped using the Acuitas tech for new drugs." However, it remains unclear how Moderna's LNP technology fundamentally differs from Acuitas', given that Moderna has never publicly disclosed the composition of its LNPs.

Arbutus and Genevant also went on to sue[525] Pfizer and its German partner, BioNTech SE, claiming that the Comirnaty vaccine used their LNP technology without a license. This led Acuitas to file a lawsuit against Arbutus claiming that there had been no infringement of the latter's patents in the development of Pfizer/BioNTech's Comirnaty vaccine. (Acuitas' lipid nanoparticle components, ALC-0315 and ALC-0159 are used in Pfizer/

BioNTech's Covid vaccine.) In May 2024, a New Jersey federal judge dismissed[526] Acuitas' lawsuit against Arbutus, which sought a declaration that the LNP technology behind the Pfizer/BioNTech Covid vaccine does not infringe Arbutus' ten patents.

The patent wars have spread beyond the realm of LNP technology to the modified mRNA molecules used in Moderna and Pfizer/BioNTech's Covid vaccines. In 2022, Moderna filed two infringement lawsuits against Pfizer and its German partner BioNTech, both in U.S. and German courts. Moderna claimed Pfizer and BioNTech used the exact same mRNA chemical modification in Spikevax for Comirnaty, which it has been developing since 2010. However, both Pfizer and BioNTech have been researching mRNA technology for medicines, with BioNTech using mRNA for melanoma immunotherapy[527] since 2012.

In May 2024, Moderna won the latest round of its long-running legal battle with Pfizer and BioNTech with the European Patent Office (EPO) upholding the validity of one of Moderna's patents for its Spikevax vaccine, while the U.S. Patent Office[528] put its lawsuit on hold.

## "We Had The Vaccine The Whole Time"

Prior to 3/11, a former Moderna employee commented how the lavishly funded biotech was in desperate need of a "Hail Mary."[529] As previously noted, hindered by the standard regulatory hurdles, Moderna's most promising products had failed to go beyond animal testing, let alone being brought to market. This was likely due to the troubling toxicity issues related to the (Arbutus-owned/sub-licensed through Acuitas) LNP-mRNA delivery system. Despite top company executives claiming the issue had been resolved and that Moderna had developed its own safer LNP system causing "less inflammation," the company's SEC filing stated otherwise. In addition, the biotech was heavily embroiled in legal disputes, which threatened its ability to capitalize on any of its future LNP-mRNA based products.

In the months running up to 3/11, Moderna found itself teetering on the precipice of financial ruin. According to *STAT*:[530] "In late 2019, executives began cutting back on research and other expenditures. Cash from investors had stopped pouring in and partnerships with some drug makers had been discontinued. In meetings at Moderna, Bancel emphasized the need to stretch every dollar and employees were told to reduce travel and other expenses, a frugality they were advised would last several years." Stephen Hoge, Moderna's president, told STAT, "We were freaked out about money."

Strikingly, also in late 2019, "thought leaders and decision-makers" gathered at the Milken Institute School of Public Health for its Future of Health Summit.[531] One of the panels discussed "the prospects of an effective universal influenza vaccine." What was said during the discussion, proved to be not only revelatory but also concerning. The speakers included then NIAID director, Dr. Anthony Fauci, then BARDA director, Dr. Rick Bright, and Michael Specter, staff writer for *The New Yorker*. They discussed the need to "blow up the system" of traditional egg-grown vaccines by an "exciting and disruptive" event, that would usher in mRNA technology not beholden to regulatory control. The following is an excerpt of a transcript from that panel discussion.[532]

Specter: Why don't we blow the system up? Obviously, we can't just turn off the spigot on the system we have and then say, "Hey, everyone in the world should get this new vaccine, we haven't given it to anyone yet" but there must be some way that… we grow vaccines mostly in eggs the way we did in 1947.

Fauci: In order to make the transition from getting out of the tried-and-true egg-growing, which we know gives us results that can be, you know, beneficial. I mean, we've done well with that, to something that has to be much better, you have to prove that this works. And then you've got to go through all of the clinical trials, phase one, phase two, phase three, and then show that this particular product is going to be good over a period of years -that alone, if it works perfectly, is going to take a decade.

Bright: There might be a need or even an urgent call for an entity of excitement out there, that is completely disruptive, does not beholden to bureaucratic strings and processes.

Fauci: So, we really do have a problem of how the world perceives influenza and it's going to be very difficult to change that unless you do it from within and say, "I don't care what your perception is. We're going to address the problem in a disruptive way and in an innovative way" because you do need both.

Bright: It is not too crazy to think that the outbreak of a novel avian virus could occur in China somewhere. We could get the RNA sequence from that, beam it to a number of regional centers, if not local, if not even in your home at some point and print those vaccines on the patches and self-administer.

When the "disruptive" events of 3/11 unfolded causing mayhem around the world, for Moderna, it was their long awaited "Hail Mary" moment by being the first vaccine manufacturer out the gate: from vaccine sequence selection to first human dosing with mRNA-1273 in 63 days.

It is important to focus on the sequence of events that led to Moderna's pivotal moment and take a closer look at its history of collaboration with the National Institutes of Health (NIH). The reported[533] version recounts how one Saturday morning in early January 2020, "Barney Graham, M.D., Ph.D, director of the VRC's Viral Pathogenesis Laboratory (VPL), and VRC research fellow Kizzmekia Corbett, Ph.D., dropped everything and immediately began working on a vaccine for the illness that would become known as COVID-19… Dr. Graham and Dr. Corbett quickly mapped out a plan to begin experiments, assigned roles to team members, and went to work designing an antigen — in this case, a copy of the spike protein found on the surface of the COVID-19 virus, which it uses to infect cells. This antigen molecule, when provided via a vaccine, would trick the body into forming a defensive arsenal against future infection. After years of prior work to unlock the mysteries of coronaviruses and, with their partners at Moderna, perfect a method to coax the body to manufacture antigens via messenger RNA (mRNA), they were prepared. Less than 48 hours after the release of the novel coronavirus' genome, the team had designed the protein that their candidate COVID-19 vaccine would use to teach the immune system to fend off the virus. Sixty-five days later, the VRC began clinical trials in collaboration with Moderna and clinical investigators from NIH's Division of Microbiology and Infectious Diseases. Ultimately, the vaccine received emergency use authorization from the U.S. Food and Drug Administration (FDA) on December 18, 2020, just one week after a similar vaccine developed by Pfizer."

It is astonishing that in less than two days after the SARS-Cov-2 genomic sequence was released, the Moderna/NIH Covid vaccine had been designed. Moreover, its design was completed before China had even acknowledged that the disease could be transmitted from human-to-human on January 20th. The vaccine had already been manufactured and shipped to the NIH for the start of its Phase 1 clinical trial, before the first American death was announced a month later. Moderna's speed was commented on in the New York Magazine article entitled, "We had the vaccine the whole time."[534]

Later, a *Washington Post* article[535] ran the headline "Serendipity and foresight prepared the world to fight the coronavirus." It reported: "The trajectory of science is often shaped by accidents, foresight and luck. And Graham's role in shifting the path of the pandemic embodied that. The right team was in the right place to fight a health calamity sparked by an invisible enemy before anyone knew it was there."

Notably, it revealed how before dawn on New Year's Eve 2019, Graham emailed Kizzmekia Corbett, leader of the coronavirus team at his lab, "FYI. Get ready for 2020," while forwarding a news report about the outbreak in China.

This raises the critical question: why did Graham, in the remaining hours of 2019, imply that the coming new year would usher in something of great significance, particularly in relation to the coronavirus team at his lab? There were no public reports from late 2019 indicating that the "mystery illness" was a coronavirus. Moreover, why in early January 2020, did NIH scientists "drop everything" and work through their weekend to design a vaccine for a virus that was not yet known to be transmissible and more than a week before the first confirmed coronavirus case in the United States. Was it merely an act of "serendipity and foresight" as described by the Washington Post, or a hint that the script of this global Covid drama was being read ahead of time by a select few?

And how fortuitous for Moderna, with its longstanding relationship with U.S. government agencies, such as DARPA and NIAID's Vaccine Research Center (VRC) to find itself perfectly positioned at the vanguard of fighting "a health calamity sparked by an invisible enemy before anyone knew it was there."

The Washington Post article highlighted how Barney Graham, his team at the VRC, and "the world's coronavirus experts" had been collaborating and "studying the nooks and crannies of spike-covered coronaviruses" in the decade leading up to 3/11. It also went on to reveal how Graham "had forged a relationship with an up-and-coming biotechnology company, Moderna, that could design vaccines fast."

In 2016, "studying the nooks and crannies of spike-covered coronaviruses" paid off for Barney Graham and his team at the VRC, including scientists from Dartmouth College and Scripps Research Institute, as they had designed a way of stabilizing the pre-fusion shape of the human coronavirus HKU1 (responsible for the common cold) by introducing a modification, referred to as "2P Mutation."[536] This mutation worked by "locking" the spike protein in a shape more likely to elicit a strong immune response by presenting a stable structure to the immune system. A "2P Mutation" patent[537] was filed the following year, ensuring that if a coronavirus vaccine were to be produced using this patent, the credited scientists and institutions such as the United States government, Dartmouth College and Scripps Research Institute would benefit from any royalties. This patent became known as the 070 patent.[538]

What is noteworthy is that Graham and his team had attempted to stabilize the spike protein for SARS and MERS but had "little success,"[539] according to Vanderbilt University's Research News, so "Graham and McLellan turned to the more common coronavirus HKU1." Interestingly, the article credits how the mRNA-based shots and the anti-viral drug, Remdesivir, (discussed in the next chapter) all had their roots in research conducted by Barney Graham and others at Vanderbilt School of Medicine in the 1990s.

How fortuitous that only a few years later, this prescient patent was eventually used and hailed as the "secret to the success" of Moderna, Johnson & Johnson, Novavax, CureVac, and BioNTech/ Pfizer's Covid mRNA vaccines. "The work of Dr. Barney Graham and Kizzmekia Corbett and others stabilized the pre-fusion spike protein which is used in virtually all, with few exceptions, of the vaccines that are now successful," then-NIAID Director, Dr. Anthony Fauci, explained at a House of Representatives hearing[540] in April 2021.

Notably, the late Adam Andrzejewski, founder and CEO of the influential government oversight group, OpenTheBooks,[541] who died unexpectedly in August 2024, wrote an explosive article in the *New York Post*[542] revealing how: "The agency [NIH] and its scientists collected $710 million in royalties during the pandemic, from late 2021 through 2023. These are payments made by private companies, like pharmaceuticals, to license medical innovations from government scientists."

Undoubtedly, royalties from the 070 patent would have contributed to the $710 million collected by the NIH. This patent among others would eventually seed significant friction between Moderna and the NIH. The dispute arose when Dr. Barney Graham's lab at the VRC contested Moderna's exclusion of key government scientists (Kizzmekia Corbett, Barney Graham, and John Mascola) from the list of co-inventors associated with Moderna's mRNA technology patent.

"Moderna has made a serious mistake here in not providing the kind of co-inventorship credit to people who played a major role in the development of the vaccine that they are now making a fair amount of money off of," NIH Director Dr. Francis Collins told Reuters.[543] By late 2021, Moderna offered the NIH co-ownership of the patent[544] to resolve the dispute and avoid any entanglements of lawsuits with the federal agency.

At the start of Moderna and the NIH's "public-private partnership," Dr. Barney Graham and his team at the VRC had been collaborating with Moderna on developing mRNA vaccines to combat Nipah virus and Middle East respiratory syndrome coronavirus (MERS-CoV) but both these projects did not progress beyond animal testing. That is until 3/11.

The main reason for the MERS-CoV mRNA vaccine to fail and progress no further than animal testing was due to a troubling phenomenon observed during the preclinical trials: the vaccinated animals exhibited Vaccine-Associated Enhanced Disease (VAED). VAED is the outcome where instead of providing immunity, the vaccine causes the subject to experience even more severe symptoms upon encountering the wild virus, compared to if they had never been vaccinated. The mechanism by which this phenomenon occurs is called Antibody-Dependent Enhancement (ADE) where pre-existing antibodies, instead of neutralizing a virus (so that it can no longer infect cells), facilitate its entry into cells, potentially leading to a more severe disease.

One of the most infamous instances of VAED occurred during a Respiratory Syncytial Virus (RSV) vaccine children's trial in the 1960s. This vaccine not only failed to protect but also led to enhanced respiratory disease in vaccinated children upon natural RSV infection, resulting in severe cases and even fatalities. VAED[545] has also been reported in animal studies and in humans for vaccine candidates against SARS-CoV-1, dengue virus (DENV), HIV-1 and simian immunodeficiency virus (SIV).

Notably, in May 2021, when the Covid vaccine rollout was well underway, the Brighton Collaboration and Coalition for Epidemic Preparedness Innovations (CEPI) redefined the term VAED.[546] It could be argued that the increased rigor and specific criteria would have excluded many cases that did not meet the full definition, despite certain individuals showing symptoms of VAED. This would have significantly lowered the case count potentially resulting in this important safety signal to go undetected.

In an interview with Stéphane Bancel by MIT Sloan finance professor Andrew Lo, a summarized article,[547] drew attention to the fact that:

"Moderna had already spent two years developing a vaccine for MERS (Middle East Respiratory Syndrome). When it saw the genetic sequence of the new coronavirus (technically SARS-CoV-2) that China published Jan. 11, Moderna scientists realized it was extremely similar to the MERS sequence and quickly shifted focus. By mid-March, the firm had a vaccine and had begun its first human trial in Seattle."

Why did Moderna scientists quickly shift focus when they saw the genetic sequence of SARS-CoV-2 on January 11, when it was not even viewed as a threat? And how serendipitous that SARS-CoV-2 happened to be "extremely similar to the MERS sequence." The very respiratory virus that Moderna and the VRC had already spent two years developing a mRNA vaccine, arising from the NIH's patent to stabilize the spike-protein.

So, what was Moderna's CEO, Stéphane Bancel, doing in early January 2020? He was vacationing in the South of France, when apparently early one morning, a headline in the Wall Street Journal about an outbreak of a mysterious illness in China, caught his attention. According to *Boston* magazine,[548] "Bancel didn't like the sound of it one bit" so he forwarded the story link in an email to Barney Graham, deputy director of the VRC, and asked "Can you make any sense of the viral outbreak going on in China?"

As per *Business Insider*,[549] Bancel spotted the Wall Street Journal article on January 6th[550] and that same day he emailed it to Graham, who responded: "If it's a coronavirus, we know what to do and have proven mRNA is effective."

Graham's hubristic statement was based purely on preliminary data published in 2019, which was reported in *STAT*,[551] from two small early Phase 1 human trials, where participants were administered with experimental mRNA vaccines targeting cytomegalovirus (CMV) infection and the DARPA-funded mosquito-borne chikungunya virus (mRNA-1647 and mRNA-1944 respectively).

Significant adverse events were reported from the chikungunya virus vaccine (mRNA1944) trial, mentioned earlier. In addition, "muscle pain, fevers, and chills were also reported in about one-third of participants" involved in the clinical trial for the CMV (mRNA-1647) vaccine. It is concerning how Graham viewed these small, early Phase 1 trials for mRNA vaccines with known safety issues, as proof that "mRNA is effective."

Later in January, Bancel attended the World Economic Forum in Davos, Switzerland, where he concluded that "the world was on the brink of the worst pandemic in more than 100 years." So, what made the salesman with no scientific background reach that conclusion? Allegedly, it was his meeting with two key scientists, who also happened to be at Davos, then-director of the Wellcome Trust, Sir Jeremy Farrar and Dr. Richard Hatchett from the Gates Foundation-funded, Coalition for Epidemic Preparedness Innovations (CEPI). As noted earlier, Hatchett was former director of BARDA before Rick Bright took over. CEPI went on to help fund Moderna's early Covid vaccine trials.

It is striking that Bancel referred to the pair as the "infectious diseases mafia." The duo apparently spent days in Davos with the Moderna CEO "sketching disaster scenarios on napkins, prompting him to realize the potential seriousness of the outbreak."

Another notable occurrence, observed from early January 2020 onwards, was the fact that Moderna's stock, which had been in steady decline, skyrocketed in value from $18.89 per share to $449.38, its peak on 10 September 2021. Controversially, in May 2020, just after Moderna announced "positive results"[552] from their early-stage Covid vaccine trial on 45 participants (although, according to Moderna, data on the second dose was not available for the 250 microgram group), two of its insiders, chief financial officer, Lorence Kim and chief medical officer, Dr. Tal Zaks, executed options and sold nearly $30 million of shares. By the summer of 2020, Moderna insiders, including Noubar Afeyan and Stephane Bancel, sold $250 million of shares as the stock soared.

*The New York Times*[553] reported "Flagship Ventures, an investment fund run by the company's founder and chairman, Noubar Afeyan, sold more than $68 million worth of Moderna shares on May 21. Those transactions were not scheduled in advance, according to securities filings."

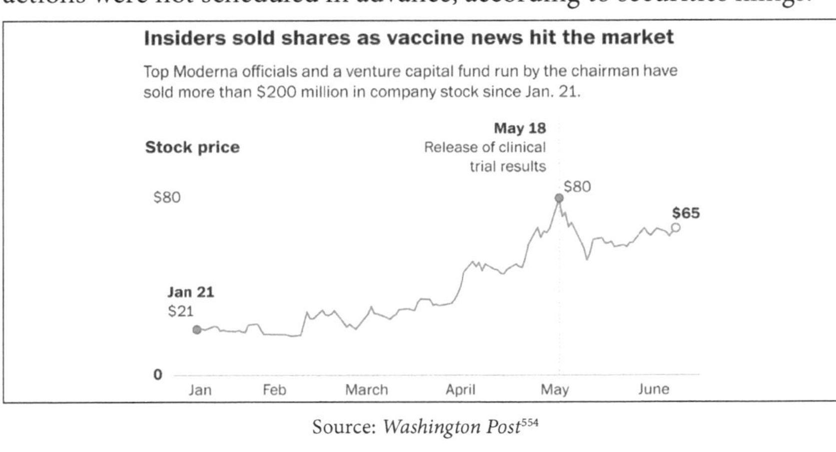


Source: *Washington Post*[554]

In September 2020, business researcher and consultant, Jim Collins penned an article for *Forbes*,[555] "Why are Moderna Insiders Selling So Many Shares?" He wrote: "The pace and frequency of sales of MRNA [Moderna] stock by Moderna insiders is shocking to me. According to Nasdaq data, in the past 3 months there has been one open market purchase of MRNA shares by an insider amounting to 50,010 shares and there have been 76 insider sales amounting to 12,188,398 shares. In the past year the discrepancy is just as wide; 4 purchases of a combined 200,341 shares by insiders and 212 sales of a combined 39,086,672 shares by insiders...This is extraordinary. I have been reading SEC documents for the past three decades and I have never seen such a mismatch between insider selling and (largely non-existent in the case of MRNA) insider buying."

From August to September 2020, well over half of Moderna's insider sale transactions were made by its CEO, Stéphane Bancel. Indeed, it had become significantly apparent that Moderna insiders were cashing out on their long-awaited "Hail Mary" moment.

• • •

In 2016, Peter Kolchinsky from RA Capital Management, an investor in Moderna, presciently stated, "We think that when the world does get to see Moderna, they're going to see something far larger in scope than anybody's seen before." His foresight was spot on. However, it took a few more years for the "disruptive" events of 3/11 to unfold, enabling the unicorn to bring to market its first ever product: a novel, gene-based "vaccine." A product that was rolled out in unprecedented fashion around the world, eerily reminiscent of former-BARDA director, Rick Bright's remark, one that was "not beholden to bureaucratic strings and processes" but through the corner-cutting channel of emergency use authorization, granted under the premise: "There is no adequate, approved, and available alternative to the product for preventing COVID-19 caused by SARS-CoV-2."

However, the following chapter investigates how that claim proved not to be the case, as in early 2020, certain repurposed generic drugs were reported to be effective, lifesaving early treatments for COVID-19.

CHAPTER TEN

# ELIMINATE THE COMPETITION

*"These drugs have been suppressed... for reasons that have nothing to do with the science and medicine."*

~Dr. Harvey Risch,
November 30, 2021, *The Epoch Times*[556]

This chapter examines how specific antimalarial and antiparasitic medications, such as hydroxychloroquine and ivermectin, which have been safely used for decades, gained worldwide attention as potential early treatments for COVID-19, only to face widespread condemnation by global health authorities, public health officials, and the mainstream media. Furthermore, physicians advocating for these drugs were subject to extreme scrutiny and backlash.

## The Hydroxychloroquine Story

Hydroxychloroquine (HCQ) traces its origin to quinine, a compound derived from the bark of the Cinchona tree, which was used by South American Indigenous peoples to treat fevers.

Quinine's derivative, chloroquine, was first synthesized in 1934 by Hans Andersag in Germany, during the nation's wartime malaria research efforts. By the 1950s, hydroxychloroquine was developed as a drug with fewer side effects than chloroquine and in 1955, the U.S. Food and Drug Administration (FDA) approved it as a malaria treatment. In the late 1950s and early 1960s, clinicians observed that chloroquine and its derivative, hydroxychloroquine, had anti-inflammatory effects. This paved the way for its application in managing auto-immune conditions like rheumatoid arthritis and lupus. By the late 70s and 80s, both these medications had been added to the World Health Organization's Model List of Essential Medicines due to their proven efficacy and safety profiles.

On January 13, 2020, France's Ministry of Solidarity and Health made the unusual decision to classify hydroxychloroquine "in all its forms under List II of poisonous substances" due to the potential genotoxic risks associated with related substances like chloroquine. HCQ was readily available over the counter in France but after the decree was issued, it was subject to compulsory medical prescription.

In March 2020, the Ukrainian-born and Brooklyn-raised, Orthodox Jewish family physician, the late Dr. Vladimir Zelenko, became the one of the first physicians to publicly advocate the use of the antimalarial as an early treatment for COVID-19. His proposed treatment protocol, which later became known as the "Zelenko Protocol," involved hydroxychloroquine, the antibiotic azithromycin, and zinc sulfate for early-stage COVID-19 patients.

Dr. Zelenko reported the use of his treatment protocol on seven hundred of his patients, asserting a 100 percent success rate in preventing hospitalizations. "I'm seeing tremendous positive results," he said in a March 21, 2020, video,[557] which was addressed to President Trump and eventually posted to YouTube and Facebook (both platforms removed it under COVID-19 misinformation policies). This was shortly followed by a fervent open-letter[558] to the President, imploring him to declare war on COVID-19 through immediate, accessible outpatient treatment protocols. Framing the crisis as "World War III—virus versus humanity," Zelenko warned that bureaucratic delays and overcautious testing were condemning millions to unnecessary suffering and death. He advocated for aggressive intervention upon the first suspicion of infection, emphasizing a narrow therapeutic window before irreversible pulmonary damage sets in.

At the heart of his proposal was a simple, affordable triad of medications (hydroxychloroquine, azithromycin, and zinc sulfate) whose risks, he argued, were grossly exaggerated by fearmongering. Obstructing such life-saving drugs, he charged, bordered on crimes against humanity.

A week after the Zelenko video went viral, on March 28, 2020, the U.S. Food and Drug Administration (FDA) issued an Emergency Use Authorization (EUA) for HCQ for the treatment of COVID-19. This authorization was specifically for use in hospitalized patients, not as an early treatment described in Zelenko's letter. However, it's important to note that the FDA later revoked their EUA on June 15, 2020, due to reasons later addressed in this chapter.

On the heels of Zelenko's open-letter, President Trump announced[559] to the world at a press conference that he was taking the antimalarial HCQ as a prophylaxis measure and that many of the front-line hospital workers were too. Trump even referenced "the doctor from New York" who had told him about the success of using this treatment in conjunction with others (zinc and azithromycin) on several hundred of his patients.

Over in France, the "Marseille Protocol" pioneered by one of the most cited microbiologists in the world, Dr. Didier Raoult, M.D, PhD, head of Méditerranée Infection University Hospital Institute in Marseille, had already become a lightning rod in the debate over HCQ as a treatment for COVID-19 even before the "Zelenko Protocol" gained traction.

By late February, Dr. Raoult announced what he said were promising results on a small sample of patients. The study by Gautret et al.,[560] with Raoult cited as co-author, entitled, "Hydroxychloroquine and azithromycin as a treatment of COVID-19: results of an open-label non-randomized clinical trial" first went online on March 17, 2020. It was later published in the International Journal of Antimicrobial Agents (IJAA)

The trial involved 20 patients who were treated with HCQ (600mg daily), for which some azithromycin (AZ) was added to their treatment, and 16 were used as controls. The study reported a significant reduction in viral load by day 6 in the treated group compared to controls.

"In France, they had a very good test," Trump later told the press, referring to this study. However, the mainstream media rushed to condemn it. *The Guardian*[561] reported: "With help from Fox News and Elon Musk, a misleading French study prompted a wave of misinformation that made its way to the president."

In March 2020, Musk tweeted "Maybe worth considering chloroquine for C19," with a link to a Google document by James Todaro, Gregory Rigano, and others. The document suggested chloroquine and hydroxychloroquine might work against COVID-19, citing early data from China and a French study by Didier Raoult. The Google document was later removed "for violating terms of service," and Twitter flagged the link, but not before it drew significant public and media attention.

## The Infamous Lancet Study

By late Spring 2020, backlash from public health officials and the mainstream media in response to Trump's support for the decades-old antimalarial drug, began to intensify. It reached fever-pitch around the time a particular study was published in one of the world's most prestigious scientific journals, *The Lancet*, on May 22, triggering a cascade of events.

The Mehra et al. study,[562] an observational analysis of hospitalized of roughly 96,000 COVID-19 patients, found that hydroxychloroquine or chloroquine regimens offered no benefit and "was associated with an increase in the risk of ventricular arrhythmias and a greater hazard for in-hospital death with COVID-19."

That same day, the BBC ran an article[563] with the headline: "Trump drug hydroxychloroquine raises death risk in Covid patients, study says."

By Monday, May 25th, the World Health Organization Director, General Tedros Adhanom Ghebreyesus announced[564] the suspension of its clinical trials on hydroxychloroquine and asked other countries to do likewise citing "safety concerns." The WHO Director General declared: "The executive group has implemented a temporary pause of the hydroxychloroquine arm within the Solidarity trial while the safety data is reviewed by the data safety monitoring board." Launched in March 2020, the WHO's Solidarity trial was a global effort to evaluate potential treatments for COVID-19.

Two days later, speaking to Jim Sciutto on CNN's Newsroom, Dr Anthony Fauci, then a key member of the White House Coronavirus Task Force, asserted, "The scientific data is really quite evident now about the lack of efficacy for it [hydroxychloroquine], and there's likelihood of adverse events with regard to cardiovascular [issues]."

However, the problem with *The Lancet* study was that it was based on "faked data" leading to its eventual retraction,[565] thirteen days later. Surgisphere, a little-known database company in Chicago, was entirely responsible for providing the large datasets (671 hospitals on six continents) for the study.

In the article, "*The Lancet* and the trashing of a cure for Covid,"[566] the physicist, Dr. Edmund Fordham wrote, "An open letter from 200 medical luminaries demanded an independent investigation. By the time Twitterati found suspicions that the CEO of the database company moonlighted as a male model and a marketing executive as an 'adult' actress, the house of cards was collapsing. The retraction had face-saving words, but the paper was exposed as based on data unverifiable at best, or outright fabricated:

classic fake news. Yet it came from a medical journal proud of its heritage and prestige, had sailed through the peer review process and *The Lancet* stood solidly on its dignity for a whole fortnight."

On June 4th *STAT News*[567] reported "*The Lancet*, one of the world's top medical journals, on Thursday retracted an influential study that raised alarms about the safety of the experimental COVID-19 treatments chloroquine and hydroxychloroquine amid scrutiny of the data underlying the paper."

"We can no longer vouch for the veracity of the primary data sources," Mandeep Mehra of Brigham and Women's Hospital, Frank Ruschitzka of University Hospital Zurich, and Amit Patel of University of Utah said in a statement issued by *The Lancet*. "Due to this unfortunate development, the authors request that the paper be retracted."

## The Flawed RECOVERY Trial

Circling back to Dr. Fordham's article, a key event is brought to light: "On cue the next day, Friday, conveniently distracting from the embarrassment, the Oxford RECOVERY clinical trials (with no full paper) announced that there was no improvement in mortality with hydroxychloroquine: a shocking quarter of patients died whether or not they were given the drug. One major problem with the RECOVERY trial of hydroxychloroquine is that patients were already in the 'inflammatory' stage of the illness, when hydroxychloroquine is not expected to help. Findings merely confirmed what successful clinicians have insisted on for months: you must treat early."

The RECOVERY trial was launched in March 2020 with the aim to evaluate multiple potential treatments for hospitalized COVID-19 patients (enrolling over 11,000) across 176 NHS hospitals in the UK. It used a randomized, controlled, open-label, multi-arm approach, and was co-led by Oxford University Professors Peter Horby, an infectious disease expert, and Martin Landray, a clinical trial specialist. Funding came from UK Research and Innovation, the National Institute for Health Research (NIHR), and other partners like the Wellcome Trust and the Bill & Melinda Gates Foundation. The HCQ arm of RECOVERY randomized 1,561 patients to receive HCQ plus standard care, compared to 3,155 patients receiving standard care alone.

On June 5, 2020, RECOVERY's independent Data Monitoring Committee reviewed interim data and recommended stopping the HCQ arm due to lack of efficacy. The study concluded that HCQ did not reduce mortality, shorten hospital stays, or prevent progression to severe outcomes in hospitalized patients. The trial results from RECOVERY's HCQ arm were eventually published in October in the *New England Journal of Medicine.*[568] According to the study, "Death within 28 days occurred in 421 patients (27.0%) in the hydroxychloroquine group and in 790 (25.0%) in the usual-care group" was reported.

By June 15, the antimalarial's fate was sealed with the FDA revoking[569] their EUA of hydroxychloroquine and chloroquine as treatments for COVID-19. Their announcement read, "In light of ongoing serious cardiac adverse events and other potential serious side effects, the known and potential benefits of chloroquine and hydroxychloroquine no longer outweigh the known and potential risks for the authorized use."

On the heels of RECOVERY's interim trial results, Fauci told the BBC:[570] "We know that every single good study - and by good study I mean randomized control study in which the data are firm and believable - has shown that hydroxychloroquine is not effective in the treatment of COVID-19."

However, not everyone swallowed the trial's results hook, line, and sinker. Among the vocal critics, one in particular stood out, the online French publication, *FranceSoir*. A series of hard-hitting articles were published raising several pointed objections[571] about RECOVERY's design and execution. *FranceSoir's* CEO, the business scientist and data analyst, Xavier Azalbert repeatedly argued that the HCQ doses used in RECOVERY- 2,400 mg on the first day (800 mg initially, 800 mg after 6-8 hours, then 400 mg at 12 and 24 hours), followed by 800 mg daily for 9 days- were dangerously high and potentially fatal, especially for the elderly, hospitalized patients. *FranceSoir* also alleged that Horby and Landray (RECOVERY's chief investigators) manipulated data, by using visually misleading survival curves to mask a 2% mortality increase in the HCQ arm, which they interpret as a trend toward harm from overdose.

In 2021, I had the opportunity to interview *FranceSoir's* Xavier Azalbert. The following is an excerpt from that interview.

XA: Now you have RECOVERY that comes in. It just says, hydroxychloroquine is not really toxic, but it doesn't work. And you have a death ratio of 26% in this study, that's one in four- one in four patients died. That's a lot! Then I'm well, let's look at the protocol. Let's look at what's being administered. And here, the same thing as with *The Lancet* study, I talk to my scientists, the medical doctors. We look at that and say, let's go and interview one of the chief investigators, and I interviewed[572] Martin Landray. You can see that when I speak to him, I just want to understand, what did you do and what were the basis for the decisions? It's really a scientific interview, where we're trying to understand the basis for the decision of 2400 mg of hydroxychloroquine on day one because for us, it was like a surprise... Our conclusion is that RECOVERY has overdosed some patients but this does not appear in their conclusion because it just says it doesn't work...And it was evident to us that all of this lacked what I would call sense of realism. And when I spoke to Martin Landray, I did ask him, why did you prescribe this? And he just told me, well, it's the same dosage that you would give in amoebic dysentery. And so you would have seen all of that- and doctors told us, we don't use HCQ for amoebic dysentery.

SE: Why did you think that Martin Landray picked the dosage at 2400 mg within the first 24 hours?

XA: It came out of this pharmacokinetic model, which is in version two of the hydroxychloroquine protocol, which has been done by somebody called Nick White. Basically, they tried to reach the level of effectiveness and efficiency of this molecule as rapidly as possible, right? That's called a loading dose and in order to reach this level, they work it out through their modeling that you're required to have 2400mg in the first 24 hours but in total- the patients, if they actually did a full course, would receive something like 9600mg. Now one of the particularities of hydroxychloroquine is that it has what's called a very long half-life. The half-life is measured as how long does it take for your body to remove 50% of this molecule. And it's a very long half-life... And when you work out what the toxic dosage is for hydroxychloroquine- the MHRA guidelines and the French guidelines are pretty much the same. They just say that around 2400mg or thereabouts is close to the toxic dose and at that level you need to go to an emergency room. You need to have some form of emergency treatment. Do you remember I said that over 10 days the patient has absorbed 9600mg of hydroxychloroquine, 2400mg on day one.

• • •

It came as no surprise for Dr. Raoult, architect of the "Marseille Protocol" to fiercely criticize the RECOVERY Trial's hydroxychloroquine (HCQ) dosing regimen, labelling it as "insane" and potentially lethal. In an interview with *FranceSoir*, he asserted the dose was "five times higher" than his protocol. He claimed such levels risked toxicity, including cardiac arrhythmias, especially in sick patients, stating, "They gave doses that could kill, not cure."

Several years on, the controversy surrounding RECOVERY's HCQ arm has not died down. In a March 2025 interview[573] with Del Bigtree, Raoult expressed outrage that the trial's design relied on mathematical models, which he blamed for dangerous overdoses, rather than drawing on the expertise of clinicians like himself. He further criticized the study for including patients without confirmed COVID-19 diagnoses, a flaw he said eroded its credibility. Pointing to the trial's results, published in the *New England Journal of Medicine*, Raoult decried them as a betrayal of scientific integrity, declaring, "It's not medicine. It's fraudulent science."

## The 16990 HCQ Deaths That Never Were

In January 2024, a paper by Pradelle et al.,[574] titled "Deaths induced by compassionate use of hydroxychloroquine during the first COVID-19 wave: An estimate" challenged HCQ's well-established safety profile. It was published in *Elsevier's Journal of Biomedicine & Pharmacotherapy* and sensationalized in the mainstream media. According to the paper, "HCQ might have been associated with an excess of 16990 deaths during the first wave of the COVID-19 pandemic in the six countries for which data were available."

Mainstream media outlets like *Politico*[575] were quick to pounce on this study in an attempt to discredit Trump. They ran the headline, "Hydroxychloroquine could have caused 17,000 deaths during Covid, study finds," juxtaposed by the line, "Former U.S. President Donald Trump said: 'What do you have to lose? Take it."

In similar fashion, *Forbes* ran the headline, "Hydroxychloroquine, A Drug Trump Promoted To Treat COVID-19, Linked To 17,000 Deaths, Estimates Show."

Uncannily, this study drew many similarities with the infamous Lancet study discussed earlier- it was based on "what critics have described as scientific fraud," "unreliable data," and eventually retracted on August 26, 2024.

The advocacy group BonSens.org, spearheaded the retraction campaign. They criticized its use of the Axfors et al. meta-analysis as overly broad, its assumption of uniform HCQ dosing (ignoring RECOVERY's excessive 2400 mg/day, detailed earlier), and its speculative extrapolation across six countries. Xavier Azalbert, also heavily criticized the study's reliance on an "unreliable" Belgian dataset, which was later deemed fraudulent.

Dr. David Gortler's critique of the study, published in the *Brownstone Institute*,[576] cast doubt on the credibility of Dr. Danyelle Townsend, professor at the University of South Carolina College of Pharmacy's Department of Drug Discovery and Biomedical Sciences, and editor-in-chief of the journal that published the fraudulent paper.

An extract reads, "These are pharmacology fundamentals that ought to be known by any pharmacist or physician – let alone to a professor serving as a Journal Editor-in-Chief at a taxpayer-funded state College of Pharmacy. Did not even one person on her editorial board of over 50 'peer-reviewers' and staff ponder the celebrated and storied history of HCQ (and its predecessors) and how incongruent this study's findings were before choosing to publish data denigrating HCQ safety? The correct answer to that might actually be: 'no'..."

## Delayed Truths

On July 4, 2025, after five long years, the UK-based PRINCIPLE[577] trial, an open-label, randomized trial led by the University of Oxford, designed to evaluate potential COVID-19 treatments in high-risk, community-based patients, published the results of their HCQ trial arm in *Scientific Reports.*[578]

The PRINCIPLE trial was primarily funded by UK Research and Innovation (UKRI) and the Department of Health and Social Care (DHSC) through the National Institute for Health Research (NIHR). It began recruiting participants on April 2, 2020. However, immediately following the publication of the infamous Mehra et al. study in *The Lancet* on May 22, 2020, which claimed that HCQ was associated with increased mortality and cardiac arrhythmias in hospitalized COVID-19 patients- the UK's Medicines and Healthcare products Regulatory Agency (MHR) immediately suspended the HCQ arm of the PRINCIPLE trial- the very same day. Despite the retraction of *The Lancet* study which was proven to be fraudulent, the MHRA did not revoke the suspension of the HCQ trial arm.

It is noteworthy that five years later, published results showed that the 207 participants from the HCQ arm, who received 200 mg twice daily for seven days, led to a statistically significant reduction in median time to first feeling recovered by two days compared to usual care alone. In addition,

HCQ was shown to be well-tolerated, with no serious safety concerns reported, consistent with its established safety profile at the doses used.

The research group behind the X account @CovidAnalysis, which was banned from the platform (formerly Twitter) for two years, focuses on COVID-19 data analysis and is associated with websites such as c19early.org, c19hcq.org, c19ivm.org, and hcqtrial.com. They provided their perspective to me on the five-year delay in publishing the HCQ arm results of the PRINCIPLE trial. They shared this in our interview:

"We find the withholding of these results unconscionable - efficacy and safety for outpatient treatment known in June 2020. The opposite of the propaganda fueled by the fraudulent Surgisphere paper and the RECOVERY trial (dosage known to be harmful, very late-stage treatment, not relevant to early treatment or prophylaxis). A combination of low-cost treatments used early could have ended the pandemic quickly, reducing risk below that of existing respiratory diseases. For example, there are many effective treatments[579] that can be applied directly to the respiratory tract. Yet we ended up with almost complete suppression of low-cost treatments in high-profit countries. HCQ was the first with significant evidence and therefore the initial target of those with substantial investments in more profitable alternatives. This is an RCT from Oxford, considered a top-tier research institution with a strong track record in conducting high-quality RCTs, which have directly supported FDA approvals in the U.S. Release of these results could have made it much harder to suppress the evidence for HCQ, and also supported coverage of results for all low-cost treatments."

Interestingly, another study run by the Mahidol Oxford Tropical Medicine Research Unit, shared the same fate as the PRINCIPLE's HCQ trial arm. The COPCOV study, funded by the Bill & Melinda Gates Foundation through the COVID-19 Therapeutics Accelerator, a collaborative initiative launched with Wellcome and Mastercard, was a double-blind, randomized, placebo-controlled trial evaluating chloroquine (CQ) and hydroxychloroquine (HCQ) for prophylaxis against COVID-19 in healthcare workers and high-risk groups, conducted from 2020 to 2022. It enrolled 4,652 participants, significantly less than the originally planned 40,000 due to "protracted delays resulting from controversies over efficacy and adverse events with HCQ use, vaccine rollout in some countries, and other factors," cited by the authors.

It took four years for the results to be eventually published on September 12, 2004, in *PLOS Medicine*.[580]

The authors stated: "In this large placebo-controlled, double-blind randomized trial, HCQ and CQ were safe and well tolerated in COVID-19 chemoprevention, and there was evidence of moderate protective benefit in a meta-analysis including this trial and similar RCTs." The drugs (HCQ and CQ) reduced all-cause respiratory illnesses and workdays lost (337 days per 1,000 participants over three months for the treatment group vs. 441 days for placebo, a reduction of about 104 days).

Isn't it interesting that the PRINCIPLE and the COPCOV study, backed by organizations, that critics argue, with vested interests that may have contributed to suppressing low-cost, effective treatments for Covid, both demonstrated HCQ's safety and efficacy in reducing recovery time and respiratory illness- yet faced years-long delays in reporting.

These delays, compounded by regulatory suspensions and media narratives, undoubtedly hindered the adoption of HCQ as an early Covid treatment, potentially at the cost of countless lives.

## HCQ Doctors Under Fire

Since 2020, Dr. Didier Raoult has faced significant backlash for his advocacy of HCQ as an early treatment for COVID-19. On April 3, 2020, shortly following the release of the Gautret et al. study, the International Society of Antimicrobial Chemotherapy (ISAC), co-publisher of the International Journal of Antimicrobial Agents (IJAA), issued a scathing critique. They declared the study "did not meet the Society's expected standard," citing ethical and methodological flaws. Remarkably, it required an additional four years for *Elsevier* to formally retract the study on December 17, 2024.

In the wake of 3/11, the 2010 Grand Prix Inserm laureate faced severe consequences for advocating hydroxychloroquine (HCQ) as an early treatment for COVID-19, ultimately leading to the retraction of 32 of his academic papers and a two-year suspension from practicing medicine.

In July 2020, the French Infectious Diseases Society (SPILF) filed a complaint[581] with the Bouches-du-Rhône Order of Physicians, accusing Raoult of spreading disinformation and breaching medical ethics by promoting an unproven treatment. In September 2021, Raoult was forced to retire from his role as IHU director. A few months later, he faced formal disciplinary action from the French Order of Physicians, culminating in the imposition of a two-year ban on practicing medicine,[582] effective

February 1, 2025, citing 11 violations of the public health code, including "charlatanism" and insufficient caution in public statements.

The late Dr. Vladimir "Zev" Zelenko did not remain unscathed either. Following his widely circulated video appeal to then-President Trump, the tight-knit Hasidic community of Kiryas Joel, of which Zelenko served as a physician for nearly two decades, wrote an open-letter imploring him to cease his endeavors. "Dr. Zelenko's videos have caused widespread fear that has resulted in the discrimination against members of the Hasidic community throughout the region," the officials wrote. Tensions escalated, and by May 2020, Zelenko announced his departure[583] from the community, citing harassment by local figures he blamed for undermining his practice.

Mainstream media outlets like The New York Times and The Washington Post portrayed him as the "simple country doctor turned right-wing fringe figure" pushing unproven treatments.

## BARDA's Derailment of HCQ

Notably, in a 2021 interview, (this interview was posted on the video-sharing platform Bitchute but due to the introduction of the UK's Online Safety Act, the platform is no longer accessible to UK users) Zelenko alleged how early COVID-19 treatments, particularly HCQ, were systematically sabotaged. He accused Dr. Rick Bright, the former director of BARDA (Biomedical Advanced Research and Development Authority) of derailing the use of HCQ for early outpatient treatment. He asserted that Bright's decision to restrict HCQ to hospital use only, prevented its widespread use in the critical early stages of COVID-19, which Zelenko claimed led to countless unnecessary deaths. The following statement was made by Dr. Zelenko in that interview.

"What I'm about to tell you is the mechanics of genocide. And the basis of what I'm about to tell you is Dr. Bright's own words in a documentary called 'Totally Under Control' and what he describes is the following: When he got the President's order to make a hydroxychloroquine available to every American, he says he felt that that was a terrible idea, and him and his team were against it. So, they crafted together with Janet Woodcock, who is now currently the acting head of the FDA, a strategy to limit access to hydroxychloroquine. And how did they do that? Well, first they were supposed to use the "Right to Try" legislation which enabled every single American to have access to certain drugs outside of clinical trials. They were supposed to use that pathway to make hydroxychloroquine available to every single American. Instead, what they did was they crafted an Emergency Use Authorization that opened the national stockpile medication to only hospitalized patients. What that did effectively, and it sent a message to every single doctor in America and their employer-that the government is only in support of hydroxychloroquine usage in the hospital setting. And certain employers set policies that if a doctor uses hydroxychloroquine in the outpatient setting, they would lose their job."

The coronavirus vaccine researcher, and former Novavax vice president, Dr. Rick Bright, was BARDA director from November 2016 until April 2020, when he was transferred to a less influential post at the National Institutes of Health. Bright alleged that the Trump administration ignored his early warnings about COVID-19 and was demoted in retaliation for his opposition to the off-label use of hydroxychloroquine, pushed by President Donald Trump at the time.

In a statement[584] released by his lawyers, Bright stated: "Specifically, and contrary to misguided directives, I limited the broad use of chloroquine and hydroxychloroquine, promoted by the Administration as a panacea, but which clearly lack scientific merit. While I am prepared to look at all options and to think "outside the box" for effective treatments, I rightly resisted efforts to provide an unproven drug on demand to the American public. I insisted that these drugs be provided only to hospitalized patients with confirmed COVID-19 while under the supervision of a physician. These drugs have potentially serious risks associated with them, including increased mortality observed in some recent studies in patients with COVID-19."

The following month, he filed a whistle-blower complaint,[585] where it stated, "Dr. Bright repeatedly urged his BARDA team and ASPR [Assistant Secretary for Preparedness and Response] leadership to invest in vaccine development proposals with strong scientific merit ... He advocated for funding vaccine candidates that could be developed and manufactured quickly and safely, such as those using novel platforms."

Yet, the paradox lies in this: the well-established safety record of the anti-malarial drug, used effectively for decades, was sidelined in favor of the "unproven," "novel platforms" of the modified mRNA vaccines associated with serious risks.

The previous chapter references Bright's career as a pharma-aligned bureaucrat directing billions of federal funds to biotech companies, such as grants to Moderna for its Zika mRNA vaccine candidate. During his tenure at Novavax, where he served as vice president of global influenza programs, the company's recombinant nanoparticle vaccine technology was developed and later used for its COVID-19 vaccine (NVX-CoV2373). In the early months of 2020, Bright oversaw billions in federal funding to partner with pharmaceutical giants like Moderna, Johnson & Johnson, and Pfizer for Covid vaccine development.

Equally notable is the striking comment made by Bright during the 2019 Future Summit of Health, referenced in the previous chapter. When pressed on whether the traditional egg-based vaccine system needed to be "blown up," he replied, "There might be a need or even an urgent call for an entity of excitement out there, that is completely disruptive, does not beholden to bureaucratic strings and processes."

Critics suggest that figures like Rick Bright were instrumental in bringing mRNA technology to the market; a technology that until 3/11 had been stalled by "bureaucratic strings and processes," such as real concerns over its unproven safety profile. It can also be said that the emergence of Covid became the "entity of excitement" Bright envisioned, propelling the experimental vaccine technology into the spotlight as a medical countermeasure. It has been argued that they may have viewed HCQ as a major hurdle to the rollout of this new technology. This is because, for the U.S. Food and Drug Administration (FDA) to issue an Emergency Use Authorization (EUA) an essential condition needs to be met: the absence of any adequate, approved, and available alternative treatment.

## The "Wonder Drug" Ivermectin

Another drug that triggered intense backlash, arguably harsher than what hydroxychloroquine faced, is the long-established anti-parasitic ivermectin (IVM). Originally derived from a Japanese bacterial culture half a century ago, this Nobel Prize-winning drug, included on the WHO's list of essential medicines, rapidly became public enemy #1 for the public health authorities and fact-checkers, when it was repurposed for early COVID-19 treatment and prevention.

The earliest reference of ivermectin's potential to treat COVID-19 came from an Australian laboratory study[586] published in April 2020, led by Leon Caly from Monash University, showing it "eliminated SARS-CoV-2 in cells in 48 hours." The researchers concluded: "Altogether the current report, combined with a known-safety profile, demonstrates that ivermectin is worthy of further consideration as a possible SARS-CoV-2 antiviral." While this was not a clinical endorsement, it sparked great interest amongst doctors who began exploring its off-label use.

Dr. Thomas Borody, the Australian gastroenterologist, emerged as one of ivermectin's early advocates. He wrote to Australian Health Minister Greg Hunt requesting funding for a "triple therapy" protocol involving ivermectin, zinc, and doxycycline. "You need drugs that block enzymes in the cell," Prof Borody told *NCA NewsWire*.[587] "When Ivermectin and zinc combine, it's very important in killing the reproductive cycle where multiplication occurs. Virtually everybody gets cured – it's so simple and in 10 days, side effects are virtually unheard of."

Dr. Pierre Kory, a critical care physician and pulmonary (lung) specialist, is cited as one of the early ivermectin advocates in the U.S. In March 2020, Dr. Kory co-founded the Front-Line COVID-19 Critical Care Alliance (FLCCC), alongside Dr. Paul Marik, then-Professor of Medicine and Chief of the Division of Pulmonary and Critical Care Medicine at Eastern Virginia Medical School.

In my 2021 interview,[588] Dr. Kory recalled how in the early days of the pandemic, he was part of a group of critical care doctors who rallied together to develop treatment protocols for "the sickest of the sick." "We weren't the FLCCC at the time, but in essence, we already were," he shared. This was the genesis of the FLCCC, a pioneer group with over 2000 peer-reviewed publications amongst its members, that formulated what became widely known as the Math +[589] hospital treatment protocol for COVID-19. They were the first to offer guidance on efficacious medications to treat hospitalized COVID-19 patients, incorporating the use of corticosteroids and other repurposed treatments. After initial criticism, their protocol was later adopted in many countries.

Dr. Kory gained worldwide attention when testifying twice in front of the U.S. Senate, first in May 2020, for advocating the use of corticosteroids. Dr Kory disclosed that ivermectin was not used in their original COVID-19 treatment protocol but was being closely followed. It took a further six months, when dramatic results came in from randomized controlled trials, showing the generic anti-parasitic drug to be "highly effective at controlling the pandemic." The results were significant enough to compel Dr. Kory to testify once again in front of the U.S. Senate Committee on

Homeland Security and Governmental Affairs on December 8 that year, advocating for its use as a lifesaving COVID-19 treatment.

In his ten-minute testimony,[590] Dr. Kory described ivermectin as a "wonder drug" attributed to "the mountains of data" that had emerged. The video footage went viral, with over a million views in the first few hours. In response to sticking his head above the parapet, the eminent ICU physician received a barrage of attacks from the mainstream media. The viral video was swiftly removed from YouTube. However, it did not deter other doctors from around the world, who having heard Dr. Kory's powerful testimony, propelled them to investigate the effectiveness of ivermectin as a COVID-19 treatment, leading many to prescribe it for their patients.

## The Censoring of Ivermectin

During my interview with Dr. Kory, I asked about the retraction of his peer-reviewed paper[591] on ivermectin by Frontiers in Pharmacology. "There is a major opposition to ivermectin and the first time that opposition raised its ugly head was with our paper," he stated.

Dr Kory's ground-breaking paper concluded that "Ivermectin, based on the risk-benefit profile and overwhelming reproducible efficacy, should be deployed immediately in the prevention and treatment of COVID-19." He explained how his paper "was peer-reviewed by three senior governmental scientists and an expert clinician; it went through three rounds of peer-review and was accepted for publication, however, the publication date kept on getting pushed back. Suddenly, we were told by the lead editor of all the Frontier journals that they were not going to publish our paper but retract it." When asked what reason they gave, Dr Kory responded, "they called in an anonymous peer-reviewer, who felt our conclusions were unsupported."

He described how his experience was not unique and that it had happened to many other authors. He listed other papers that were retracted, initially accepted but later rejected, or outright rejected from the beginning.

- Dr. Puya Dehgani-Mobaraki MD, a head and neck surgeon, wrote a science review on the mechanisms of action of ivermectin in COVID-19. It was published in one of the Nature journals (had over 500,000 views) but then was suddenly retracted[592] by the Editor-in-Chief, against the objections of the peer-reviewers.

- Dr. Tess Lawrie MD, Ph.D., a world expert in systematic reviews and meta-analysis, conducted a peer-reviewed systematic meta-analysis of ivermectin, as Lawrie claims,[593] it was accepted for publishing by Lancet Respiratory Medicine journal but was later rejected, based on the editor not believing the evidence was strong enough.
- Dr. Eli Schwartz MD, from Sheba Medical Centre in Israel, conducted a placebo double blinded randomized controlled trial on ivermectin[594] showing massive reductions in the time to viral clearance, proving it to be a powerful anti-viral drug. It was rejected outright by all the high-impact journals.
- Dr. Waheed Shouman, from Zagazig University in Egypt, did a major prophylactic trial[595] on ivermectin. TrialSite covered this trial in an article.[596] Shouman had to stop the trial early because the difference between the control and the treatment group was so vast that it would have been unethical to carry on. No high impact journal wanted to publish his findings.

Kory made the poignant argument: "The enemy isn't ivermectin. It's the cheap repurposed drugs that would compete in a marketplace with profitable patented drugs." He claimed that in 2020 the scientific journals and the agencies, "conspired to kill hydroxychloroquine" and in 2021, "they went after ivermectin."

He also spoke about the drug, Proxalutamide (an androgen suppressant), and the fact that his colleague, Dr. Flávio Adsuara Cadegiani from Brazil, conducted a large placebo double-blinded, randomized controlled trial[597] showing significant benefits to COVID-19 mortality and hospitalization. His paper was submitted to the *New England Journal of Medicine* and passed peer-review, soon after a letter was received by the authors stating that the journal would not be publishing it.

## The FDA's Smear Campaign

In my view, by the summer of 2021, the smear campaign targeting ivermectin was well underway. Its peak came with a viral FDA social media post, which became one of the agency's most widely shared tweet, analyzed later in this chapter.

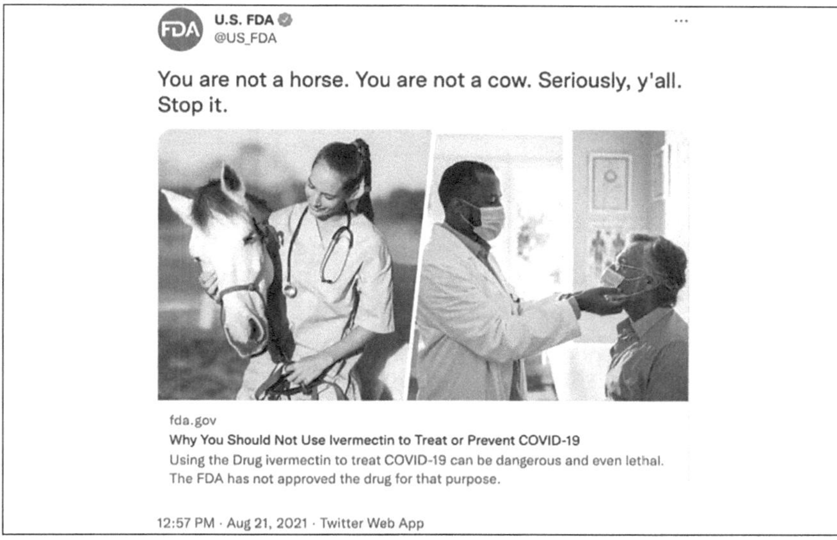
U.S. FDA
@US_FDA
You are not a horse. You are not a cow. Seriously, y'all. Stop it.
fda.gov
Why You Should Not Use Ivermectin to Treat or Prevent COVID-19
Using the Drug ivermectin to treat COVID-19 can be dangerous and even lethal. The FDA has not approved the drug for that purpose.
12:57 PM · Aug 21, 2021 · Twitter Web App

The discrediting of this anti-parasitic drug, led me to write the October 2021 investigative report, "How Ivermectin became a Target for the Fraud Detectives", published in *Trial Site News.*[598]

Firstly, the report highlighted the drug's real-world track record in significantly reducing mortality, hospitalization rates, and infection risk for COVID-19. Mexico City saw a 75% drop in hospitalizations with early treatment of 50,000 patients versus 70,000 untreated. Peru's mass distribution cut excess deaths by 74% in a month. The Indian state of Uttar Pradesh with over 240 million people, implemented a large-scale ivermectin distribution program as part of its COVID-19 response. The state distributed home treatment kits containing ivermectin, doxycycline, zinc, and other medications to combat early-stage infections. By September 2021, only 11 cases were reported with no deaths. Besides the real-world data, to date there have been 52 randomized controlled trials (RCTs) and multiple meta-analyses conducted on ivermectin showing the effectiveness of the drug against Covid.

The report's focus was on a group of researchers, including Jack Lawrence, Gideon Meyerowitz-Katz, Nick Brown, Kyle Sheldrick, and James Heathers, who have been described as "fraud detectives" and who scrutinized certain ivermectin studies, contributing to the retraction of the Elgazzar et al. randomized placebo-controlled trial from *Research Square*.[599] Lawrence, a student at the time, alleged fraud, plagiarism, and data manipulation, claiming he accessed Elgazzar's raw data with a guessed "1234" password. Elgazzar refuted these accusations, insisting the data was not his, while the retraction occurred without his input. The Guardian and BBC reported on these claims, including Lawrence's description of some ivermectin supporters as "a mix of right-wing figures, anti-vaxxers and outright conspiracy theorists."

> Critics have noted that the group known as the "fraud detectives" seemed to focus on studies showing benefit for ivermectin, while not addressing flaws in studies like Lopez-Medina et al. and the TOGETHER trial. The following is an extract of the adapted report.
>
> Even though "the fraud detectives" seemingly found no problems with the Lopez-Medina study, more than 100 physicians did. They signed an open letter[600] concluding that the Lopez-Medina study was fatally flawed.
>
> Some have found it noteworthy that this group, which specializes in investigation ivermectin studies, did not highlight the flaws in these studies that others have identified.
>
> The TOGETHER Clinical Trials[601] (one of the largest randomized clinical trials in the world evaluating the effectiveness of repurposed drugs, including ivermectin) is another study that has been criticized for potential flaws and conflicts of interest. The trial is associated with MMS Holdings. The same company that assists pharmaceutical firms like Pfizer[602] in study design and approval processes. Critics suggest this may have influenced the results showing no benefit for ivermectin.
>
> The co-lead investigator of the TOGETHER trial is Dr. Edward Mills,[603] an associate professor in the Department of Health and Research Methods, Evidence, and Impact at McMaster University in Canada. He also serves as a clinical trial advisor at the Bill & Melinda Gates Foundation.

The fraud detectives are of the collective opinion that if the Elgazzar study is removed from the meta-analyses – "the revision will show no mortality benefit for ivermectin." In contrast, scientists with decades of experience disagree, such as Dr. Tess Lawrie M.D., Ph.D., Andrew Bryant, and Dr. Edmund Fordham. They wrote a letter to the editor of the *American Journal of Therapeutics*[604] and explained when the Bryant et al. study was re-analyzed to exclude the Elgazzar study, the results showed a "49% reduction in mortality in favor of ivermectin."

Dr. Pierre Kory, MD, (winner of the British Medical Association's 2015 President's Choice award) along with Dr. Paul Marik MD, also wrote a letter to the editor[605] of the American Journal of Therapeutics stating "we decided to redo the original meta-analyses excluding this study [Elgazzar et al]. The summary point estimates were largely unaffected when the study by Elgazzar et al was removed."

Another mainstream media report targeting ivermectin is the BBC article,[606] written by Rachel Schraer and Jack Goodman. It reads: "The scientists in the group – Dr Gideon Meyerowitz-Katz, Dr James Heathers, Dr Nick Brown, and Dr Sheldrick – each have a track record of exposing dodgy science."

The article incorporates commonly used derogatory phrases such as "pushing anti-vaccine sentiments," "hype around ivermectin," and "conspiracy theories of ivermectin cover-ups" in referring to those who support the use of ivermectin as a COVID-19 treatment. The referenced scientists who are stated as being "pro-ivermectin" are not described in favorable terms. Dr. Pierre Kory is considered by the BBC to have "an exaggerated influence" and Dr. Tess Lawrie is accused of making "unsubstantiated claims regarding the Covid vaccines adverse events." Perhaps the BBC is unaware that Covid vaccine adverse events (including deaths) have been recorded on databases such as VAERS[607] and the UK's Yellow Card[608] scheme, since their rollout.

The BBC article stated: "The BBC can reveal that more than a third of 26 major trials of the drug for use on Covid have serious errors or signs of potential fraud." Critics argue this reveals bias and lacks independently verified evidence, potentially amounting to unsubstantiated claims.

Both the BBC and *The Guardian* published articles assuming the Elgazzar study was fraudulent, based on the group's claims and the initial retraction.

## The TOGETHER Trial

As noted in the report, the TOGETHER trial was a randomized, placebo-controlled trial conducted in Brazil to evaluate treatments, including ivermectin, for early COVID-19 in high-risk outpatients. The ivermectin arm, published in the *New England Journal of Medicine*[609] in March 2022, involved 1,358 patients, with 679 receiving ivermectin (400 μg/kg daily for 3 days) and 679 receiving placebo.

The TOGETHER trial was supported by FastGrants and the Rainwater Charitable Foundation, an investment fund largely in Vanguard index funds. Vanguard holds significant shares in Pfizer. While these associations do not necessarily imply bias, that have been noted by critics.

Before the trial's publication, co-investigator Edward Mills presented its findings at an NIH symposium in August 2021, claiming ivermectin had "no effect whatsoever." On cue, global media outlets amplified the narrative of ivermectin's "failure," influencing public health policy. *The Los Angeles Times*[610] published a headline stating, "Major study of ivermectin, touted by anti-vaccine groups, finds 'no effect whatsoever' for COVID."

Dr. Pierre Kory, a vocal critic of the trial, posted on social media:[611] "I'm calling it. TOGETHER's IVM study is likely the most corrupt in history. Read all about the over 40 fraudulent actions taken in the design & conduct of this trial. Authors are now refusing to answer questions or share the patient-level data."

The polymath, Alexandros Marinos, was another who raised serious concerns. He wrote[612] a series of articles on his Substack, where he was "able to establish that the trial had underdosed its highest-risk ivermectin patients. It also suffered from randomization failure which- given the deadly gamma variant wave which was ongoing at exactly that time- quite likely helped the fluvoxamine arm at the expense of ivermectin." Marinos also cited several other flaws: unethical recruitment, non-independent DSMC, and data access delays that compromised the trial's validity.

Researchers, Dr. David Scheim, Dr. Edmund Fordham, and Professor Colleen Aldous in collaboration with the World Council for Health, wrote a letter[613] to the TOGETHER trial authors and the *New England Journal of Medicine* editor-in-chief, calling for the immediate release of the trial's data or retraction of the paper. They highlighted that the trial misdirected inquiries to a data repository (ICODA) that never hosted the data, calling it a "flagrant breach of scientific ethics." They also pointed to discrepancies in outcome measures, such as per-protocol death and hospitalization rates, which were not disclosed despite requests.

## The FDA's Smoking Gun

Turning to the FDA's infamous "You're not a horse" tweet, in my investigative report "FDA's Smoking Gun: Disinformation Campaign Targeting Ivermectin," published in *TrialSite News*,[614] in November 2021, I highlighted internal FDA communications that, in my view, suggested the agency led efforts to strongly deter off-label ivermectin use via its viral "You are not a horse" tweet and related messaging.

The email, secured via a FOIA request by journalist Linda Bonvie, involves members of the world's top regulatory body boasting about how well the "You're not a horse" tweet did with engagement.

**From:** Jefferson, Erica [redacted]
**Sent:** Sunday, August 22, 2021 11:35 AM
**To:** Woodcock, Janet [redacted]
**Cc:** Tierney, Julia [redacted]; Safford, Melissa [redacted]
Rebello, Heidi [redacted] Mulieri, Chris [redacted]
Kimberly, Brad [redacted]; Walsh, Sandy [redacted]
Felberbaum, Michael [redacted]
**Subject:** Sharing: FDA Ivermectin / COVID-19 Tweet Goes Viral

Hi Dr. Woodcock,

I hope you are having a great weekend. I know we are all eager for tomorrow.

Separately and as you know, the OEA team and I have been meeting over the past several weeks to discuss ways in which we can more effectively use our social media platforms to share important public health information with consumers. I'm sure you saw some of the news coming out of Mississippi on Friday regarding the use of ivermectin to treat / prevent Covid-19 and the increase in adverse events (poisonings) the state highlighted as a result of its use. I expressed to the team late Friday night that we take the opportunity to remind the public of our own warnings for ivermectin and by early Saturday morning the social media team had posted the following tweet:

Needless to say, the direct, straight-forward and clever (humorous) communication, paired with a follow-on tweet that provided additional answers to common questions about ivermectin, saw the tweet quickly going viral and being shared across multiple social medium platforms (where it was amplified by other influencers) and resulted in additional news coverage by: NYT, CNN, NBC News and Rolling Stone to name a few. Notably, the official Today Show Instagram account (3 million followers) also featured an original post on the account. We also took the opportunity to highlight a Consumer Update on ivermectin, that was prepared and distributed earlier this year. I'm pleased to report that as a result of the tweet, the update was accessed 177k times yesterday alone.

By comparison, the tweet currently ranks as our 2nd most popular tweet of all time in terms of the number of people we've reached with the content:

J&J Pause tweet - 20.4M
**Not a Horse tweet – 14.5M**
Immunocompromised EUA FB - 10.8M
J&J Pause tweet inside original thread - 6.8M
Pfizer4Kidz tweet - 4.5M

As you know, I am committed to identifying unique (for FDA) ways for us to reach the "everyday" American to "brand" FDA. I am grateful the OEA team is enthusiastically supportive of this goal and in particularly, I want to recognize Brad, Chris and Sandy, for mobilizing quickly Friday night and Saturday morning to create a unique viral moment at such a critical time for the FDA's image and in our fight against Covid-19. While we won't *always* be able to take this approach (we are still a government entity), we will seek to develop content that allows the agency to feel both accessible and informative in a time of incredible misinformation. We will be meeting with OCC soon to discuss our new recommended approach for social media engagement. We look forward to sharing more about these efforts in the weeks ahead, including an ambition effort to counter much of the vaccine information out there as we prepare to approve Comiraty.

Please let me know if you have any questions in the interim. Thanks for your support on our efforts to evolve FDA's communications with consumers.

Best,
Erica

**Erica V. Jefferson** (she/her)
Associate Commissioner for External Affairs
**U.S. Food and Drug Administration**
Tel: [redacted]

F

An excerpt from my investigative report reads:

Showcasing the agency's front and central role in promoting propaganda, the author, Erica Jefferson, an associate commissioner for the FDA's external affairs, boasts to Dr. Janet Woodcock, the FDA's acting commissioner, how the "Not a Horse Tweet" got 14.5 million tweets.

Jefferson expresses her excitement of the "FDA ivermectin/COVID-19 tweet" going viral. She writes, "needless to say the straightforward and clever (humorous) communication ..saw the tweet quickly going viral and being shared across multiple social medium platforms (where it was amplified by other influencers) and resulted in additional news coverage by: NYT, CNN, NBC News and Rolling Stone to name but a few."

Jefferson's reference to other influencers on social media amplifying the message and helping it go viral is very revealing, including the role of mainstream media. It can be said that this speaks to a larger network of entities involved in the disinformation campaign against ivermectin-like the Trusted News Initiative, a consortium of Big Tech (Twitter, Facebook, Microsoft) and Big Media set up to combat anti-vaccine "disinformation" and from what is becoming evidently clear, early-treatments for COVID-19, too.

The tweet posted by the FDA (see below) was published on August 21, 2021, with the email from Erickson to Woodstock, sent the following day. Copied in were many high-ranking FDA officials, such as Julia Tierney, acting chief of staff, Melissa Safford, senior advisor to the commissioner.

Yes, a version of ivermectin is used for veterinary purposes, but the massive increase in prescriptions that concerned the FDA was the human variety, prescribed by licensed physicians with consent from their patients. But the messaging was meant to confuse people to think that they were one and the same. Of course, those people that were involved with self-medication needed education, but what the FDA does here is try to kill two birds with one stone. The FDA doesn't go out of its way to educate but instead spread disinformation.

Jefferson reveals in her email that the Office of External Affairs (OEA) team had spent "the past several weeks" planning on how to effectively use their social media platforms "to share important public health information." She references the news coming out of Mississippi regarding the use of ivermectin to treat COVID-19 "and the increase in adverse events (poisonings)."

It seems the FDA seized the opportunity in the Mississippi State Department of Health's network alert[615] sent out on August 20 stating that "70% of the recent calls have been related to the ingestion of livestock formulations of ivermectin." This is confirmed in her email, as Jefferson writes, "I'm sure you saw some of the news coming out of Mississippi on Friday night [August 20]..I expressed to the team late Friday night that we take the opportunity to remind the public of our warnings for ivermectin.."

Strong concerns have been raised about the FDA's communications strategy regarding ivermectin and that the reported "poisonings" were based on inaccurate data.

Nonetheless, the mainstream media jumped on the poisonings' bandwagon, citing the Mississippi department of health data. *The Guardian* ran with the headline, "A human is not a horse. So why is a livestock drug sweeping America?" However, the department later clarified it was only 2% of recent calls to the center that have been about people ingesting ivermectin, and that 70% of those calls related to livestock or animal formulations.

The Rolling Stone, The New York Times, The Washington Post, the Associated Press, and *The Guardian*,[616] all had to print corrections regarding the false information.

It's worth noting that the journalist, Linda Bonvie, responsible for sourcing the FOIA-released FDA email, further investigated the 70 percent claim made by the Mississippi State Department of Health. Bonvie constructed a timeline[617] published by Citizens for Health, covering the two weeks in 2021, during which time the "You're not a horse" tweet was issued. Her investigation revealed that only about 11 inquiries (2% of calls) involved veterinary ivermectin. Despite a retraction, the false narrative persisted, amplified by outlets like The New York Times and NPR, and fueled further by the FDA and CDC, which misrepresented call volumes and risks.

• • •

On March 21, 2024 a settlement[618] was reached, leading to the U.S. Food and Drug Administration (FDA) agreeing to remove social media posts and webpages discouraging the use of ivermectin for treating COVID-19. Needless to say, the infamous "You are not a horse" campaign was one of them.

The landmark case was initiated by plaintiffs, Drs. Mary Talley Bowden, Robert I. Apter, and Paul E. Marik, who filed a lawsuit against the agency under the leadership of Commissioner Robert Califf, MD. The lawsuit was prompted by the FDA's dissemination of misleading information about ivermectin.

The following day, Dr. Bowden took to social media to post: "FDA loses its war on ivermectin and agrees to remove all social media posts and consumer directives regarding ivermectin and COVID, including its most popular tweet in FDA history. This landmark case sets an important precedent in limiting FDA overreach into the doctor-patient relationship."

An FDA spokesperson told *The Epoch Times* [619]that the agency "has chosen to resolve this lawsuit rather than continuing to litigate over statements that are between two and nearly four years old."

## IVM Doctors Under Fire

Just as prominent doctors advocating for hydroxychloroquine (HCQ) faced intense scrutiny, those promoting ivermectin (IVM) also endured significant professional and personal consequences.

Take for instance, Dr. Paul Marik, an eminent critical care physician and former professor at Eastern Virginia Medical School, who co-founded the Front-Line COVID-19 Critical Care Alliance (FLCCC) with Dr. Pierre Kory. In August 2023, the American Board of Internal Medicine (ABIM) revoked Marik's board certifications, citing his promotion of ivermectin and statements questioning the safety and efficacy of COVID-19 vaccines as conduct that "poses serious concerns for patient safety and undermines public trust" in medical certification. Earlier in 2021, Marik was forced to resign from his positions at Eastern Virginia Medical School and Sentara Norfolk General Hospital, reportedly due to his advocacy for ivermectin.

Like Marik, Dr. Pierre Kory's ABIM certifications were also revoked in August 2023 for spreading "misinformation." In May 2020, he resigned from the University of Wisconsin Hospital in May 2020, citing frustration with colleagues' reluctance to adopt his treatment protocols, including ivermectin and corticosteroids.

Dr. Mary Talley Bowden, an ENT specialist based in Houston, Texas, member of the FLCCC, and vocal advocate for ivermectin as a COVID-19 treatment, had her admitting privileges suspended by Houston Methodist Hospital in November 2021. The hospital stated she was spreading "dangerous misinformation"[620] on social media about COVID-19 treatments and criticism of vaccine mandates.

Dr. Shankara Chetty, a South African family doctor, treated over 14,000 COVID-19 patients using his early-intervention "8th day" protocol, which heavily featured off-label repurposed drugs including ivermectin and hydroxychloroquine. He reported a 100 percent success rate, with no hospitalizations, oxygen requirements, or deaths under his care.

Despite these claimed outcomes, in 2023 Professor Francois Venter filed a complaint[621] with the Health Professions Council of South Africa (HPCSA), accusing Chetty of "practicing pseudo-science" and "using unproven remedies." This led to formal charges of unprofessional conduct, including prescribing ivermectin and hydroxychloroquine, failing to act in patients' best interests, and mischaracterizing the disease and spike protein toxicity. Disciplinary hearings began in April 2024 but were deferred, with the substantive proceedings now scheduled for May 2026.

Dr. Jackie Stone, a family medicine physician in Harare, Zimbabwe, was a prominent advocate for ivermectin. She reported dramatic reductions in mortality following its use in her practice and claimed Zimbabwe saw a tenfold drop in COVID-19 deaths after the Medicines Control Authority of Zimbabwe (MCAZ) authorized ivermectin in January 2021.

In September 2022, Stone was found guilty on two of four charges by the Medical and Dental Practitioners Council of Zimbabwe (MDPCZ) for prescribing ivermectin and nanosilver, which were not aligned with official guidelines. She faced professional sanctions, including threats to her medical license, which she claimed were attempts to suppress ivermectin use. Stone described her disciplinary hearing as "persecution" to make an example of her and deter other doctors from prescribing ivermectin. She alleged that junior doctors feared sharing data due to threats from regulatory bodies. The proceedings were widely followed by ivermectin supporters globally, including the FLCCC.

On October 3, 2024, Stone reportedly died by suicide. Physician and writer, Dr. Meryl Nass, posted about Stone's death on the social media platform X: "Jackie Stone was one of the first doctors in southern Africa to treat COVID with ivermectin and teach others how to do so. She was hounded so badly she committed suicide yesterday."

CHAPTER ELEVEN

# RUSH TO MARKET

*"We are speeding up as much as possible,*
*but we also need to make sure that our scientific assessment*
*is as robust as possible. Let's not forget the responsibility/accountability*
*attached to the recommendation to the EC to grant a CMA."*

~Noel Wathion, EMA Deputy Executive Director,
Leaked Email, November 22, 2020

The "warp speed" development of the COVID-19 vaccines brought novel products to market at an unprecedented pace. While many praised the collaborative effort and regulatory flexibility that made it possible, others have raised serious questions about whether the accelerated Emergency Use Authorization processes placed greater emphasis on urgency than on comprehensive safety review.

In March 2021, *The BMJ*[622] obtained leaked internal European Medicines Agency (EMA) documents relating to the Pfizer-BioNTech vaccine review. These showed that reviewers identified significantly lower mRNA integrity in early commercial batches compared with those used in the clinical trials. The documents indicated that EMA assessors flagged this as a "major objection" and sought further explanation from the manufacturer regarding potential impacts on safety and efficacy.

*TrialSite News* was given access to the data leak in the form of internal EMA emails and confidential Pfizer documents from November 10–25, 2020 period. I analyzed them and wrote a two-part investigative report that examined how the EMA, FDA, MHRA, and Health Canada all scrambled to approve, amid serious warnings. It also highlights how the "red flags" in manufacturing were ultimately "resolved."

The following is an adapted version of my 2022 investigative series: "What the Leaked EMA Emails & Docs Reveal: Major Concerns with Pfizer C-19 Vaccine Batch Integrity and The Race to Authorize."[623]

## "The Rush into EUA"

The November 16, 2020, email from Marco Cavaleri, EMA's Head of Biological Health Threats and Vaccines Strategy at the time, reveals that the U.S. FDA was "going to rush into EUA."

Classified as internal/staff & contractors by the European Medicines Agency

Cavaleri Marco
Mon 11/16/2020 12:34 PM
Inbox
FDA has a call with MHRA in 3 hours to discuss Biontech CMC aspects. They are going to rush into EUA.
FDA still unclear and not so easy for them to be faster than Xmas, but pushed hard by Azar and US GOV
Marco

Classified as internal/staff & contractors by the European Medicines Agency

Cavaleri refers to this rush being "pushed hard by Azar and US GOV." Under the Trump administration, Alex Azar, former pharmaceutical executive, was the United States Secretary of Health and Human Services (HHS) from 2018-2021. The FDA is an agency that falls directly under the HHS.

It's worth noting that when Azar was former president of the pharmaceutical company Lilly USA LLC, a division of Eli Lilly, drug prices skyrocketed[624] under his leadership. The company was embroiled in a class-action lawsuit under his tenure, where it was accused of exploiting the drug pricing system to increase profits for its insulin drug.

Cavaleri's email speaks to the extent of how politics (and the U.S. government) was driving the FDA's regulatory process. And of course, on that note Trump's Operation Warp Speed[625] was to ensure all vaccine development records would be shattered.

However, across the Atlantic in Europe's regulatory agency tension mounted as the pressure to accelerate deadlines made the air and general mood tense. The pressure and anxiety were palpable in the reviewed email exchanges. Persons of high integrity and clarity as to their roles and commitments as stewards of public health emerged. For example, one individual demonstrated significant concern over accelerated timelines to ensure they would meet the "deadline" for vaccine authorization at the expense of a robust assessment. He was Noel Wathion, at the time the EMA's deputy executive director (who retired in June 2021 and died two years later).

In the leaked email from Wathion dated November 22, 2020, he importantly points out, "We are speeding up as much as possible, but we also need to make sure that our scientific assessment is as robust as possible. Let's not forget the responsibility/accountability attached to the recommendation to the EC to grant a CMA."

**From:** Wathion Noel
**Sent:** Sunday, 22 November 2020 17:19
**To:** SOLOMON Olga (SANTE) ; Boone Hilde ; Cavaleri Marco
**Cc:** RYS Andrzej Jan (SANTE) ; SCHMIDT Florian (SANTE) ; Cooke Emer
**Subject:** RE: Covid vaccines: information flow in the coming weeks

Dear Olga,

Of course we can discuss on Monday how to best provide updates to the EC on real time developments for these first vaccines. Let's see how to best achieve this.

Three comments I would like to make in addition:

- The likelihood that FDA (and also MHRA) will issue an EUA before a CMA is granted is extremely high. So we have to prepare for this. Certainly the lay public and the media will not understand the nuance...for them an "authorisation" is an authorisation. We have options to address this going from damage limitation to proactive expectation management. We have to choose which option is the best taking into account the exact circumstances.
- We are speeding up as much as possible but we also need to make sure that our scientific assessment is as robust as possible. Let's not forget the responsibility/ accountability attached to the recommendation to the EC to grant a CMA. And we need the (Co)-Rapps' and the CHMP's support for achieving this. Without them it will not happen.
- The fact that the company now suddenly wants to get a full MA instead of a CMA may even make things more challenging...

Kind regards,

Noel

Classified as confidential by the European Medicines Agency

Wathion assumed the FDA (and the MHRA's) EUA would be issued before the EMA granted its own CMA, which turned out to be correct. What's interesting is his concern to address the "damage limitation" resulting from the probable outcome of the EMA finishing last in this regulatory race and his fear that this would result in public opinion and the media turning against the agency. Speed seemingly superseded concerns of quality based on a careful review of these emails.

In an earlier email dated November 19, he reveals a "rather tense" TC (teleconference call) with the European Commissioner (Ursula von der Leyen) which was "at times even a bit unpleasant." This reflects the mounting pressure which the EMA staff were under to issue CMA quickly following an EUA granted by the FDA/MHRA for the Pfizer-BioNTech vaccine. Von der Leyen is implicated in potentially being responsible for this tense environment with "a delay of several weeks...not easily acceptable for the EC [European Commission]."

-----Original Message-----
From: Wathion Noel
Sent: Thursday, 19 November 2020 19:12
To: Cooke Emer; Sweeney Fergus; Nolte Alexis; Boone Hilde; Dias Monica; Cavaleri Marco
Subject: Some reflections after today's TC with the Commissioner

Dear all,

Since Alexis and Monica were no longer connected when we had our short discussion after today's TC with the Commissioner, a brief summary of what I already said together with some additional reflections.

As a minimum we can say that the TC was interesting, the atmosphere was rather tense, at times even a bit unpleasant, and provides a hint on what EMA may expect if the expectations are not being met, irrespective if such expectations are realistic or not.

The real added value of today's TC in my view is that we have more clarity now on what may not be easily acceptable for the EC, ie a delay of several weeks between an authorisation granted by the FDA/ MHRA (under whatever form) and a CMA opinion issued by EMA. The political fall-out seems to be too high, even if the "technical" level at the MSs (as it was referred to by the Commissioner) could defend such a delay in order to make the outcome of the scientific review as robust as possible.

Although we know that whatever we do (speeding up the process to align as much as possible with the "approval" timing by FDA/MHRA versus taking the time needed to have robust assurance in particular as regards CMC and safety) EMA will have a very big challenge addressing questions and criticism from various parties (EC, MSs at political level, EP, media, the general public) in case of a delay of several weeks.

Even if it can not be excluded now that at the end we are aligned with the FDA/MHRA (both in the outcome of the scientific review and the timing), the opposite certainly can not be excluded at this moment so we need to prepare for the worst case scenario. So how do we go from here? Are the current measures enough? In my view, probably not. We will be overwhelmed from all fronts and be in the middle of the storm. And on who's support will we be able to count? I hope it will not be a rethorical question...

What can we do on top, without creating the perception that we are interfering outside our "technical" mandate?
A non-exhaustive list:
1. Explaining the EMA process and what it will deliver:
- A public event is organised on 11/12: I think we need to critically review if we will achieve what is needed, taking into account the already brought forward date and the content related aspects.
- Making better use of social media tools as referred to by Emer today: we urgently need a dedicated strategy. However the resources in Comms are so stretched already that they have at this moment enormous difficulties to cope with the high influx of (media) queries. Reaching out to a specialist company to help out?
2. Explaining the differences between US/U.K. EUA and CMA: although the general public and the media will not (necessarily) understand the nuances between the 2 concepts we have to finalise this exercise which is currently ongoing ASAP, and then, more importantly, decide how to make best use of it. CMC, responsibility and accountability are certainly elements to be considered in my view.
3. Making the CMA process adapted as much as possible to the current pandemic situation: this exercise is ongoing but (1) the time gained may be limited and (2) any changes may be too late for the Pfizer/BioNTech vaccine. Nevertheless I think we should finalise ASAP if only to demonstrate that we did our utmost.

I hope these reflections can contribute to coming to a decision how to best address the important challenges ahead.

KR,

Noel

In early 2022, *TrialSite News*[626] reported how von der Leyen was embroiled in scandal, when a group of independent MEPs demanded her immediate resignation and full disclosure of a series of private text messages between her and Pfizer's CEO, Albert Bourla. Only a small portion of these texts were ever disclosed. Of the ones that were, they revealed her negotiating portions of a European-wide vaccine deal, (1.8 billion doses of the Pfizer-BioNTech COVID-19 vaccine, valued at approximately €35 billion), unilaterally with Bourla via a series of texts.

Turning back to the email, Wathion lays bare his reflections after this particular TC, and shockingly writes how "the political fall-out seems to be too high even if the 'technical' level at the MSs [Member States] could defend such a delay in order to make the outcome of the scientific review as robust as possible."

In addition, Wathion points out that a potential delay of several weeks to secure "robust assurance in particular as regards CMC and safety" will be met with "criticism from various parties," including media, EC (European Commission) and EP (European Parliament). Wathion speaks of his fear that if the deadline "to align as much as possible with the 'approval' timing by FDA/MHRA" cannot be met- "we will be overwhelmed from all fronts and be in the middle of the storm." However, this potential delay appeared to be necessary "in order to make the outcome of the scientific review as robust as possible." This implies that speed at the expense of safety was the order of the day to avoid "political fallout." Politics, appeared to be dictating COVID-19 vaccine authorization protocol, not science.

In the following email from Marco, the EMA official reveals that Pfizer's CEO Albert Bourla "lobbied" Peter Marks. This could be interpreted as highly controversial, given Marks is the director of the Center for Biologics Evaluation and Research (CBER) at the FDA. Pfizer's apparent access into the federal watchdog raises significant questions at the least, if not introduces the possibility for disturbing entanglements between industry and a purportedly independent, scientific federal agency.

> Few highly confidential news after talking with FDA:
>
> Pfizer:
> - they need to sort out CMC aspects which will require a bit of time.
> -They are in negotiation with Pfizer to postpone submission for EUA until end of NOV (planned NOV 21).
> -Mature efficacy data will be ready likely beg of DEC (earlier than expected)
> -FDA may target an AC 18 DEC for issuing EUA before end of the year
> - we agreed to keep channels open and share views so to avoid misleading messages going through (Pfizer CEO lobbied Peter Marks telling him EMA wants the data earlier!!)
> -we may discuss together with FDA (and HC) the CMC package once ready
> - we concurred that a conclusion roughly at the same time, if at all possible, would be fantastic
>
> Moderna:
> -they plan to submit EUA application end of NOV and could follow a similar pattern or even faster as CMC seems to more straight forward
> -for us this may take a bit longer but colleagues are pushing hard to compress review timeframe
>
> Can tell you more at tomorrow's SG
>
> Marco

## Major Batch Integrity Concerns

An email from Cavaleri reveals at that time the FDA knew of "some issues" associated with the CMC which needed to be sorted out and may "end up being the difficult bit." CMC refers to the Chemistry, Manufacturing and Controls, which covers various procedures used to assess and ensure the safety and consistency between pharmaceutical product batches.

> Cavaleri Marco
>
> Tue 10/11/2020 14:00
>
> Deleted Items
>
> Thanks Irene
>
> I just learned from FDA that there are some issues on CMC to be sorted out so I guess that if we can try to catch up would be good. I fear CMC will end up being the difficult bit
>
> FDA may conclude on EUA by Xmas (not earlier); any chances we can issue CMA at the same time?
>
> Marco
>
> Classified as internal/staff & contractors by the European Medicines Agency

An email from Evdokia Korakianiti (an EMA scientific administrator) explains in more detail what these "issues" were and how they were in fact major concerns to do with the Pfizer- BioNTech vaccine.

> Korakıanıtı Evdokia
> Mon 23/11/2020 10:38
> Inbox
>
> Dear Colleagues,
>
> This email is for awareness and to flag an important comparability issue with the BioNTech vaccine that needs to be addressed prior to approval.
>
> **Issue:** A significant difference in %RNA integrity / truncated species has been observed between the clinical batches ( ~ 78% mRNA integrity) based on which the Interim analysis was performed and the proposed commercial batches (~ 55%).
>
> The company claims that the efficacy of the drug product is dependent on the expression of the delivered RNA, which requires a **sufficiently intact RNA molecule.** The root cause for for the lower %RNA integrity at commercial batches has not yet been identified
>
> **Impact:** The potential implications of this RNA integrity loss in commercial batches compared to clinical ones in terms of both safety and efficacy are yet to be defined. Whether or not the observed comparability issues could be a blocking point will depend on the relevance of these observations to safety and efficacy and the company will be requested to fully justify the lower %RNA integrity (and other differences noted).
>
> Point for discussion will be whether the comparability issues can be solved only by Quality data (additional functional/ in vitro biological data + available non-clinical) or that further clinical data (bridging studies are/will be performed) will be needed. It is difficult to make any projections on this.
>
> **Way forward:** This issue and other MO ( but in our view not blocking to a potential approval) have been raised at ETF and are being discussed at BWP this week and in a TC with FDA on Wednesday
>
> With many thanks to Ton who's is the Quality specialist for this vaccine together with Brian looking after the chemical elements
>
> Best regards
>
> *Evdokia*

Alarmingly, significant differences in the levels of mRNA integrity between Pfizer-BioNTech's commercial (large scale) and clinical vaccine batches (small scale) were observed. "~78% mRNA integrity" in the clinical ones and "~ 55% in the proposed commercial batches" with the "root cause" not yet identified. Safety and efficacy implications due to this concern were also noted in the email "as yet to be defined."

In a confidential Pfizer report, which was also leaked along with the EMA emails, the company states that according to Acuitas Therapeutics' (the biotech company who developed the lipid nanoparticle platform for the Pfizer vaccine) own general experience, "a minimum threshold is approximately 70%." (See screenshot below)

> RNA molecules that are not fully encapsulated and protected by the LNP are considered inactive, as they are exposed to nucleases and further degradation after administration. RNA must be sufficiently intact to be successfully translated to the target protein, hence a minimum level of encapsulation efficiency needs to be achieved for a candidate RNA-LNP system. This minimum threshold is approximately 70% based on Acuitas Therapeutics general experience.

Then on page 30 it states: "The efficacy of the product is dependent on expression of the delivered RNA, which requires a sufficiently intact RNA molecule."

**3.2.P.2.2.3.4.1. RNA Integrity**

The RNA integrity of BNT162b2 drug product samples is assessed using a capillary gel electrophoresis-based (CGE) method, also called the Fragment Analyzer (FA) method, to separate components based on the differential migration of RNA of different molecular size in an applied electric field. In contrast to drug substance sample analysis, RNA from drug product is analyzed following disruption of the LNP in detergent and ethanol. Under fully denaturing conditions, the RNA is expected to unfold and migrate through the gel matrix, as a function of length and size, toward the anode. An intercalating dye binds to RNA and associated fragments during migration allowing for fluorescence detection. All other peaks that migrate prior to or after the main peak are integrated separately and will lower the overall RNA integrity percent, ie. intact RNA. The efficacy of the product is dependent on expression of the delivered RNA, which requires a sufficiently intact RNA molecule.

PFIZER CONFIDENTIAL
Page 30

This exact phrase "requires a sufficiently intact RNA molecule" was used in the email from EMA staffer, Evdokia Korakianiti, which I included above, sent on November 23, 2020- now we likely know where Korakianiti referenced it from.

For the commercial batches (which were going to be rolled out across the globe) to have such a significantly lower level of mRNA integrity (intact RNA molecule) is concerning given its intrinsic tie to the efficacy and potential safety of the product.

The next day Veronika Jekerle, Head of Pharmacy Quality Office, writes to Evdokia.

**From:** Jekerle Veronika [redacted]
**Sent:** 24 November 2020 12:02
**To:** Korakianiti Evdokia [redacted]
**Cc:** Facchini Claudio [redacted]; Moseley Jane [redacted]; van der Stappen Ton [redacted]; Dooley Brian [redacted] Rager Irene [redacted] Seguin Vanessa [redacted]
**Subject:** update from BWP meeting on BioNTech

Dear Evdokia,

The BWP has just discussed the BioNTech BWP and below you will find the main conclusions:

The Dossier is generally of good quality considering the speed in development and compilation.

- 3 major objections are agreed:

- **MO1**: GMP distant assessments for US manufacturing sites (Note: Distance assessment on the Wyeth, Andover site (DS, QC DS, QC DP) and on the Pfizer, Chesterfield site (QC DS, QC DP) are ongoing → interim reports expected 11 Dec 2020, MO reworded to allow statement of GMP)
- **MO2**: Differences in the level of mRNA integrity; comparability between clinical and commercial material, DS and DP is questioned (Note: root cause analysis ongoing an 2 additional PPQ batches manufactured with a slightly adjusted process – waiting for results, if RNA integrity is improved back to initial levels this could be accepted / characterisation data requested to understand protein variability from mRNA fragments → potential impact on safety).
- **MO3**: Pending PPQ batches for DP: comparability, process validation and stability (Note: as above: 2 PPQ batches manufactured and currently undergoing testing).
- Note that full information on two novel excipients (lipid in the nanoparticles) is not yet provided. This data is expected in the next CMC wave.

**Conclusions:** a number of major concerns remain that impact the benefit/risk of the vaccine (efficacy/safety) most notably the comparability issue around % mRNA integrity. These concerns are shared by most member states. **An approval by the end of the year could potentially be possible, if these concerns + GMP will be resolved.** Any remaining Quality issues will need to be considered in the context of overall B/R (& could potentially be addressed via specific obligations/Annex II conditions/recommendations).

The BWP report reflecting these conclusions is undergoing written adoption today.

With thanks to Ton, Brian and Claudio,

Kind regards,

Veronika

Veronika Jekerle, PhD
Head of Pharmaceutical Quality Office
Quality and Safety of Medicines

The difference in the level of mRNA integrity was again noted as a major concern "shared by most member states" and its "potential impact on safety." Jekerle highlights in bold, "An approval by the end of the year could potentially be possible, if these concerns + GMP will be resolved."

This gives rise to the critical question: how were all these concerns resolved when CMA was granted only a few weeks later, on December 21? A possible way it was resolved is explained later in this report.

In contrast to the concerns of some of the other EMA officials, Marco Cavaleri writes around the same time in the following email (see below) that the mRNA content is not a major concern, according to the FDA- "the issue on the mRNA content not perceived as major." He also shockingly states, "unclear if GCP inspections ever done." This revelation is concerning given that GCP refers to Good Clinical Practice, which is "an international ethical and scientific quality standard for designing, conducting, recording and reporting trials that involve the participation of human subjects."

What's even more alarming is his following statement: "no major interest from FDA." This reveals the regulatory agency's lack of interest on whether GCP inspections were completed, in the context of Pfizer's clinical trials, which was relied on by the FDA to grant EUA for the Pfizer-BioNTech vaccine. It should be noted that historically, the FDA has inspected less than one percent[627] of all US clinical trial sites.

Cavaleri Marco

Mon 23/11/2020 16:14

Deleted Items

An update from FDA:

Pfizer/Biontech:

Advisory committee on 10 December and opinion for EUA likely one week later.

CMC issues would affect authorisation but not EUA. In any case, the issue on the mRNA content not perceived as major. Gaps are around comparability and process validation for drug substance.

For EUA, commercial lots will be used but maybe also clinical lots (to be confirmed)

Unclear if GCP inspections ever done (TBC), but no major interest from FDA

Moderna:

Advisory committee on 17 December for an EUA opinion by end of the year.

CMC seems more streamlined. Interim clinical report awaited

AZ:

FDA very sceptical on data from the ongoing studies outside US and data are indeed quite puzzling as released today. They are not encouraging any submission for EUA at this stage

We may go first on this one, but it would still take a bit longer even in the best case scenario

Marco

Classified as internal/recipients only by the European Medicines Agency

Further troubling information is revealed (see following screenshot) when multiple regulatory agencies: Health Canada (HC), EMA, MHRA and FDA are all aware of the issue with percentage mRNA integrity, yet FDA and Health Canada make an unsubstantiated claim that "safety concerns associated. Are more of a theoretical concern."

**From:** Jekerle Veronika <
**Sent:** 25 November 2020 16:28
**To:** Korakianit Evdokia <; Prilla Stefanie<
Nolte Alexis
**Subject:** RE: Ad-hoc MLT minutes for comment by 16:30 today

Dear Evdokia,

Please see the additional points resulting from the TC with FDA we just had:

FDA shared with us the following information:

- FDA have received 7 commercial DS and 6 additional DP lots (2 additional GMP lots which EU hasn't received yet). The latest lots indicate that %intact RNA are back at around 70 – 75%, which leaves us cautiously optimistic that additional data could address the issue

- FDA and Health Canada indicated that the safety concerns associated with variable species of mRNA/protein are more of a theoretical concern as 5' caped intact species appear to stay comparable (which equates to fully functional mRNA)

- FDA/HC/EMA agreed that alignment on specifications % mRNA integrity are key in order to avoid that one regions gets all the suboptimal material (in particular a concern by Health Canada), specifications should be clinically qualified

- FDA mentioned an amendment of the CT protocol to compare immunogenicity of process 1 and 2 material; however unclear whether patients have received these doses yet; this info would be valuable to bring clinical bridge in the range of the specs for % of mRNA integrity; very likely to not be available though before end of the year

- FDA indicated that for a full BLA they would require 3 PPQ lots each for DP and DS

- Applicant has shared with FDA and us/MHRA only today an issue with visible particles in the DP (appears to be lipid nanoparticle components). FDA has posed questions to applicant, we will also FU on this issue.

Kind regards,

Veronika

Health Canada then appears to contradict itself because it is later described as showing particular concern about one region receiving "all the suboptimal material." Obviously, it did not want to be that region.

The end of the email shockingly reveals: "Applicant [Pfizer] has shared with FDA and us [EMA]/MHRA only today and issue with visible particles in the DP [drug product] appears to be lipid nanoparticle components.)" This is highly concerning due to this significant issue being made known to the three key regulatory agencies on November 25, only a few weeks away before the EMA granted CMA and the FDA granted EUA for the Pfizer vaccine, and just days before the MHRA granted authorization in the UK on December 2, 2020.

Veronika's assumption that the "visible particles" could be LNPs (lipid nanoparticles) is hard to accept given nanoparticles are not visible to the naked eye. So what were these visible particles?

## How % mRNA Integrity was Apparently Resolved

The discrepancy between batches appears to have been resolved when it is mentioned that the "latest lots [received by the FDA] indicate the % intact RNA are back around 70-75%." However, a leaked report of a meeting with Pfizer and the EMA on November 26, 2020, a day after Veronika's email, reveals that the RNA integrity specification was revised down to >=50% for drug product shelf life, significantly lower than the minimum threshold of 70% that Acuitas Therapeutics had stipulated and the average 78% of the clinical batches. Was this the EMA's (and potentially FDA/MHRA/HC) way of "resolving" the issue to ensure "an approval by the end of the year"?

**Major Objection #2 (Comparability)**

2. Comparability between clinical and commercial material has not yet been demonstrated, which raises uncertainties about consistency of product quality and hence uncertainties as regards product safety and efficacy of the commercial product. Significant differences between batches manufactured by DS Process 1 and 2 are observed for the CQA mRNA integrity. In addition, the characterisation of BNT162b2 DS is currently not found acceptable in relation to this quality attribute. This is especially important considering that the current DS and DP acceptance criteria allows for up to 50% fragmented species. Therefore, the dossier should be updated with additional characterisation data on mRNA integrity in sections 3.2.S.2.6 (comparability) and 3.2.S.3 of the dossier.

***Response***:
A comprehensive drug substance comparability study was performed and summarized in roll #2 of the MAA, which includes updated data in 3.2.S.2.6. In addition, we are revising the RNA integrity specification for drug substance to >=60%, drug product release to >=55%, and drug product shelf life to >=50%. The sponsor agrees to update the 3.2.S.3 section with additional characterization data concurrent with the establishment of primary/working reference material.

Confidential

Mention is made of "uncertainties about consistency of product quality and hence uncertainty as regards product safety and efficacy of the commercial product." However, it is baffling how lowering the RNA integrity specification would remedy that major objection.

Another slide states, "Truncated [shortened] and modified RNA species should be regarded as product- related impurities." This confirms that these shortened mRNA species, which lowered the level of %mRNA integrity, were classed as impurities. A further serious concern arising from these impurities is flagged "the possibility of translated proteins other than intended spike protein (S1 S2) resulting from truncated and/or modified mRNA species should be addressed." (See following screenshot)

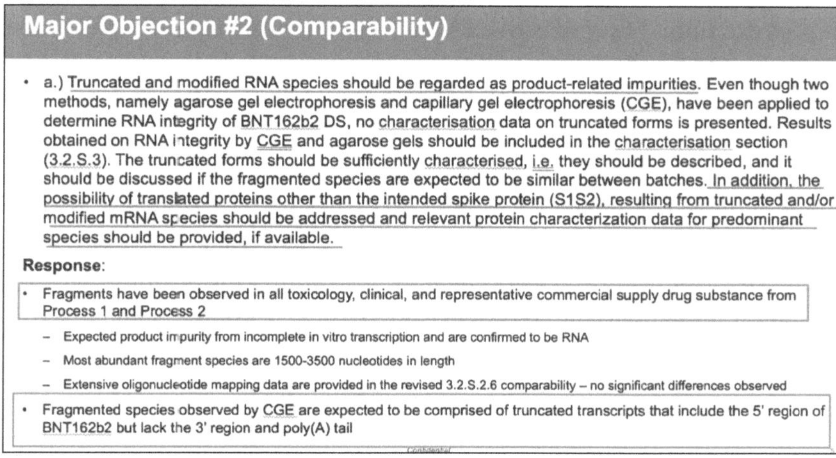

**Major Objection #2 (Comparability)**

- a.) Truncated and modified RNA species should be regarded as product-related impurities. Even though two methods, namely agarose gel electrophoresis and capillary gel electrophoresis (CGE), have been applied to determine RNA integrity of BNT162b2 DS, no characterisation data on truncated forms is presented. Results obtained on RNA integrity by CGE and agarose gels should be included in the characterisation section (3.2.S.3). The truncated forms should be sufficiently characterised, i.e. they should be described, and it should be discussed if the fragmented species are expected to be similar between batches. In addition, the possibility of translated proteins other than the intended spike protein (S1S2), resulting from truncated and/or modified mRNA species should be addressed and relevant protein characterization data for predominant species should be provided, if available.

**Response**:

- Fragments have been observed in all toxicology, clinical, and representative commercial supply drug substance from Process 1 and Process 2
  - Expected product impurity from incomplete in vitro transcription and are confirmed to be RNA
  - Most abundant fragment species are 1500-3500 nucleotides in length
  - Extensive oligonucleotide mapping data are provided in the revised 3.2.S.2.6 comparability – no significant differences observed
- Fragmented species observed by CGE are expected to be comprised of truncated transcripts that include the 5' region of BNT162b2 but lack the 3' region and poly(A) tail

The leaked documents indicate that regulatory bodies, including the FDA, MHRA, EMA and Health Canada were aware of differences in mRNA integrity between clinical trial batches and early commercial batches and because of that the effect on "safety and efficacy" was unknown. The leaked Pfizer/EMA meeting reports highlight concerns that were documented during the assessment process, including questions about whether adjustments to RNA integrity specifications fully addressed the observed differences.

One resource that has attracted attention for examining batch-to-batch variations in COVID-19 vaccines in reported adverse events following vaccination is howbadismybatch.com.[628] This site aggregates publicly available VAERS data, allowing users to input batch codes and view associated reports of deaths, disabilities, and illnesses. It could be suggested that controversies surrounding mRNA integrity and other Chemistry, Manufacturing and Control (CMC) issues, could explain the elevated adverse event rates observed in specific batches.

• • •

The following is an adaptation of the final instalment on the leaked EMA emails and other confidential documents investigation, published in *TrialSite News*[629] on October 5, 2022. It explores further leaked internal emails highlighting European Commissioner, Ursula von der Leyen's efforts to steer member states (MSs) away from using Article 5 (2), their national Emergency Use Authorization for the COVID-19 vaccines, in favor of an EU-wide Conditional Marketing Authorization (CMA). The report examines other sensitive EMA documents including the November 24, 2020, Quality Office Chemistry, Manufacturing, and Controls (CMC) presentation by the Biologics Working Party (BWP) and Rapporteur's Rolling Review assessment report, which provide further evidence supporting the "major objections" raised in the original investigation. Additionally, it analyses unredacted Pfizer vaccine contracts and the European Commission's Advance Purchase Agreement signed in November 2020 with Pfizer and BioNTech "for the development, production, priority-purchasing options and supply of a successful COVID-19 vaccine for EU Member States."

## No Stranger to Scandal

Ursula von der Leyen has been under intense public scrutiny over her private negotiations of a multi-billion-euro vaccine deal (the EU's biggest contract) via secret texts and phone calls[630] made with Pfizer's CEO, Albert Bourla, contravening the Commission decision for a steering board to "provide guidance throughout the evaluation process." Furthermore, she refused to grant public access to the secretive text messages exchanged between Bourla and herself, when called to do so. A European Court of Auditors published an alarming report,[631] which stated "we asked the Commission to provide us with information on the preliminary negotiations for this agreement (scientific experts consulted and advice received, timing of the talks, records of the discussions, and details of the agreed terms and conditions). However, none was forthcoming."

The fire has also been heating up for Pfizer's Bourla, when he was called to testify before the European Parliament's Special Committee on COVID-19 to face questions over those secretive vaccine deals but last minute pulled out[632] from facing the committee.

## More Leaked Emails

Below is an email from Hilde Boone of the EMA, stating that "she [von der Leyen] will be prepared to call relevant health ministers personally to avoid the use of Art 5(2)."

**From:** Boone Hilde [redacted]>
**Sent:** Thursday, November 12, 2020 3:57 PM
**To:** SOLOMON Olga (SANTE) <[redacted]; SCHMIDT Florian (SANTE) [redacted]
**Cc:** GIRARD Thomas (EMA) <[redacted]>; CAVALERI Marco (EMA) <[redacted]; WATHION Noel (EMA) <[redacted]>
**Subject:** Art 5(2) vs CMA

Dear Olga & Florian

Just a heads-up: we just finished the TC between the Commissioner and ECDC/EMA in which the Commissioner asked questions about the expected approval of the Pfizer vaccine, and timing of FDA vs EU approval. So, automatically the issue of national Art 5(2) vs CMA came up, which Noel explained in detail and also how we plan to further discuss it with the NCAs next week and in HMA. Guido also suggested to consider raising it with the Health Ministers at EPSCO.

Sandra and Giorgios said that they would further discuss also within SANTE, so, hence my email to you.

(Andrzej was also present)

Also of note:
The Commissioner said that, since EC made a commitment to the MSs and EP that the vaccines will be available to all MSs at the same time – and that therefore it will be important that MSs will not be 'forced' to use that national route due to "delays" in the formal approval procedure.

She also said that she will be prepared to call relevant health ministers personally to avoid the use of Art 5(2).

Best regards,
Hilde

## Article 5 (2) vs CMA

Article 5 (2) of Directive 2001/83 states "Member States may temporarily authorize the distribution of an unauthorized medicinal product in response to the suspected or confirmed spread of pathogenic agents, toxins, chemical agents or nuclear radiation any of which could cause harm." In other words, it's the equivalent of an Emergency Use Authorization at the member state level. It can be done very quickly because the medicinal product doesn't need to go through the standard national authorization process.

An expert on EU law explained to *TrialSite News* the downside of member states using Art. 5 (2). It would have given rise to competition amongst member states, leading to an inequitable access/distribution of the COVID-19 vaccines, particularly for those MSs who preferred to wait for the EU's CMA, which takes longer since it is supposed to follow a controlled and robust framework providing safeguards. An EU CMA helped ensure that the vaccines would have been available to all member states, at the same time, which was one of the objectives of the EU COVID-19 strategy.

However, could there have also been other reasons why von der Leyen was desperate for the MSs to avoid Art 5 (2) by her being "prepared to call health ministers personally"?

In the email below from Noel Wathion, he states "since the 1st option still is to aim for a CMA rather than an Art 5 (2) coupled or not with an Art 5 (3).."

**Fra:** Wathion Noel <[redacted]>
**Sendt:** 20. november 2020 10:16
**Til:** Thomas Senderovitz [redacted]
**Cc:** Cooke Emer <[redacted]>
**Emne:** RE: von der Leyden statements

Dear Thomas,

I cc Emer in my response.
As such not that much has changed since she clearly states "if everything goes well". And yes, this is aligned with EMA and the statements we have made in several interviews since the moment the interim analysis results for the Pfizer/ BioNTech vaccine (confirmed this week by the final analysis results) and the interim analysis results for the 2nd mRNA vaccine for Moderna have been made public.
What is new in my view is that she clearly identifies the 2 vaccines that could be approved before the end of the year. There are still issues with both (CMC seems to be a concern for the Pfizer/ BioNTech, and the rolling review for Moderna just started giving less time to review) so its needs to be seen if all this can be sorted out on time, whilst not compromising the robustness of the review.
Acknowledging that the legal tools in the US versus the EU are different, and since the 1st option still is to aim for a CMA rather than an art 5(2) coupled or not with an Art 5(3), we are trying to make the CMA process as adapted as possible to the pandemic situation since so far it was primarily used for oncology medicines. The discussion at the EU Exe SG on Wednesday was very useful and we are speeding up this work.
This brings me to the next point, i.e. how to best ensure continuation of the alignment within the Network; we have now the following meetings scheduled over the next weeks to discuss COVID-19:

- HMA on Thursday: 10 minutes update by EMA and a specific topic on clinical trials if I am not mistaken, to be presented by PEI.
- EU Exe SG the week after next, where the point on making the CMA process as efficient as possible is again on the agenda.
- MB on 16-17/12.

As a point for reflection, since we are dealing with an extraordinary situation of utmost importance for the Network and its credibility, to be addressed over the next 6 weeks (we will be in the hotspot for the 1st vaccines, the pressure should be much less certainly with this level of efficacy and on condition that there are no major quality and safety issues), shouldn't we organize an urgent ad-hoc meeting HMA, EMA, EC (for some 3 hours) to have a more in-depth discussion on all bottlenecks for speeding-up the CMA process and also to align ourselves on the communication for the different scenarios (earlier approval by FDA/ MHRA, similar timelines, balance speed versus robustness)? Or alternatively to extend the HMA meeting next Thursday, or the EU Exe SG the week thereafter? But I wouldn't wait much longer than Wednesday next week.
Looking forward to your feedback.
KR,

Noel

Article 5(3) states: "Member States shall lay down provisions in order to ensure that marketing authorization holders, manufacturers and health professionals are not subject to civil or administrative liability for any consequences resulting from the use of a medicinal product."

The fact that Wathion points out that an Art. 5 (2) can be "coupled or not with an Art. 5 (3)," raises the important question whether member states would have had the option to not give indemnity to the marketing authorization holders (in this case BioNTech) and manufacturers (BioNTech and Pfizer).

## The Predatory Pfizer Contracts and Advance Purchase Agreements

According to the non-profit consumer advocacy organization Public Citizen's[633] analysis of leaked contracts, Pfizer has seemingly "bullied" countries into silence; can go after sovereign state assets (under the waiver of sovereign immunity); made the "Purchaser grant on Pfizer's[634] behalf all exemptions and waivers of country specific requirements for the Product or permitted by the Government authority (including but not limited to serialization, applicable laboratory or quality testing..)" and enjoy full indemnity- exemption from legal liability that may result from their product. In fact, it is the Purchaser who is made liable on their behalf. This means governments have had to pay compensation to citizens who have suffered from vaccine adverse events, not the vaccine manufacturers.

Pfizer and supporters have described these terms as necessary risk protections for rapid emergency development and distribution during the pandemic.

The screenshot below is taken from the unredacted version of the advance purchase agreement (APA) between the European Commission (EC), acting on behalf and in the name of member states, Pfizer Inc. and BioNTech (collectively "the Contractor") signed in November 2020 (around the same time the leaked EMA emails were generated). It states, "each Participating Member State shall indemnify and hold harmless the Contractor, their Affiliates. From and against any and all liabilities incurred…relating to harm, damages and losses….arising from or relating to the use and deployment of the Vaccines.."

> **I.12 INDEMNIFICATION**
>
> I.12.1 The Commission, on behalf of the Participating Member States, declares that the use of Vaccines produced under this APA will happen under epidemic conditions requiring such use, and that the administration of Vaccines will therefore be conducted under the sole responsibility of the Participating Member States. Hence, each Participating Member State shall indemnify and hold harmless the Contractor, their Affiliates, sub-contractors, licensors and sub-licensees, and officers, directors, employees and other agents and representatives of each (together, the **"Indemnified Persons"**) from and against any and all liabilities incurred, settlements as per Article I.12.6, and reasonable direct external legal costs incurred in the defence of Third Party Claims (including reasonable attorney's fees and other expenses) relating to harm, damages and losses as defined in Article I.12.2 (together, the **"Losses"**) arising from or relating to the use and deployment of the Vaccines in the jurisdiction of the Participating Member State in question. This Article I.12 applies to Losses which arise from or relate to the Vaccines

However, information posted on the EC's website[635] states that under an EU Conditional Marketing Authorization (CMA), "liability is with the holder of the marketing authorization" (which in this case is BioNTech). This directly conflicts with the APA that the EC signed with Pfizer and BioNTech (for 200 million vaccine doses priced at 15.50 Euros per dose excl.VAT), a month before CMA was granted. It is noteworthy that the EC published a heavily redacted version[636] of the identical APA, any section related to indemnity/liability or simply considered "sensitive" has been censored.

Another important point to consider when it comes to Art 5 (2) vs an EU CMA, is that given some European countries mandated the vaccine for adults, at-risk age groups and certain job sectors, it is highly unlikely those MSs would have been able to do that with an unauthorized medicinal product, which these vaccines would have been classified under Art 5 (2).

## The Chemistry, Manufacturing and Controls Issues

Returning to Noel Wathion's November 20, 2020, email, which raises several concerning points: "there are still issues with both (CMC seems to be a concern for the Pfizer/BioNTech and the rolling review for Moderna just started giving less time to review) so it needs to be seen if all this can be sorted out on time, whilst not compromising the robustness of the review."

The original TrialSite News report discussed what those CMC (Chemistry, Manufacturing and Controls) issues were with Pfizer/BioNTech, particularly the loss of RNA integrity in the commercial batches and the unknown visible particles observed.

Wathion tellingly states, "there are still issues" implies that these were not solved but still ongoing. His concern of "compromising the robustness of the review" because of the need to authorize on time is emphasized, as well as the worry of speed over safety.

It is particularly noteworthy that on the same day that Wathion outlined his concerns, copying in Emer Cooke, head of the EMA, to his email- the first advance purchase agreement was signed between Pfizer, BioNTech and the EC.

The report also contained a leaked email from Veronika Jekerle, EMA's Head of Pharmaceutical Quality Office, where she outlined the three agreed major objections and the conclusion of the BWP (Biologics Working Party) regarding the Pfizer-BioNTech vaccine. Her email was sent on November 24th the same day as the BWP presentation. Below, are a series of screenshots of the actual leaked BWP power point presentation (which Jekerle references in her email), entitled "EMA Quality Office CMC Observations." At the end of her email she thanks, "Ton, Brian and Claudio." Ton van der Stappen and Brian Dooley are named in the following screenshot of the slide..

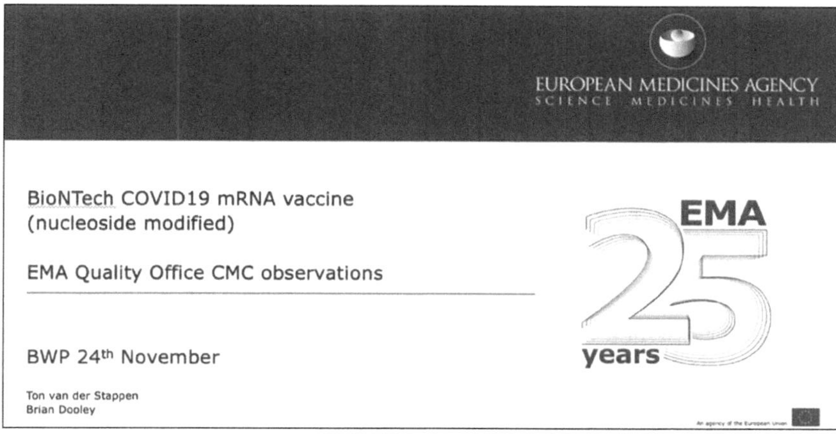


The screenshot below presents wide-ranging data, which backs up one of the major EMA objections in reference to the significant drop in %RNA integrity between the clinical and commercial batches. It's noteworthy that batches from Pfizer's Andover, USA (~62%) and Puurs, Belgium (~55%) sites were reported as having significantly lower %RNA integrity than batches provided by BNT (BioNTech) and Polymun.

**Overall Batch Analyses %RNA integrity**

| Company | Drug Substance batch number | %RNA integrity | Mean %RNA integrity | Drug Product batch number | %RNA integrity | Company | Mean %RNA integrity |
|---|---|---|---|---|---|---|---|
| | ? | | | COVVAC/270320 69 | 69 | | |
| | R427-P020.2-DS | 77 | | BCV40420-A | 75 | | |
| | R438-P020.2-DS | 80 | | BCV40620-A | 85 | | |
| | R438-P020.2-DS | 80 | | BCV40620-B | 86 | | |
| | R438-P020.2-DS | 80 | | BCV40620-C | 83 | | |
| | R438-P020.2-DS | 80 | | BCV40620-D | 77 | Polymun | 78 |
| BNT | R438-P020.2-DS | 80 | 81 | BCV40620-E | 85 | | |
| | R443-P020.2-DS | 81 | | BCV40720-A | 71 | | |
| | R443-P020.2-DS | 81 | | BCV40720-B | 72 | | |
| | R443-P020.2-DS | 81 | | BCV40720-C | 69 | | |
| | R443-P020.2-DS | 81 | | ED3938 | 62 | Pfizer, Puurs (S2S2) | 63 |
| | R445-P020.2-DS | 86 | | EE3813 | 63 | | |
| Pfizer, Andover | 20Y513C101 | 62 | 62 | EE8492 | 55 | Pfizer, Puurs (WSLS) | 55 |
| | 20Y513C101 | 62 | | EE8493 | 55 | | |

The screenshot below is taken from the unredacted APA signed by the EC. It specifies that the majority of Europe's vaccine supply will "come from Pfizer's manufacturing site in Puurs, Belgium." This is concerning given the data shows that the %RNA integrity of batches from that site were the lowest at 55%, compared to other sites.

**I.6.3 Supply mechanism**

Vaccine supply in Europe will primarily come from Pfizer's manufacturing site in Puurs, Belgium and shall incorporate RNA produced at BioNTech controlled manufacturing sites including sites operated by the following sub-contractors in Germany:

12

The screenshot below shows the acceptance criteria of various BNT 162B2 Drug Product lots. Drug Product refers to "medication in its marketed form, including its fillers, coloring agents, and other active or inactive agents." The acceptance criteria for Emergency Supply is greater or equal to 50%, which happens to be just below the batches with the lowest %RNA integrity supplied by Pfizer, Puurs. For some reason, the acceptance criteria for the clinical Drug Product Lots differs and is set higher at greater or equal to 60%.

Batch Analyses Drug Product

EUROPEAN MEDICINES AGENCY

**Batch Analyses for Nonclinical and Clinical BNT162b2 Drug Product Lots**

| Quality Attribute | Analytical Procedure | Acceptance Criteria[a] | Lot Number | | | | | |
|---|---|---|---|---|---|---|---|---|
| | | | BCV40420-A | BCV40620-A | BCV40620-B | BCV40620-C | BCV40620-D | BCV40620-E |
| | | | Results | | | | | |
| RNA integrity | Capillary gel electrophoresis | ≥ 60%[b] | 75 | 85 | 86 | 83 | 77 | 85 |

**Batch Analyses for Clinical BNT162b2 Drug Product Lots**

| Quality Attribute | Analytical Procedure | Acceptance Criteria[a] | Lot Number | | | | |
|---|---|---|---|---|---|---|---|
| | | | BCV40720-A | BCV40720-B | BCV40720-C | ED3938 | EE3813 |
| | | | Results | | | | |
| RNA integrity | Capillary gel electrophoresis | ≥ 60%[b] | 71 | 72 | 69 | 62 | 63 |

**Batch Analyses for Emergency Supply BNT162b2 Drug Product Lots**

| Quality Attribute | Analytical Procedure | Acceptance Criteria[a] | Lot Number | |
|---|---|---|---|---|
| | | | EE8492 | EE8493 |
| | | | Results | |
| RNA integrity | Capillary gel electrophoresis | ≥ 50% in the peak corresponding to intact RNA | 55 | 55 |

EMA

CMC (Chemistry, Manufacturing and Controls) "involves defining manufacturing practices and product specifications that must be followed and met in order to ensure product safety and consistency between batches." Given the data shown above, it's evident there were significant CMC issues regarding the inconsistency of the %RNA integrity between batches, which is reflected in the leaked EMA emails and documents. What's concerning is that the manufacturer (Pfizer/BioNTech) claimed, "The efficacy of the drug product is dependent on the expression of the delivered RNA, which requires a sufficiently intact RNA molecule."

It is deeply concerning that lowering the specification down to 50% was potentially how this major objection was solved. According to a leaked Rapporteur's Rolling Review Assessment (revised report date: 25 November

2020) compiled by the CHMP and PRAC rapporteurs- they found the "current acceptance criteria" particularly troubling. The report states, "no characterization data on RNA integrity and truncated forms is presented and the potential safety risks associated with truncated RNA isoforms are not addressed. This is especially important considering that the current DS and DP acceptance criteria allows for up to 50% fragmented species."

> In addition to double stranded RNA, there are more product-related impurities, i.e. truncated RNA, also referred to as fragmented species. Truncated RNA is reflected in the DS specification in terms of RNA integrity. However, the characterisation of BNT162b2 DS is currently not found acceptable in relation to the CQA RNA integrity. Significant differences between batches manufactured by Process 1 and 2 are observed for this specific attribute. Even though two methods, namely agarose gel electrophoresis and capillary gel electrophoresis, have been applied to determine RNA integrity of BNT162b2 DS, no characterisation data on RNA integrity and truncated forms is presented and the potential safety risks associated with truncated RNA isoforms are not addressed. This is especially important considering that the current DS and DP acceptance criteria allows for up to 50% fragmented species. Therefore, the dossier should be updated with additional characterisation data and discussion on mRNA integrity, **this is considered a major objection.**

Truncated (shortened by missing either top or end section) RNA is defined as a "product-related impurity" and the fact that potential safety risks arising from this fragmented species "are not addressed" is highly alarming.

Reference is made to "the current DS and DP acceptance criteria," this implies that it was not always set at that level and perhaps it had been changed (lowered). The question is why? Could it have been that process 2 (the manufacturing of the commercial batches) was just not replicable at the same specification level to the clinical batches (small scale) of process 1, therefore a lower standard was set in order for CMA to be granted?

I asked the EMA for comment regarding the content of the leaked emails and documents. Their press office's response has been published below in its entirety.

"The investigation of the published material revealed that the correspondence was manipulated by the perpetrators prior to publication. Not all of the documents were published in their integral, original form and may have been taken out of context. Whilst individual emails were authentic, data from different users were selected and aggregated, screenshots from multiple folders and mailboxes were created and additional titles were added by the perpetrators.

These documents do not present a full picture of the assessment of Comirnaty, the COVID-19 vaccine developed by BioNTech/Pfizer. They show the situation up to the beginning of December 2020, when the hack was discovered, but do not mention the considerable amount of additional data, information and clarifications submitted by BioNTech/Pfizer up to 21 December 2020, the day when EMA's committee for human medicines (CHMP) gave its recommendation to grant a marketing authorization for this vaccine.

Comirnaty works because the mRNA it contains provides instructions for producing a spike protein which triggers an immune response. Its efficacy therefore depends on the presence of suitable amount of intact mRNA, which is known to be relatively unstable. What the documents show is how the assessment of any medicine works: following scrutiny of the data submitted by the company, the CHMP had questions about the integrity of mRNA and raised them formally as a 'major objection.' This is an integral part of the assessment of any medicine. If major objections remain unresolved, they preclude the granting of the marketing authorization. In this case, the company addressed the issues raised satisfactorily and subsequently supplied the required information and data after beginning of December 2020, which allowed EMA to move towards a positive opinion for this vaccine.

The public assessment report of Comirnaty summarizes the conclusions of the CHMP on this issue and details the steps taken during the marketing authorization procedure of Comirnaty as well as the obligations placed on the marketing authorization holder to carry out additional studies to closely monitor the pharmaceutical quality of vaccine. These obligations were also included in the Product Information published at the time of the CHMP opinion.

Even in a public health emergency as COVID-19, there has always been consensus across the EU not to compromise standards and to base any recommendation on the available scientific evidence on a vaccine's safety, pharmaceutical quality and efficacy, and nothing else. Authorizations are only granted when the evidence shows convincingly that the benefits of vaccination are greater than any risks posed by a vaccine."

• • •

In July 2024, the European General Court ruled that the European Commission, helmed by Ursula von der Leyen, violated European law by failing to provide the public with "sufficiently wide access"[637] to COVID-19 vaccine contracts. It should be noted that von der Leyen called for countries to discuss Covid vaccine mandates in Europe because "too many people still refuse to get shots voluntarily."[638]

The court highlighted "irregularities" in the Commission's practice of redacting crucial sections of these agreements. It firmly asserted that the Commission could not substantiate its claims that broader access would harm pharmaceutical companies' commercial interests.

The case was instigated by Green MEPs seeking transparency on vaccine contracts, highlighting the Commission's refusal to disclose crucial documents despite public interest. This refusal triggered legal action, culminating in the damning verdict against the Commission's secrecy.

However, just a day after the European Court of Justice's ruling, following a secret ballot among MEPs, von der Leyen secured the backing of 401 Members of the European Parliament and was re-elected[639] as President of the European Commission for a further five years.

And what was the outcome of the 2023 lawsuit brought by *New York Times* journalist Matina Stevi-Gridneff seeking access to all text messages between European Commission President Ursula von der Leyen and Pfizer CEO Albert Bourla, during negotiations for Covid vaccine contracts worth €35 billion? Two years later, the General Court ruled[640] that the Commission had violated transparency rules by refusing the request without adequately explaining why the messages could not be located or retrieved. The court found this breached EU "good administration" standards and overturned the refusal.

However, following the ruling, the Commission re-adopted a refusal claiming exhaustive searches (including von der Leyen's phones) "found nothing." It admitted exchanges occurred but classified them as "short-lived" for call coordination, not warranting retention. According to the Commission, Von der Leyen reportedly replaced her phone multiple times post-2021 without full data transfers, "leading to loss."

To this day the texts remain undisclosed.

CHAPTER TWELVE

# BEYOND THE LABEL

*"I sequenced all the DNA that was in the vaccine... it's surprising that there's any DNA in there. I'm alarmed about the possible consequences... but you should be alarmed about the regulatory process that allowed it to get there! This DNA could be causing some of the rare but serious side effects like death from cardiac arrest... It can and likely will integrate into the genomic DNA of cells... a real hazard for genome modification... and a very real theoretical risk of future cancer."*

~Phillip Buckhaults, Ph.D.,
Testimony to South Carolina Senate,
September 13, 2023

From 2023 onwards, independent laboratories in the United States, Canada, Europe, and elsewhere conducted genomic sequencing on vials of Pfizer-BioNTech and Moderna mRNA COVID-19 vaccines. These analyses reported the presence of residual bacterial plasmid DNA fragments in both products at levels ranging from billions to hundreds of billions of copies per dose. Figures that exceed regulatory guidelines by hundreds of times when measured by fluorometry. Pfizer-BioNTech vaccine vials were also found to contain sequences from the SV40 promoter/enhancer region, a genetic element historically used in laboratory settings to enhance gene expression and known to have oncogenic (cancer-causing) potential.

Regulators such as Health Canada and the European Medicines Agency acknowledged the presence of residual DNA and Pfizer's failure to specifically disclose the SV40 sequence. However, they maintained there was no proven risk, while experts warned of genomic integration, insertional mutagenesis, autoimmune attack, cancer, and the contamination of future generations.

This chapter examines the manufacturing switch that independent researchers associate with elevated residual DNA levels, the non-disclosure of SV40 sequences acknowledged by regulators and the decision by agencies including the MHRA not to conduct vial-level testing. It also explores manufacturers' own patents and scientific publications acknowledging potential oncogenic risks of residual plasmid DNA contamination, along with the growing body of independent evidence that has led some scientists and legal observers to conclude the world's most widely administered products may meet the technical definition of adulteration and misbranding under federal law, characterizations manufacturers and regulators dispute.

What began as a promise of precision medicine has, according to critics including molecular biologists and regulatory experts, functioned as what they characterize as one of the largest undeclared genetic experiments in modern human history.

The following is an adaptation of my investigative report "Thou Shalt Not Adulterate,"[641] published in November 2023.

## The DNA Contamination Scandal

In early 2023, Kevin McKernan, R&D lead of the Human Genome Project and genomics expert, made a concerning discovery while analyzing vials of Pfizer-BioNTech and Moderna's mRNA COVID-19 vaccines at his Boston laboratory. His analysis revealed the presence of billions of fragments of plasmid (bacterial) DNA in both vaccines, along with sequences from the SV40 promoter/enhancer region (a genetic element known for its cancer-promoting potential) detected only in the Pfizer-BioNTech product.

Bacterial plasmid DNA is not listed as an approved ingredient in the Pfizer-BioNTech shot.

> **WHAT ARE THE INGREDIENTS IN THIS VACCINE?**
> Pfizer-BioNTech COVID-19 Vaccine contains the following ingredients: messenger ribonucleic acid (mRNA), lipids (((4-hydroxybutyl)azanediyl)bis(hexane-6,1-diyl)bis(2-hexyldecanoate), 2 [(polyethylene glycol)-2000]-N,N-ditetradecylacetamide, 1,2-distearoyl-sn-glycero-3-phosphocholine, and cholesterol), tromethamine, tromethamine hydrochloride, and sucrose. Pfizer-BioNTech COVID-19 Vaccine may also contain sodium chloride.

Source: FDA website[642]

It is also absent from the list of ingredients for Moderna's product.

| **WHAT ARE THE INGREDIENTS IN THESE VACCINES?** SPIKEVAX (COVID-19 Vaccine, mRNA), Moderna COVID-19 Vaccine, and Moderna COVID-19 Vaccine, Bivalent contain the following ingredients: messenger ribonucleic acid (mRNA), lipids (SM-102, polyethylene glycol [PEG] 2000 dimyristoyl glycerol [DMG], cholesterol, and 1,2-distearoyl-sn-glycero-3-phosphocholine [DSPC]), tromethamine, tromethamine hydrochloride, acetic acid, sodium acetate trihydrate, and sucrose. |
|---|

Source: FDA website[643]

The fact that independent laboratories have reported such significant levels of plasmid DNA fragments (billions to hundreds of billions per dose, vastly exceeding regulatory guidelines when measured by fluorometry) in both these products has led critics to argue that these levels may meet the technical definition of adulteration.

So, what is plasmid DNA and how did it get into the shots? Plasmid DNA is a double-stranded, circular DNA molecule that is common to bacteria.

In order to understand how it got into the shots, my interview[644] with Joshua Guetzkow PhD., is highly revealing. Guetzkow succinctly explained how Pfizer/BioNTech conducted a "bait-and-switch" of their biological product that went on to be injected into the arms of billions.

A key takeaway from the interview was that the Pfizer/BioNTech mRNA product rolled out to the masses, was not the same one tested in Pfizer's pivotal clinical and non-clinical trials (animal studies). This is because the commercially rolled out product was made using an entirely different process. Guetzkow, categorically stated, when it comes to biological products: "The process is the product."

The product used in the clinical trial was made via Process 1. These small-scale clinical batches were made using the more expensive PCR process to amplify the DNA template used to make the modified mRNA for the vaccines. A highly efficient filtration mechanism was also employed using magnetic beads.

However, the product, which was sold and distributed around the world, was manufactured using Process 2. This involved large-scale batches manufactured using a much cheaper process: E. coli bacteria, which were selected to replicate the DNA used as a template for the mRNA.

This introduced contamination both from the residual (plasmid/bacterial) DNA and the E. coli membranes called endotoxins, which are also highly inflammatory. The significant drop in RNA integrity (a measure of how intact the RNA molecule is) was a direct result from this switch from

Process 1 to Process 2. (These two different manufacturing processes were referenced in the previous chapter.)

The contamination scandal does not stop there. McKernan found that in the Pfizer/BioNTech shots, the bacterial DNA contains bioactive gene sequences: SV40 promoter and enhancer.

## What is SV40?

According to an article[645] published in PubMed, "The polyomavirus simian virus 40 (SV40) is a known oncogenic [tumor causing] DNA virus which induces primary brain and bone cancers, malignant mesothelioma, and lymphomas in laboratory animals."

Traditionally, SV40 has been used on lab animals to induce the formation of cancer cells (tumor growth). In 1960, Simian Virus 40 (SV40) was discovered in the oral form of the poliovirus vaccine. It was said to have contaminated up to 30 percent of the poliovirus vaccines in the U.S. It was found in the vaccines produced between 1955-1961, when monkey kidney cell cultures (harboring Simian Virus) were used in the production process. Lederle, a subsidiary of Wyeth, was the manufacturer at the time. Wyeth was later purchased by Pfizer in 2009.

The difference between SV40 found in the poliovirus vaccine and its presence in the Pfizer-BioNTech shots- is that the complete virus was found in the former. In the latter, two viral components: SV40 enhancer and promoter, were discovered. Enhancers are short nucleotide sequences that enhance the transcription rate in the genome. Promoters are larger nucleotide sequences that initiate the process of transcription.

The work of David Dean, Ph.D.[646] is highly relevant here. His lab[647] at the University of Rochester, "studies the mechanisms and applications of plasmid and DNA-binding protein nuclear localization."

An extract taken from his university lab's website reads: "We have demonstrated that portions of the 72 bp SV40 enhancer are required for the nuclear entry of plasmid DNA in all eukaryotic cells tested to date; plasmids not containing this sequence remain in the cytoplasm until cell division, whereas plasmids containing the enhancer migrate to the nucleus within several hours."

Dean states very clearly just how integral the presence of the SV40 enhancer is for enabling plasmid DNA to migrate and enter the nucleus of a cell (genome integration).

## Other Labs Replicate the Concerning Findings

McKernan's findings were later replicated in other independent labs, such as that of the cancer genomics professor at the University of South Carolina, Phillip Buckhaults, Ph.D.

On September 13, Buckhaults testified in front of the South Carolina Senate about his discovery. The following screenshot is taken from one of his slides shown at the hearing.

> The Pfizer mRNA vaccine is contaminated with the plasmid DNA vector that was used as the template for in vitro transcription reaction.
>
> this DNA could be the cause of some of the rare but serious side effects like death from cardiac arrest.
>
> The DNA can and likely will integrate into the genomes of transfected cells.
>
> There is a very real hazard for genome modification of long-lived somatic cells, which could cause sustained autoimmune attack toward that tissue.
>
> There is also a theoretical risk of future cancer, depending on the piece of DNA and site of integration.

Source: SC Senate Hearing,[648] USC Professor Dr. Phillip Buckhaults

During the hearing, Buckhaults stated: "I sequenced all the DNA that was in the vaccine and I can see what's in there and it's surprising that there's any DNA in there... I'm alarmed about the possible consequences of this both in terms of human health and biology, but you should be alarmed about the regulatory process that allowed it to get there! So, this DNA in my view, it could be causing some of the rare but serious side effects like death from Cardiac Arrest. There's a lot of cases now of people having suspicious deaths after the vaccine. It's hard to prove what caused it...This DNA is a plausible mechanism. This DNA can and likely will integrate into the genomic DNA of cells that got transfected with the vaccine...This is a real hazard for genome modification of long live somatic cells, like stem cells and it could cause theoretically- this is all a theoretical concern, but it's pretty reasonable, based on solid molecular biology that it could cause a sustained autoimmune tact toward that tissue. It's also a very real theoretical risk of future cancer in some people, depending on where in the genome this foreign piece of DNA lands."

## "The Higher DNA Content, The Increase in Frequency of Serious Adverse Events"

On October 9, 2023, the World Council for Health organized an urgent expert hearing[649] on the topic of bacterial (plasmid) DNA and genetic sequences in the mRNA vaccines. The hearing which took place virtually, featured immunologists, geneticists, specialist physicians and research scientists from the United States, Canada, France, Germany and Australia. The evidence presented led to the panel calling for an "immediate moratorium on these novel genetic vaccines."

The panelists included, Kevin McKernan, Jessica Rose Ph.D., David Speicher Ph.D., Maria Gutschi and David Wiseman Ph.D., who co-authored the study:[650] "DNA fragments detected in monovalent and bivalent Pfizer/BioNTech and Moderna modRNA COVID-19 vaccines from Ontario, Canada: Exploratory dose response relationship with serious adverse events." Their paper was published on October 19, 2023, on the OSF preprint server.

The authors stated: "These data demonstrate the presence of billions to hundreds of billions of DNA molecules per dose in these vaccines. Using fluorometry all vaccines exceed the guidelines for residual DNA set by FDA and WHO of 10 ng/dose by 188 – 509-fold." They went on to reveal: "we found preliminary evidence of a dose response relationship of the amount of DNA per dose and the frequency of serious adverse events (SAEs)."

This means that vials with higher doses of DNA content could cause more adverse reactions. I turned to Jessica Rose Ph.D., computational biologist and co-author of the paper for comment. "Health Canada recently confirmed the presence of SV40 promoter in the Pfizer products. In fact, this was confirmed on the same day that our paper hit the OSF preprint server. We found residual DNA in all 27 (Pfizer and Moderna) vials that we tested, including Adult monovalent XBB.1.5 (at levels that exceed EMA standards) meaning that this is an ongoing and potentially serious problem that warrants an immediate moratorium on these products, and an investigation into the effects of this residual DNA. Some of the potential effects include genomic (and possibly germ-line) integration that may lead to genomic instability, DNA damage and cancer. We also plotted a dose response curve using serious adverse event reports for the specific vials tested from VAERS (Canadian reports) and this is important because dose response is one of the Bradford Hill criteria for causality. More vials need to be tested, and people need to be tested for integration events as well."

## Health Canada & European Medicines Agency Confirm Presence of Plasmid DNA

It is interesting that on the same day the Speicher et al. paper was published, Health Canada confirmed the presence of SV40 enhancer-promoter based on the plasmid DNA sequence in the mRNA vaccines. *The Epoch Times*[651] broke the story: "The regulator said that after scientists Kevin McKernan and Dr. Phillip J. Buckhaults publicly raised the presence of SV40 enhancers in the vaccines earlier this year, "it was possible for Health Canada to confirm the presence of the enhancer based on the plasmid DNA sequence submitted by Pfizer against the published SV40 enhancer sequence."

The report went on to quote an email sent by Health Canada to The Epoch Times: "Health Canada expects sponsors to identify any biologically functional DNA sequences within a plasmid (such as an SV40 enhancer) at the time of submission. Although the full DNA sequence of the Pfizer plasmid was provided at the time of initial filing, the sponsor did not specifically identify the SV40 sequence."

If Health Canada (and other regulators) had tested the novel mRNA shots at the vial level, they would have found the contaminants, just as other independent scientists had. Instead, they relied solely on the sponsor's (BioNTech's) submissions and later cited the lack of specific highlighting of the SV40 sequence as part of their response.

The same excuse was touted by the European Medicines Agency (EMA) as stated in their email to The Epoch Times: "While the full DNA sequence of the plasmid starting material was provided in the initial marketing authorization application for Comirnaty, the applicant [BioNTech] did not specifically highlight the SV40 sequence."

## The MHRA's Response

On the heels of Health Canada and EMA admissions, I submitted a Freedom of Information request to the UK's Medicines and Healthcare products Regulatory Agency (MHRA) via WhatDoTheyKnow[652] on 20 October 2023, asking:

1. Has the MHRA ever independently tested the Pfizer/BioNTech vaccine at the vial level?
2. Does the MHRA intend to test the Pfizer/BioNTech COVID-19 mRNA vaccine for the presence of fragmented DNA and SV40 enhancer?

Their full response is reproduced below:

In the context of fragmented DNA and SV40 enhancer MHRA has not tested the Pfizer/BioNTech vaccine at the vial level. Independent laboratory testing of vaccines is carried out by the MHRA's Official Medicines Control Laboratory (OMCL) (with a NIBSC certificate being applied to compliant batches).

The independent testing does not verify the composition of the vaccine, rather it assesses key parameters that focus on biological quality of the product. Independent assessment also confirms that the manufacturer has reported on its wide-ranging tests on the product. Batches of vaccine that meet the specifications in the approval are certificated allowing the manufacturer to market them in the UK for use before the batch expiry date. In terms of the Pfizer/BioNTech vaccines tests conducted at the MHRA include: Potency/sequence ratio, identity, RNA encapsulation, RNA content, RNA integrityAll vaccine manufacturers must operate to Good Manufacturing Practices and their facilities are licensed, and are inspected periodically. These procedures help to ensure that no batches of vaccine that may be contaminated get released in the UK.

There are currently no intentions to test the Pfizer-BioNTech COVID-19 mRNA vaccine for the presence of fragmented DNA and SV40 enhancer. We trust that you will find this information of use.

The MHRA's disclosure is highly revealing. Firstly, it confirms they have never tested the vaccine at the vial level. Independent testing by the MHRA's Official Medicines Control Laboratory (OMCL) focuses on key parameters: potency/sequence ratio, RNA content, RNA integrity and RNA encapsulation.

This limited scope is particularly notable in light of my earlier investigative report for TrialSite News, which examined the leaked EMA emails revealing a sharp drop in mRNA integrity between clinical (Process 1) and scaled-up (Process 2) batches. Regulators, including EMA and MHRA classified it as a major objection but ultimately approved the product by accepting a lowered standard.

Moreover, what is particularly troubling is the MHRA's admission that: "There are currently no intentions to test the Pfizer-BioNTech COVID-19 mRNA vaccine for the presence of fragmented DNA and SV40 enhancer."

I asked lead author of the Speicher et al. paper, molecular virologist David Speicher Ph.D., for his view on the MHRA's disclosure. He explained: "While the MHRA has responded in a similar manner to Health Canada, the EMA and TGA, it is clear by their response that they did not test for residual DNA or SV40 sequences. While the MHRA may not have the lab capacity themselves and blindly take Pfizer and Moderna at their word based on documents submitted about their products, they should have an independent laboratory assess unopened vials for residual DNA and the SV40 promoter-enhancer sequences. Both Health Canada and the EMA have since confirmed the presence of residual DNA and the SV40 promoter-enhancer but are adamant that the vaccines are still safe and effective without providing any scientific reasoning.

The published literature is clear that DNA fragments with an SV40 enhancer entering the cytoplasm will translocate to the nucleus and integrate. This could have untold effects for generations. While integration at this point is still hypothetical, it needs to be disproven before we can be certain these vaccines are indeed safe. We simply cannot dismiss these shots as "safe and effective" without clear scientific proof and discussion. Therefore, I think it's essential that we have a moratorium on the modRNA technology until these issues are resolved."

Returning to the World Council for Health expert panel hearing, Associate Professor of Viral Immunology in the Department of Pathobiology at the University of Guelph, Dr. Bridle stated: "Anybody who's received plasmid DNA in these shots, they have never given informed consent for that," he explained. "Those of us who know the manufacturing process … were assured that there would not be plasmid DNA present. There's no excuse [for] companies like Pfizer and Moderna, with all of their money and all of their expert scientists, to leave the plasmid DNA in the vaccines," Bridle said. "The fact that they didn't get rid of this is egregious."

Bridle was the first to publicly analyze Pfizer's biodistribution study,[653] released by the Japanese regulatory agency in 2021. Pfizer's data showed how the modified mRNA and expressed spike protein were widely distributed in the body within hours, contradicting early assurances that the vaccine "stays in the arm."

## Moderna Knew the Risks of Injecting Plasmid DNA

On November 9th, a post from the account @findogg,[654] drew wide-spread attention on the social media platform, X.

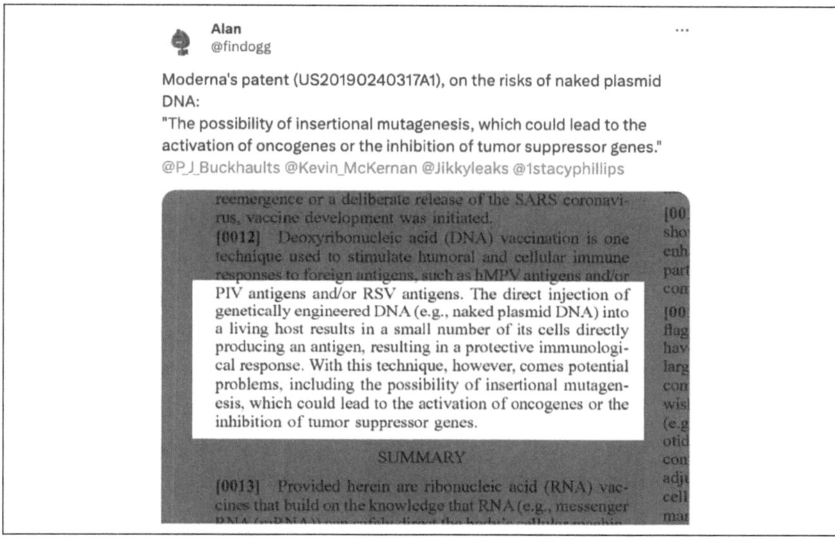


The post relates to Moderna's 2019 patent[655] for "respiratory virus ribonucleic acid (RNA ) vaccines [eg. mRNA] and combination vaccines."

Just to remind the reader, plasmid (bacterial) DNA was detected, in not only the Pfizer/BioNTech mRNA shot, but also in Moderna's. Moderna's patent shows how the biotech company was fully aware of the "potential problems" associated with the "direct injection of genetically engineered DNA (e.g., naked plasmid DNA)," such as "the possibility of insertional mutagenesis, which could lead to the activation of oncogenes or the inhibition of tumor suppressor genes," i.e., increased risk of cancer.

According to Ranzani et al.'s[656] definition: "Insertional mutagenesis is the phenomenon by which an exogenous [of external origin] DNA sequence integrates within the genome of a host organism." The authors go on to state: "When insertional mutagenesis induces the deregulation of oncogenes or tumor suppressor genes (TSG), it can cause cell transformation." An oncogene is a mutated gene that has the potential to cause cancer.

## Dr. Campbell's Interview Of Professor Dalgleish

The 2023 interview[657] of Prof. Angus Dalgleish (Consultant Medical Oncologist and professor of oncology at St George's, University of London) by Dr. John Campbell is particularly notable. A transcript of an interview segment, can be read below:

Prof. Dalgleish: Not only is the quality control awful [of the COVID-19 mRNA vaccines] but it's contaminated with DNA plasmids. One report up to 350 times with sequences from the SV40 promoter. Well, the SV40 is an oncogenic promoter used in cancer development in mice. So what the hell is that doing in an RNA vaccine, you have to ask? Because the presence of that and the presence of DNA means it can integrate. You don't have to go very far into the literature to find people reporting that the spike protein is integrated into all sorts of different tissues. They said that "it stays at the point of the injection site and there's no way it spreads." This turns out to be a complete lie! It's been identified at autopsy. It's been identified everywhere. And this is the other thing with patients- I can't get autopsies on these patients to prove this. It's quite incredible but a colleague who had an explosive cancer- colorectal. At surgery, sent the pieces away- the metastases away- and Spike messenger RNA from the vaccine insertion was confirmed. This to me is quite frightening that this is occurring. And also, there's been this- "we don't need to do post-mortems on patients dying from this." It's like it's from on high and they just won't do it. I pleaded for one, on the patient who died from explosive melanoma who said, "I never felt well after the booster, I just felt chronically unwell and then the melanoma came exploding back."

Dr. John Campbell: Had the relatives consented to a post-mortem?

Prof. Dalgleish: Oh yes!

Dr. John Campbell: Hang on a minute- you're one of the most senior doctors in the country. You wanted a post-mortem and the relatives had consented to a post-mortem, but that was refused?

Prof. Dalgleish: Yes, it was overruled.

## Moderna's "Superior" DNA Removal Method

It is important to mention that the process of residual DNA removal was not unknown to the vaccine manufacturers. As it happens, Moderna had even invented a "superior" method to remove it.

An earlier patent filed by Moderna: US10077439B2[658] with a patent date of September 18, 2018, discloses an invention relating to the "Removal of DNA fragments in mRNA production process." The background surrounding this invention, is as follows: "The DNA template used in the mRNA manufacturing process must be removed to ensure the efficacy of therapeutics and safety, because residual DNA in drug products may induce activation of the innate response and has the potential to be oncogenic [potential to cause cancer] in patient populations. Regulatory guidelines may also require the quantification, control, and removal of the DNA template in RNA products. Currently available or reported methods do not address this deficiency."

Moderna uses explicit statements, how the residual DNA "must be removed" because of their "potential to be oncogenic" (cancer causing). The patent application goes on to describe a superior practice for residual plasmid DNA removal which "can be conveniently scaled up for larger batches."

> The new methods are superior to previous practice in that no DNase I enzyme is required, and the purification/DNA removal process is done by a single step column. It can be conveniently scaled up for larger batches. The mRNA should be recovered with high yield and not suffer additional loss as in other purification or partitioning methods. If labeled cDNA is removed without enzyme digestion, there are no concerns of secondary contamination of smaller DNA fragments or oligonucleotides.
>
> Example 6: Quantitation of RNA Transcript for Detection of Impurities
>
> After removal of the DNA (either by DNase digestion or removal of labeled DNA), the RNA transcript sample is subjected to a total nuclease digestion using nuclease P1. Thus, the presence of any deoxythymidine (dT), deoxyadenine (dA), deoxycytidine (dC), and deoxyguanosine (dG) are detected and their levels quantified by LC-MS/MS.
>
> Then, the sample is subjected to liquid chromatography-tandem mass spectrometry analysis to detect the presence of individual residual deoxynucleotides (impurities).

Source: Patent US10077439B2

This indicates that an advanced method for the removal of residual plasmid DNA for "larger batches" existed prior to the mass-production of the mRNA COVID-19 shots. The CEO of Moderna, Stéphane Bancel, is cited as one of the inventors.

(12) **United States Patent**
**Issa et al.**

(54) **REMOVAL OF DNA FRAGMENTS IN MRNA PRODUCTION PROCESS**

(71) Applicant: **ModernaTX, Inc.**, Cambridge, MA (US)

(72) Inventors: **William Joseph Issa**, Roslindale, MA (US); **Yuxun Wang**, Cambridge, MA (US); **Stephane Bancel**, Cambridge, MA (US)

(73) Assignee: **ModernaTX, Inc.**, Cambridge, MA (US)

Source: Patent US10077439B2

The evidence shown here suggests that vaccine manufacturers were aware of potential risks from residual plasmid DNA, including innate immune activation and oncogenicity.

## BioNTech Knew Too

In a 2014 review article[659] titled "mRNA-based therapeutics developing a new class of drugs," published in *Nature Reviews Drug Discovery*, lead author Ugur Sahin (who is also the co-founder and CEO of BioNTech) wrote: "In addition, IVT mRNA-based therapeutics, unlike plasmid DNA and viral vectors, do not integrate into the genome and therefore do not pose the risk of insertional mutagenesis."

This can be interpreted as an admission by Sahin that plasmid DNA does integrate into the genome, posing the risk of insertional mutagenesis. This raises an important question about why residual plasmid DNA levels in Comirnaty (reported in independent analyses as reaching billions to hundreds of billions of molecules per dose) were not removed.

## The Case for Willful Misconduct?

The manufacturers of the novel COVID-19 vaccines were granted indemnity status,[660] meaning they benefited from protection against any and all liabilities arising from their products. In the case of Pfizer and BioNTech, it was built into their advance purchasing agreements and contracts signed by nations around the world.

Moderna was also given indemnity status. The screenshot below reveals Moderna's indemnity "as part of the contract between HMG" (Her Majesty's Government, at that time).

> The agreement to provide an indemnity as part of the contract between HMG and Moderna creates a contingent liability on the covid-19 vaccination programme. It has been and remains the Government's strategy to manage covid-19 until an effective vaccine/s can be deployed at scale. Putting in place appropriate indemnities to be given to vaccine suppliers has helped to secure access to vaccines much sooner than may have been the case otherwise.

Source:[661] 13 April 2021 UK Parliament debate- Statement from Minister for Covid Vaccine Deployment (Nadhim Zahawi)

Similarly, the unredacted advance purchase agreement[662] (APA) between the European Commission, (acting on behalf of member states), Pfizer Inc., and BioNTech SE (signed November 2020) included the following indemnity language: "each Participating Member State shall indemnify and hold harmless the Contractor, their Affiliates...from and against any and all liabilities incurred...relating to harm, damages and losses...arising from or relating to the use and deployment of the Vaccines.."

> **I.12 INDEMNIFICATION**
>
> I.12.1 The Commission, on behalf of the Participating Member States, declares that the use of Vaccines produced under this APA will happen under epidemic conditions requiring such use, and that the administration of Vaccines will therefore be conducted under the sole responsibility of the Participating Member States. Hence, each Participating Member State shall indemnify and hold harmless the Contractor, their Affiliates, subcontractors, licensors and sub-licensees, and officers, directors, employees and other agents and representatives of each (together, the **"Indemnified Persons"**) from and against any and all liabilities incurred, settlements as per Article I.12.6, and reasonable direct external legal costs incurred in the defence of Third Party Claims (including reasonable attorney's fees and other expenses) relating to harm, damages and losses as defined in Article I.12.2 (together, the **"Losses"**) arising from or relating to the use and deployment of the Vaccines in the jurisdiction of the Participating Member State in question. This Article I.12 applies to Losses which arise from or relate to the Vaccines

Source: Advance Purchasing Agreement between EC, Pfizer and BioNTech (page 24)

Many of these contracts contain exceptions for cases of willful misconduct or gross negligence. Some critics and independent observers have suggested that if manufacturers failed to fully disclose certain manufacturing-related findings, such as the presence of residual plasmid DNA fragments and SV40 promoter-enhancer sequences, this could potentially fall outside the scope of the indemnity protections.

> **II.6.5 No limitation of liability**
>
> (i) Nothing in this APA excludes or limits the liability of either party for:
>
> (a) wilful intent, fraud or fraudulent misrepresentation;
>
> (b) any breach of Article II.9 (Confidentiality);
>
> (c) in the case of the Commission, failure to pay the Advance Payment;
>
> (d) in the case of a Participating Member State, failure to pay the price for the Product or any other sums properly owing to the Contractor or a Participating Contractor Affiliate under this APA and Vaccine Order Form;
>
> (e) in the case of a Participating Member State, the indemnity given by it under Article I.12;
>
> 31

Source: Advance Purchasing Agreement between EC, Pfizer and BioNTech (page 31)

BioNTech's May 2023 SEC filing also include standard risk disclosures, noting that the discovery of previously unknown safety issues with approved products could lead to loss of marketing authorization, suspension of sales, product liability claims, and material harm to the company's business and reputation.

> ***If we discover safety issues with our products, including our COVID-19 vaccine, that were not known at the time of approval, commercialization efforts for our products could be negatively affected, approved products could lose their approval or sales could be suspended, we could be subject to product liability claims and our business and reputation could be materially harmed.***

Source: BioNTech's US SEC filing, May 2023[663]

As stated earlier, several independent laboratories have reported detecting residual plasmid DNA in some tested vials of mRNA COVID-19 vaccines at levels ranging from billions to hundreds of billions of DNA molecules per dose (using methods such as fluorometry and sequencing). Health Canada and the European Medicines Agency have acknowledged the presence of residual plasmid DNA fragments, including SV40 promoter-enhancer sequences, in Pfizer-BioNTech vaccine batches. Both agencies, along with other regulators, continue to state that these levels are within acceptable limits, that the fragments are non-functional, and that there is no evidence of harm or integration into human DNA after billions of doses administered worldwide.

The UK's Medicines and Healthcare products Regulatory Agency (MHRA) has stated in FOI responses (referenced earlier) that it has not conducted vial-level testing, and it has no plans to test for fragmented DNA or SV40 enhancer sequences. Critics have questioned whether this level of independent verification is sufficient given the theoretical concerns raised in some studies about residual DNA. They also argue why have regulators so readily dismissed this major safety red flag that could carry unknown risks for generations.

## The Trojan Horse

In early 2025, I interviewed[664] consultant pharmacist, Maria Gutschi, with decades of experience in hospital infectious disease work and regulatory affairs for Health Canada. Gutschi became deeply skeptical of the COVID-19 mRNA vaccines the moment she read the European Medicines Agency's European Public Assessment Report in February 2021.

"My jaw fell," she recalls, "because I've never seen a report of that character ever in my ten years of reading them, where there were so many specific obligations which are required under law to be met, especially for manufacturing." For biologics, she stresses repeatedly, "the process is the product." By 2025, she says almost none of those legally binding obligations have been fulfilled. Independent testing she helped coordinate in Canada confirmed excessive residual plasmid DNA and massive lot-to-lot variability. The biggest shock was Pfizer's undisclosed SV40 promoter/enhancer sequence. "This is an outright lie," Gutschi states bluntly, "what I call hard fraud... a right-out non-disclosure of significant active fraud."

Gutschi further stated that according to FOIA documents, Health Canada scientists were horrified when they discovered it and began a risk-assessment process that looked headed toward withdrawal, yet the effort was quietly squashed after consultations with the FDA and EMA.

Gutschi explains that the lipid nanoparticles are not inert carriers but pharmacologically active delivery bombs: "They are like a knife or like a bomb that goes into the cell membrane... everything that's in the lipid nanoparticle is now in the cytosol." She likens the payload to "a whole army that came in like a Trojan horse" that the cell was not ready for. Combined with the SV40 promoter and the sheer quantity of DNA fragments, the risk of genomic integration and oncogenesis is, in her view, unacceptably high.

In early 2025 she co-authored an open letter[665] to every Canadian MP, senator, and provincial chief medical officer demanding immediate suspension. "We have enough evidence at this point to show that the risks do not outweigh the benefits," she says. "The contamination, particularly with the SV40, is a risk too high… they should no longer be considered vaccines and taken off the market." Her ultimate goal is not merely recall but rigorous, transparent research.

• • •

On 3 January 2024 the Florida Surgeon General, Dr. Joseph Ladapo became the first senior public health official in the world to demand these products be withdrawn because of plasmid DNA contamination. The rest of the world's regulators pretended not to hear him.

The following is an adaptation of my early 2024 article[666] "Beyond Contamination" that I wrote on the heels of Ladapo's announcement.

## Dr. Ladapo's Warnings

An increasing number of prominent medical professionals have been calling for an immediate halt in the use of the alleged, "safe and effective" COVID-19 mRNA shots. On January 3, 2024, the Florida State Surgeon General, Dr. Joseph Ladapo, joined the ever-growing list.

An excerpt from the Florida Department of Health's bulletin[667] reads: "The Surgeon General outlined concerns regarding nucleic acid contaminants in the approved Pfizer and Moderna COVID-19 mRNA vaccines, particularly in the presence of lipid nanoparticle complexes, and Simian Virus 40 (SV40) promoter/enhancer DNA. Lipid nanoparticles are an efficient vehicle for delivery of the mRNA in the COVID-19 vaccines into human cells and may therefore be an equally efficient vehicle for delivering contaminant DNA into human cells. The presence of SV40 promoter/enhancer DNA may also pose a unique and heightened risk of DNA integration into human cells."

The bulletin included the following statement from Dr. Ladapo:

"DNA integration poses a unique and elevated risk to human health and to the integrity of the human genome, including the risk that DNA integrated into sperm or egg gametes could be passed onto offspring of mRNA COVID-19 vaccine recipients. If the risks of DNA integration have not been assessed for mRNA COVID-19 vaccines, these vaccines are not appropriate for use in human beings."

The Florida Surgeon General's warnings centered around the potential health risks associated with insertional mutagenesis (the integration of foreign DNA with the subject/host's genome). But he did not stop there, he also raised a further concern about the risk of generational mutagenesis. Where the "DNA integrated into sperm or egg gametes could be passed onto the offspring of mRNA COVID-19 vaccine recipients."

The basis of Dr. Ladapo's warning regarding the presence of the "SV40 promoter/enhancer DNA" in the mRNA shots, is founded on the bombshell findings of a recent pre-print study[668]. Significant levels (billions to hundreds of billions of fragments of plasmid DNA) were found in both Moderna and Pfizer/BioNTech's monovalent and bivalent mRNA shots, vastly exceeding regulatory standards.

The study's lead author, molecular virologist, Dr. David J. Speicher offered me his response to Dr. Ladapo's statement: "It is encouraging to see the courageous stand by Dr. Joseph Ladapo to call for a halt to the COVID-19 vaccines, and an honor to know that our study was instrumental in making that decision. Our Canadian study confirmed previous reports of Kevin McKernan and Dr. Philip Buckhaults, which showed high levels of residual plasmid DNA within the lipid nanoparticles in the COVID-19 modRNA vaccines. The SV40 enhancer-promoter in the Pfizer vaccines is a risk for genomic integration as well as interfering with the p53 gene (the guardian of the genome). Both could drive an increased risk for cancer. Our data on the adulteration coupled with Mulroney et al.'s *Nature* paper showing an aberrant immune response due to ribosomal frameshifting should be sufficient data for these vaccines to be halted globally. We need immediate research into the effects of these vaccines on human health. I applaud Dr. Ladapo for his stance and hope that other places, like Alberta, will follow suit."

In stark contrast to Speicher's praise of Ladapo, Dr. Paul Offit, member of the Food and Drug Administration (FDA) Vaccines and Related Biological Products Advisory Committee, responsible for the rubber stamping of the COVID-19 mRNA injections, said in an interview:[669] "It is hard to believe that Dr. Ladapo actually issued that statement" and went on to dismiss all of the Florida Surgeon General's concerns.

A month prior, the FDA responded[670] to a letter sent by Dr. Ladapo stating, "with over a billion doses of the mRNA vaccines administered, no safety concerns related to residual DNA have been identified."

The FDA letter was written by Dr. Peter Marks, then-Director of Center for Biologics Evaluation and Research (CBER), who also dismissed Ladapo's claims as "quite implausible" and "misleading."

## Were They Really Vaccines?

Despite being marketed as "vaccines" to promote uptake, critics argue that the Moderna and Pfizer-BioNTech shots align more closely with gene therapy definitions due to their mechanism of action.

In BioNTech's U.S. Security and Exchange Commission (SEC) filings,[671] (and similar Moderna disclosures), the companies noted: "Currently mRNA is considered a gene therapy product by the FDA. Unlike certain gene therapies that irreversibly alter cell DNA and may cause certain side effects, mRNA-based medicines are designed not to irreversibly change cell DNA." They further stated: "No mRNA immunotherapy has been approved, and none may ever be approved, in this new potential category of therapeutics. mRNA drug development has substantial clinical development and regulatory risks due to the novel and unprecedented nature of this new category of therapeutics."

Traditional gene therapy has been around for several decades and involves the use of viral vectors to deliver genes into cells, with historical risks including toxicity, inflammation, and insertional mutagenesis (e.g., leukemia cases in early trials).

mRNA products represent a "novel and unprecedented" class of their own. Given this experimental classification in earlier company disclosures, some observers have questioned whether more rigorous long-term safety assessments, such as dedicated genotoxicity and carcinogenicity studies, should have been required before widespread rollout. However, regulators classified and approved them as vaccines, justifying no such studies based on the components' expected lack of genotoxic potential and short-term use. My investigative reports for *TrialSite News*[672] (2021-2022) on the released Pfizer/BioNTech documents (initially sought by the FDA to remain sealed until 2096) highlighted that these specific studies were not conducted and were deemed unnecessary under the vaccine regulatory pathway.

## The Novel Ingredients Not Intended for Human Use

Two of the four compounds that make up the lipid nanoparticles (LNPs) encapsulating the modified (synthetic) mRNA had never been used before in a medicinal product: ALC-0315[673] (ionizable lipid) and ALC-0159[674] (PEGylated lipid) both licensed from Acuitas Therapeutics (discussed in chapter 9). Acuitas' LNPs are confirmed components of the

Pfizer/BioNTech Covid shot. Similarly, Moderna's proprietary ionizable cationic lipid, SM-102, had never been used in any approved medicinal product before Moderna's Covid (Spikevax/mRNA-1273). Scientific literature shows these LNPs can be toxic and "highly inflammatory."[675]

During pathologist Dr. Ryan Cole's address at the UK parliamentary office (which I reported[676] on), he shared the following: "In the lipid nanoparticles' data sheet it states these are not for human and not for veterinary use. These are for research purposes only. Yet they went into 5 billion people around the world!"

Page 1/10

**Safety Data Sheet**
**acc. to OSHA HCS**

Printing date 01/03/2024 | Revision date 01/03/2024

**1 Identification**

· **Product identifier**

· **Trade name:** ALC-0315
· **Synonym** 2-hexyl-decanoic acid, 1,1'-[[(4-hydroxybutyl)imino]di-6,1-hexanediyl] ester

· **Article number:** 34337
· **Application of the substance / the mixture**
This product is for research use - Not for human or veterinary diagnostic or therapeutic use.

· **Details of the supplier of the safety data sheet**
· **Manufacturer/Supplier:**
Cayman Chemical Co.
1180 E. Ellsworth Rd.
Ann Arbor, MI 48108
USA

· **Information department:** Product safety department
· **Emergency telephone number:**
During normal opening times: +1 (734) 971-3335
US/CANADA: 800-424-9300
Outside US/CANADA: 703-741-5970

Source:[677] Cayman Chemical Safety Data Sheet

## The Comparison Study That Was Never Done

In response to the switch from Process 1 to Process 2 (implemented to enable larger-scale manufacturing, discussed earlier), Pfizer added a protocol[678] amendment on October 6, 2020, explicitly committing to conduct a dedicated comparative study. This study would assess safety and immunogenicity in participants aged 16–55 who received either Process 1 or Process 2 material. A seemingly prudent step given the manufacturing change and the known differences in mRNA integrity and the introduction of additional plasmid DNA elements.

- Added an additional exploratory objective to describe safety and immunogenicity in participants 16 to 55 years of age vaccinated with study intervention produced by manufacturing "Process 1" or "Process 2."

- Removed the objective to describe the safety and immunogenicity of prophylactic BNT162b2 in individuals 16 to 55 years of age vaccinated with study intervention produced by manufacturing "Process 1" or "Process 2" because of the volume of BNT162b2 now distributed and administered globally using manufacturing "Process 2," making this comparison unwarranted.

Yet this promised comparison was later abandoned. Pfizer's rationale, as documented in Protocol Amendment 20[679] (dated 15 September 2022), was that "the volume of BNT162b2 now distributed and administered globally using 'Process 2' [made] this comparison unwarranted."

PF-07302048 (BNT162 RNA-Based COVID-19 Vaccines)
Protocol C4591001
Final Protocol Amendment 20, 15 September 2022

**Protocol Amendment Summary of Changes Table**

| Document History | | |
|---|---|---|
| **Document** | **Version Date** | **Summary and Rationale for Changes** |
| Protocol amendment 20 | 15 September 2022 | • Added language pertaining to early completion of this clinical trial as agreed with FDA and EMA.<br>• Updated schedules of assessments and protocol text to identify study visits that no longer need to be completed.<br>• Updated Study Procedures to describe site actions following approval of protocol amendment 20.<br>• Removed the objective to describe the safety and immunogenicity of prophylactic BNT162b2 in individuals 16 to 55 years of age vaccinated with study intervention produced by manufacturing "Process 1" or "Process 2" because of the volume of BNT162b2 now distributed and administered globally using manufacturing "Process 2," making this comparison unwarranted.<br>• Removed corresponding endpoints.<br>• Removed corresponding wording throughout the protocol text.<br>• Added rationale for removal of this objective.<br>• Added wording regarding return of e-diary devices or removal of application from participants' personal devices at the end of the study. |

The implications are deeply troubling: Process 1 underwent full animal toxicology studies and human clinical evaluation, while the Process 2 version, which became the globally distributed product, relied solely on analytical comparability data, without additional dedicated bridging animal studies or the direct human safety/immunogenicity head-to-head trial originally planned.

Billions of people worldwide ultimately received the Process 2 version (the one used in global distribution) without the direct comparative human safety and immunogenicity data that Pfizer had originally committed to collecting, effectively turning the global rollout into a global experiment.

## Dame Raine's Testimony: A Revealing Exchange

On 22 January 2025, Dame June Raine, Chief Executive of the UK's Medicines and Healthcare products Regulatory Agency (MHRA), gave oral evidence under oath at Module 4 of the UK COVID-19 Inquiry.

During questioning by lead counsel Hugo Keith KC, the discussion turned to whether the batches authorized and tested by the MHRA were the same as those ultimately supplied to the public. The exchange[680] (reproduced below) has attracted significant attention among independent observers and critics, who argue it reveals a critical failure at the highest level of the agency responsible for vaccine authorization in the UK.

Mr. Keith: Some have suggested that the batches which were delivered to the United Kingdom for use amongst its population, which were then handed out, were not the same batches, or rather were batches that were produced by a different manufacturing process on the part of the manufacturer, as has been – as had been tested by the MHRA? So bluntly, the suggestion has been made, you tested and authorized and certified a certain number of vaccines made by process, manufacturing process A, and then the manufacturers actually delivered vaccines to the British population produced as a result of a different manufacturing process, and one, by inference, which had not been tested. Is that right?

Dame Raine: Well, my understanding is that the manufacturing process would have been the same.

Mr. Keith: When manufacturers engage in the development of a vaccine or a medicine, and they're carrying out initial research and development, will they necessarily have built up to scale the manufacturing process which might be needed in the event of a successful development of that product?

Dame Raine: They might not have, but our inspectorate, who look at the manufacturing sites in great detail for the standards that will be applied, were working with likely manufacturers very early on, so that those issues could be dealt with at the time of scale-up.

Mr. Keith: And when the manufacturing processes came to be scaled up in the case of the vaccines which did prove to be successful, and therefore could be authorized and rolled out, was the MHRA alert to any changes in the manufacturing processes?

Dame Raine: Yes, we would have been.

Mr. Keith: And therefore, does it follow that if there were any changes which had any potential at all of impacting upon the quality, the effectiveness or the safety of the vaccine, you were aware of it and alert to it?

Dame Raine: Yes.

This exchange from Dame June Raine's testimony at the UK Covid-19 Inquiry is a striking example of how carefully worded answers can appear responsive while sidestepping the central distinction between the two manufacturing processes.

When Hugo Keith KC asked whether the batches tested and authorized by the MHRA were the same as those delivered to the public, Dame Raine replied: "Well, my understanding is that the manufacturing process would have been the same."

As the Chief Executive of the agency that authorized the vaccine for use across the United Kingdom, her response is deeply concerning. The reality (as previously set out in this chapter) is that the clinical-trial material (Process 1) was the basis for initial authorization and batch certification, while the version administered to the population was produced using Process 2. The fact that the MHRA's most senior official seemed unaware of this fundamental shift raises serious questions about the depth of oversight and the transparency provided to the public about what they were actually receiving.

Chapter 13 goes deeper into the unresolved problems at the heart of the mRNA technology: ribosomal frameshifting spawning off-target proteins (a risk the European Medicines Agency flagged even before authorization), and the controversy dubbed "Blotgate" over BioNTech's Western blot data submitted to regulators to demonstrate product fidelity.

CHAPTER THIRTEEN

# FAULTY MRNA TECH AND DISPUTED DATA INTEGRITY

*"There is a possibility that aberrant proteins will be expressed with possibilities for unwanted immunological events."*

~European Medicines Agency, internal report, 19 February 2021

In the glow of scientific acclaim, the 2023 Nobel Prize in Physiology or Medicine honored Katalin Karikó and Drew Weissman for their "discoveries concerning nucleoside base modifications that enabled the development of effective mRNA vaccines against COVID-19." Yet, just weeks later, a pivotal *Nature* study by Mulroney et al. shattered the narrative, revealing that the very modification, N1-methylpseudouridine, induces ribosomal frameshifting, spawning aberrant proteins and unintended immune responses. While media outlets swiftly downplayed the findings as a mere "tiny slip" with "no evidence of harm," the implications loom large.

This chapter investigates the "Blotgate" scandal, exposing discrepancies in BioNTech/Pfizer's Western blot submissions to regulators and material that suggests fraudulent looking data for protein expression fidelity. Drawing on leaked EMA documents, expert analyses, and early investigations, it uncovers how known risks of frameshifting were not resolved, raising profound concerns about transparency in one of history's largest medical rollouts.

## From Nobel Acclaim to Frameshifting Fallout

In October 2023, the Nobel Prize in Physiology or Medicine[681] cast a spotlight on Katalin Karikó and Drew Weissman, the pioneering duo whose breakthroughs in modified messenger RNA (modRNA) technology paved the way for humanity's "operation warp speed" response to 3/11. Their innovation, replacing uridine with N1-methylpseudouridine (abbreviated as 1-methylΨ) to disguise synthetic RNA from the body's immune defenses, promised a "revolution in vaccines," noted earlier in chapter 8.

However, just a few months later, that glow dimmed under the weight of a landmark study from Cambridge University by Mulroney et al., published in *Nature*[682] on December 6, 2023.

The findings exposed a subtle, insidious flaw: ribosomal frameshifting during the translation process (triggered by the synthetic 1-methylΨ), resulting in the production of abnormal proteins inducing an "off-target" immune response in the human body.

The study authors appeared to downplay any concerns that the findings might raise, by stating there was "no evidence of adverse outcomes" for the 21 patients vaccinated with the Pfizer-BioNTech shot, of which more than a quarter, experienced an immune response to the abnormal "off-target" proteins.

They went on to state: "These findings are of particular importance to our fundamental understanding of how ribonucleotide modification affects mRNA translation, and for designing and optimizing future mRNA-based therapeutics to avoid mistranslation events that may decrease efficacy or increase toxicity."

Remarkably, the same day the study was published, the BBC[683] described the modified mRNA as "revolutionary technology" that could be "fine-tuned for even greater accuracy" because of its "tiny slip."

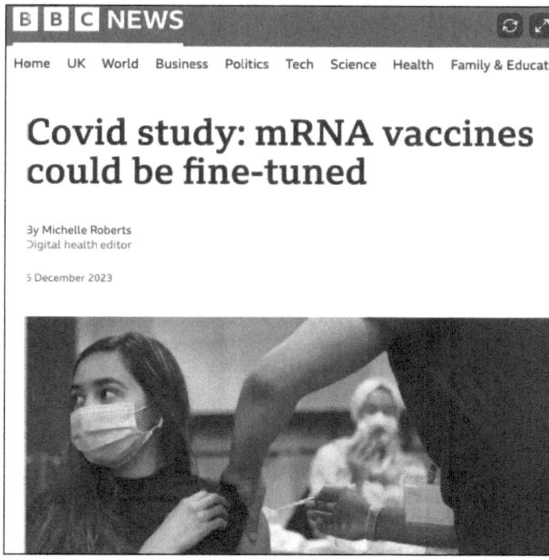
BBC NEWS

Home UK World Business Politics Tech Science Health Family & Educati

# Covid study: mRNA vaccines could be fine-tuned

By Michelle Roberts
Digital health editor

5 December 2023

Science Magazine[684] echoed the line "mRNA vaccines may make unintended proteins, but there's no evidence of harm."

The researchers themselves noted that the effects of modified ribonucleotides "on mRNA translation fidelity have not been fully explored." An accurate admission with serious implications given that these experimental shots had already been injected into 70.6%[685] of the world's population. Even the Cambridge study offers little detail on the "premature polypeptide products" produced from 1-methylΨ-containing mRNAs.

A group of researchers and scientists published[686] a detailed response to the Mulroney et al. paper. An extract from their critique reads: "The premise for the study reveals a developmental and regulatory failure to ask fundamental questions that could affect the safety and effectiveness of these products. This is no better exemplified by Pfizer's retired head of vaccine R&D who was quoted in *Nature* as saying: 'We flew the aeroplane while we were still building it.'"

This leads to my investigation[687] for TrialSite News, published in early 2023, which examined two major anomalies: BioNTech's Western blot submissions to regulators failed to confirm expression of the intended vaccinal spike protein, while analysis by an independent expert of blots submitted to the FDA revealed what they characterized as evidence of potential image duplication across multiple batches and concentrations.

## The "Blotgate" Controversy

Western blots are a standard technique to detect specific proteins, confirming presence, quantity, and size, critical for verifying that modified mRNA expresses only the expected spike protein, not aberrant ones, and that expression is consistent across batches.

BioNTech was aware of ribosomal frameshifting risks from the modified mRNA. They attempted to mitigate it by incorporating multiple stop codons in the development process to try and prevent this from happening but failed to fix the problem. This is discussed in detail later in this chapter, drawing on my March 2023 interview with genomics expert, Kevin McKernan.

Instead of raising red flags, regulators gave the green light to this flawed technology as the foundation for the COVID-19 modified RNA (modRNA) shots. What is particularly damning is that a significant safety risk associated with the modRNA was raised by the European Medicines Agency (EMA) before authorization.

In their leaked November 2020 Rolling Review Report (alongside the internal emails discussed in chapter 10), the EMA raised concerns on page 61[688] about potential autoimmune responses induced by the modRNA:

"The modRNA contains a substitution of 1-methyl-pseudouridine for uridine. This substitution decreases recognition of the vaccine RNA by innate immune sensors. Nevertheless, no further discussion was provided regarding the risk of autoimmune responses induced by the modRNA. The Applicant is invited to further discuss the possibility that the mRNA vaccine can trigger potential autoimmune responses and how does it plan to possibly evaluate their occurrence."

The Rapporteurs noted BioNTech (the applicant) provided "no further discussion" and invited them to address it. It remains unknown whether BioNTech ever evaluated the risk of autoimmune responses from the modified uridine, 1-methylpseudouridine, or translated off-target proteins, by August 2021, the July 2021 deadline had passed, and the issue was still unresolved (see snapshot of page 13 from EMA's CHMP August 2021 report.)

> predominant species should be provided. Any homology between translated proteins (other than the spike protein) and human proteins that may, due to molecular mimicry, potentially cause an autoimmune process should be evaluated. Due date: July 2021. Interim reports: March 2021, and on a monthly basis.

The following excerpt is taken from my 2023 investigative report:[689] "Startling Evidence Suggests BioNTech/Pfizer Falsified Key Data & Further Scandals." It exposes a further alarming revelation from the leaked

Rapporteur's Rolling Review report, in reference to BioNTech's Western Blot submitted to the European Medicines Agency, indicating the presence of other "off-target" proteins, which has risen to prominence because of the Cambridge University Study.

"The following criticisms were made of BioNTech's study 20-0211 "regarding the results obtained from the Western Blot," noted below:

2. In study 20-0211, regarding the results obtained from the Western Blot, a semi quantitative analysis of the results to improve the readability of the protein expression should be provided and in the analysis of the blot, some missing scientific information and explanations should be added by the applicant **(CoRapp 8)**:
   a. The presence of the two bands for BNT162b2 ARN (at 100 KDa and 190 KDa respectively)
   b. The 76.5 kDa bands are not observed in both BNT162b2 nor in S1 control lanes, and the full S protein at 141.14 kDa is also not observed in BNT162b2 lane.
   c. The lack of an important expression for the S1 protein ctrl at 76.5 Kda

Source: Leaked EMA Rapporteur's Rolling Review assessment report (page 61)

In February 2023, the document entitled "R&D DATA REPORT No. R-20-0211"[690] was released as part of the court-ordered trove of Pfizer documents. The highly revealing Western blot from BioNTech's 20-0211 R&D study is exhibited below, which the EMA assessment report criticizes.

BIONTECH

R&D Report R-20-0211 | Version 02 | Page 15 of 22

**4 TABLES AND FIGURES**

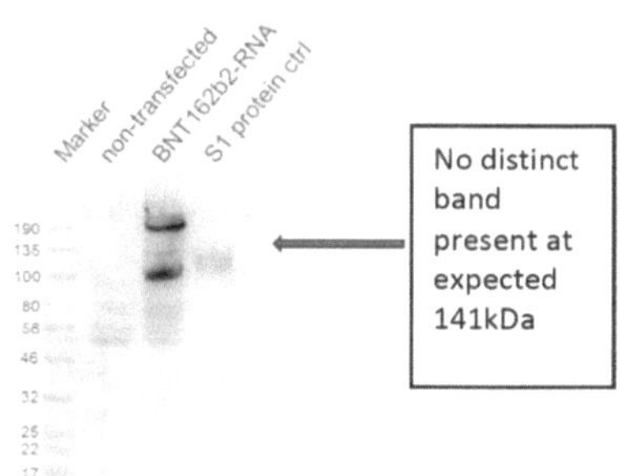


**Figure 1: Western blot analysis for detection of BNT162b2 antigen expression**
Cells were transfected with DS BNT162b2-RNA, and harvested after 18 h to allow antigen expression. Cells were lysed and lysates were subjected to a sodium dodecyl sulfate (SDS)–polyacrylamide gel electrophoresis (PAGE) system using a 4–15% gradient polyacrylamide gel followed by Western blot analysis. BNT162b2 has a predicted size of 141.14 kDa. A recombinant SARS-CoV-2 S1 Subunit protein (76.5 kDa) was used as a positive control.

From the leaked EMA's Rapporteur's Rolling Review Assessment Report (November 2020), it is clear the agency flagged the unexpected molecular weights (measured in kDa) of the two protein bands shown in the

Western Blot test, at approximately 190kDa and 100 kDa. The full spike protein (S1S2) has a predicted molecular weight of ~141 kDa, while the S1 subunit control is ~76.5 kDa.

As the figure shows, no protein bands appear at these expected positions in the BNT162b2 lane, and the S1 control lane also lacks the anticipated 76.5 kDa band. These anomalies prompted the EMA to request an explanation from BioNTech. However, the sponsor's description of the blot was highly inaccurate, in fact, the exact opposite of what the image depicts: "BNT162b2 has a predicted size of 141.14 kDa" and "SARS-CoV-2 S1 subunit protein (76.5 kDa) was used as a positive control."

This discrepancy strongly suggests that the intended S1S2 spike protein may not have been properly expressed by the vaccinal modified mRNA, or that other aberrant proteins were being expressed instead. This raise a critical question: How did the regulator, authorize these experimental modified mRNA shots just weeks later, despite raising such significant concerns in their November 2020 report?"

## Were Copy-and-Pasted Western Blots Submitted to the FDA?

Another troubling anomaly that my investigation exposed was surrounding BioNTech/Pfizer's Western blots submitted[691] to the FDA in response to the agency's queries around November 2020.

COVID-19 Vaccine (BNT162, PF-07302048)
BB-IND 19736
S.2.6 Manufacturing Process Development (modRNA)

**Figure S.2.6-42. BNT162b2 Expressed Protein Size by Western Blot**

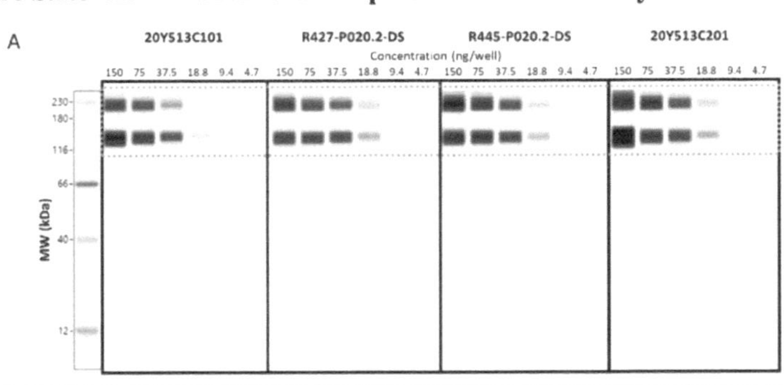


Source: "20-Nov-2020-FDA-Query-Responses," (page 107)

An independent imaging analyst with expertise in Western blot interpretation (who requested anonymity due to professional concerns) conducted software analysis of the band patterns in Pfizer/BioNTech's submitted Western blots. The quantitative analysis revealed what the analyst characterized as highly unusual similarity across bands from four separate batches tested at six different concentrations (see diagram below). The analyst noted that the probability of such identical band patterns occurring naturally across multiple independent batches and concentrations are next to nil.

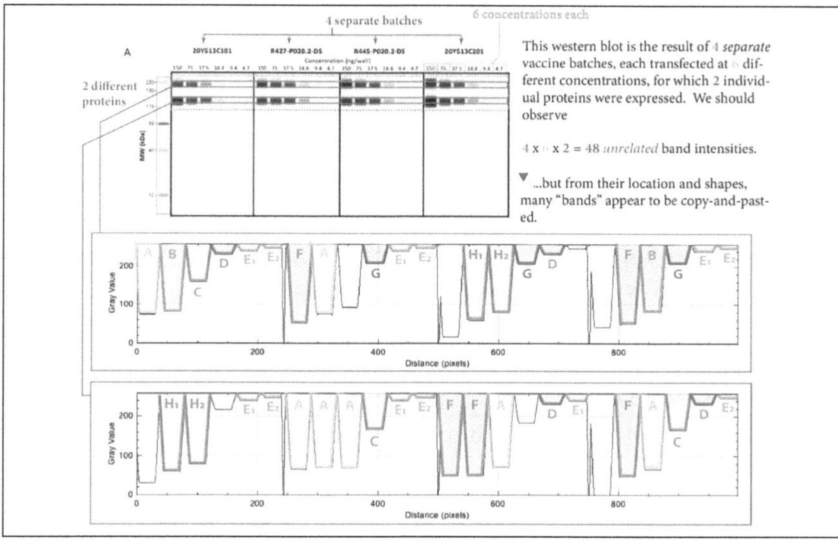


## "BioNTech Knew modRNA Would Skip But Didn't properly Fix It"

In March 2023, as part of my investigation into BioNTech's unusual Western blots, I interviewed[692] genomics scientist Kevin McKernan.

His insights directly connect to the 2023 Cambridge study by Mulroney et al. that exposed ribosomal frameshifting in the modified mRNA. McKernan highlighted the risks of N1-methylpseudouridine (1-methylΨ), the base substitution used in Pfizer/BioNTech's mRNA shots: "We have an mRNA now where every single uridine has been replaced with N1-methylpseudouridine. The body has never seen this before. That means when ribosomes go to read it, they're really confused over what it means."

He referenced the Fernandez at al., [693] 2013 paper on pseudouridine, the closest relative to 1-methylΨ, which showed ribosomes frequently misincorporate amino acids (3 to 10 percent rate in certain positions) and sometimes skip stop codons, causing frameshifting. McKernan explained that BioNTech engineers were aware of this read-through risk and attempted to mitigate it by inserting multiple stop codons. However, the chosen sequences, ΨGAΨGA in Pfizer/BioNTech (instead of UGAUGA) and ΨGAΨAAΨAG in Moderna, were among the most notorious for allowing frameshifting. "They knew it was a problem," he said, "but didn't properly fix it." The Cambridge study later confirmed this failure: N1-methylpseudouridine induces +1 frameshifting, producing off-target proteins.

In a 2021 pre-print[694] co-authored with Dr. Peter McCullough and Anthony Kyriakopoulos ("Differences in Vaccine and SARS-CoV-2 Replication Derived mRNA: Implications for Cell Biology and Future Disease"), McKernan's team flagged related issues: "The use of N1-methylpseudouridine in these mRNAs will further complicate the folding predictions as N1-methylpseudouridine (m1Ψ) has promiscuous base pairing with G and A and is known to create errors in translation."

They also noted pseudouridine's known role in ribosomal frameshifts, with the Pfizer/BioNTech stop codon sequence placing an out-of-frame human amino acid sequence of unknown function immediately upstream. The authors concluded that codon optimization in mRNA vaccines can alter protein conformation, disrupt translation speed and efficiency, and lead to immune dysregulation, epi-transcriptomic effects, and potential disease progression.

While the Cambridge study confirmed production of off-target antigens from frameshifting, it did not address the broader detrimental consequences outlined by McKernan et al., including impaired cellular functions, autoimmune disease, cancer development, and neurological disorders.

## The Regulator Knew Aberrant Proteins Could Trigger Immune Damage

On 19 February 2021, the European Medicines Agency's Committee for Medicinal Products for Human Use (CHMP) recorded the following assessment in its report[695] on the BioNTech/Pfizer mRNA shot (page 35): "Truncated and modified forms of the mRNA are present as impurities...

When present in the cell there is a possibility that aberrant proteins will be expressed with possibilities for unwanted immunological events."

This was not speculation. It was a formal safety concern raised by the Agency's own assessors after Conditional Marketing Authorization was already granted on December 21, 2020. They required the manufacturer to investigate this risk. The manufacturer never did. For some reason, the EMA determined the risk to be "low." Two years later, a landmark study published in *Nature* (Mulroney et al., December 6, 2023) confirmed the regulators' original fear: N1-methylpseudouridine causes ribosomal frameshifting in vivo, leading to production of aberrant proteins and immune responses in a subset of recipients.

• • •

The evidence laid in this chapter: from the EMA's early warnings of aberrant proteins and unwanted immunological events, to the anomalous Western blot data that raised questions among independent analysts, to the unresolved ribosomal frameshifting despite known risks, paints a troubling portrait of modRNA technology rushed to market with fundamental flaws.

However, this is merely the prelude to a deeper betrayal. If the foundational science was compromised and the data potentially manipulated to secure approval, what happened when those same regulators confronted the real-world avalanche of harm?

CHAPTER FOURTEEN

# THE BLIND WATCHDOGS

*" Who will guard the guards themselves?"*

~Juvenal, Satires 6.347–348

Several years have passed since regulators worldwide such as the FDA, MHRA, EMA, and TGA first granted Emergency Use Authorizations or equivalents for the COVID-19 gene-based injections. In that time, safety reporting systems worldwide have recorded a substantial volume of serious adverse events, including deaths, following vaccination with these products. This stands in sharp contrast to the assurances from health authorities and mainstream media that the injections were "safe and effective."

The material detailed in earlier chapters, and expanded upon here, reveals that regulators were aware of certain potential risks and manufacturing issues prior to authorization. This chapter reviews the information available before Emergency Use Authorization, with particular focus on Pfizer's pivotal clinical trials in adults (16+) and adolescents (12–15 years).

It also examines criticisms surrounding post-authorization pharmacovigilance systems, such as VAERS in the United States and EudraVigilance in Europe, and analyzes the manufacturers' own post-EUA safety reports submitted to regulators, which documented harms that emerged quickly and were often assessed as unrelated or not requiring action.

## What They Knew Before Emergency Use Authorization

From late 2021, I began poring over thousands of court-ordered disclosures of Pfizer's confidential documents from their pivotal phase III clinical trial (C4591001) and their non-clinical (animal) studies submitted to the FDA.

What emerged was a glaring pattern of omissions, systematic irregularities, and safety oversights raising serious questions about trial integrity and informed consent. Below, I have summarized key findings from my four-part series for *TrialSite News* published in 2022.

Firstly, my forensic analysis[696] of the Case Report Forms (CRFs), which are the foundational records from trial sites that capture standardized clinical data from each patient including adverse events, uncovered numerous anomalies suggestive of post hoc data modifications. These included conflicting timestamps, incomplete documentation of serious adverse events (SAEs), and evidence of extensive data "cleaning" processes.

These serious findings align with the allegations made by Brook Jackson, former regional director at Ventavia Research Group (a Pfizer trial contractor), who reported to *The BMJ* [697]that "the company falsified data, unblinded patients, employed inadequately trained vaccinators, and was slow to follow up on adverse events reported in Pfizer's pivotal phase III trial." After repeatedly notifying Ventavia of these problems, Jackson emailed a complaint to the FDA on September 25, 2020. Ventavia fired her later the same day.

In March 2022 I interviewed[698] Jackson, who detailed further claims, including: improper vaccine storage, mislabeled lab specimens, fabricated informed consent signatures, and untested potentially COVID-19-positive participants due to supply shortages.

My second report[699] examined Pfizer's confidential "Nonclinical Overview." I exposed the troubling results from the repeat-dose toxicity studies in rats: inflammatory responses (enlarged lymph nodes and spleen), sharply elevated fibrinogen (up to 3.1× control levels, a known clotting risk factor), and massive accumulation of the novel lipid nanoparticles in the liver, with lower but still significant amounts reaching the spleen, adrenal glands, and ovaries. Most alarming to me is that Pfizer explicitly stated it conducted no safety pharmacology studies, no pharmacokinetic studies, and no genotoxicity or carcinogenicity studies, claiming they were "not necessary" under 2005 WHO guidelines for vaccines. However, those same guidelines say such studies should be considered case-by-case when novel adjuvants or excipients are used, and the proprietary lipid nanoparticles (LNPs), ALC-0315 and ALC-0159, are undeniably novel and highly inflammatory.[700]

By February 2021, when this overview was approved, Pfizer and the FDA already had reports of widespread neurological, cardiovascular, and respiratory adverse events, making the decision to skip these critical safety studies even more indefensible in my view. Despite these red flags, the FDA went on to grant full licensure of Comirnaty.

The third report[701] analyzed the 3,611-page "sensitive" Pfizer document "C4591001-fa-interim-narrative-sensitive," released on 1 July 2022, which details hundreds of trial subjects withdrawn due to death, serious adverse events, pregnancy, or other reasons. I found multiple deaths shortly after vaccination: a 56-year-old woman suffered fatal cardiac arrest two months after dose 2 (no autopsy performed), a 60-year-old man died of "atherosclerotic disease" three days after his first dose (condition not listed in his medical history, no autopsy), and a 72-year-old man died after a syncopal episode judged "coincidental" despite unknown cause of death. In every instance, both the investigator and Pfizer ruled out any relation to the vaccine.

Whenever a trial investigator assessed a serious adverse event (such as life-threatening ventricular arrhythmia the same evening after dose 2, or extensive lymphadenopathy deemed "most likely" vaccine-induced by an oncologist) as reasonably possibly related to BNT162b2, Pfizer disagreed with the causality assessment. The following screenshots highlight this.

> In the opinion of the investigator, there was a reasonable possibility that the ventricular arrhythmia was related to the study intervention based on the temporal relationship since the arrhythmias began within 24 hours of Dose 2, but not related to concomitant medications or clinical trial procedures. Pfizer did not concur with the investigator's causality assessment. Additionally, Pfizer commented that there was not enough evidence to establish a causal relationship with the study intervention apart from a chronological association at this time of the report. In absence of evidence for an inflammatory response to study intervention, it was more likely that the ventricular arrhythmia was associated with the subject's underlying known cardiac conditions.

The case narrative for subject #11421247 (a 71-year-old woman) who developed severe, life-threatening ventricular arrhythmia within 24 hours of receiving her second dose of Pfizer's BNT162b2. The trial investigator assessed: "reasonable possibility that the ventricular arrhythmia was related to the study intervention." However, "Pfizer did not concur with the investigator's causality assessment" and commented that there was "not enough evidence to establish causal relationship."

**Compound: PF-07302048; Protocol: C4591001** **Page 38 of 149**
**Reason(s) for Narrative: Related Serious Adverse Event, Safety-Related Subject Withdrawal**
**Unique Subject ID: C4591001 1178 11781107; Country: USA**
**Vaccine Group (as Administered): BNT162b2 (30 μg)**
**Date of First Dose: 04SEP2020; Date of Last Dose: 04SEP2020**

**Narrative Comment**

Subject C4591001 1178 11781107, a 48-year-old white female with a pertinent medical history of drug hypersensitivity to Pitocin, received Dose 1 on 04 Sep 2020 in her left deltoid. The subject was diagnosed with lymphadenopathy on 16 Sep 2020, 12 days after receiving Dose 1.

Concomitant medications reported within 2 weeks before the onset of the event included cetirizine hydrochloride (since 2015) for seasonal allergies, ibuprofen (since 2000) for headache and osteoarthritis, and crisaborole (since 2017) for eczema.

On 04 Sep 2020 (Day 1), approximately 6 hours after Dose 1 administration, the subject reported mild injection site erythema and warmth, and moderate injection site pain. On 05 Sep 2020 (Day 2), she reported mild chills. That same day (Day 2), the injection site erythema, warmth, and chills were considered resolved, and on 06 Sep 2020 (Day 3), the injection site pain resolved. On 21 Sep 2020 (Day 18), the subject called and reported discomfort in her right arm, shoulder, and chest region on 16 Sep 2020 (Day 13), which she described as feeling like a pulled muscle even at rest. She was treated with ibuprofen 400 mg orally as needed starting on 16 Sep 2020. Additionally, the subject reported that she had called her physician, who referred her to the regional hospital emergency room (ER) for further evaluation. On 20 Sep 2020 (Day 17), the subject visited the ER, at which time her right axilla was examined, and a subsequent ultrasound of the right axilla on the same day revealed at least 4 enlarged lymph nodes, largest 2.5 × 1.1 × 2.4 cm. The laboratory results on the same day showed a white blood cell count of 7.0 k/μL (NR: 4.0 - 10.0 k/μL) with 35.2% lymphocytes (normal range [NR]: 20% - 40%), and an absolute lymphocyte count of 2.4 k/μL (NR: 1.0 - 4.0 k/μL). The subject denied any injuries, cuts, or puncture wounds to the right arm or having a similar problem previously. It was reported that no other areas other than the right axilla were assessed for lymphadenopathy. The subject received ketorolac 10 mg intravenously once (on 20 Sep 2020) while in the ER for lymphadenopathy. The lymphadenopathy was considered medically significant by the investigator. The biopsy was completed on 05 Oct 2020 (Day 32) without issue. On 12 Oct 2020, the subject communicated via phone the results of her work-up stating that her blood tests returned to normal and the biopsy showed no markers for lymphoma or other cancer. Per subject report, the oncologist considered the vaccine as the most likely etiology for her lymphadenopathy. A follow-up oncological visit is planned in 3 months with a possible repeat of the axillary ultrasonogram. The medical records have been requested by the investigator.

The subject was discontinued from the study intervention on 25 Sep 2020 because of the lymphadenopathy that was ongoing at the time of the last available report and remains in the study to be evaluated for safety, immunogenicity, and efficacy.

In the opinion of the investigator, there was a reasonable possibility that the lymphadenopathy was related to the study intervention. Pfizer did not concur with the investigator's causality assessment.

The case narrative report for subject #11781107 (a 48-year-old woman) who developed extensive lymphadenopathy with at least 4 enlarged lymph nodes after her first dose of BNT162b2. The treating hospital oncologist stated: "most likely etiology is the Pfizer vaccine." The trial site investigator opined: "reasonable possibility that the lymphadenopathy was related to the study intervention." But "Pfizer did not concur with the investigator's causality assessment" even when the cancer specialist and Pfizer's own site investigator pointed to the vaccine, the company simply overruled them.

I also found several women who became pregnant after their first dose and were withdrawn from vaccination but supposedly kept in follow-up; given prior whistle-blower revelations of protocol violations at Ventavia sites, it is unclear if these pregnancies were ever properly monitored.

Furthermore, I documented two previously healthy women suffering from cerebrovascular accidents (strokes) approximately one month after their second dose, again unanimously declared as "unrelated" by Pfizer and the trial investigators. The following screenshot shows the case report narrative of one of the women.

**Narrative Comment**

Subject C4591001 1021 10211190, a 66-year-old white female with no pertinent medical history, received Dose 1 on 10 Sep 2020 and Dose 2 on 01 Oct 2020 (Day 22). The subject was diagnosed with a cerebrovascular accident on 02 Nov 2020, 32 days after receiving Dose 2.

Concomitant medications reported within 2 weeks prior to the onset of the cerebrovascular accident included ranitidine hydrochloride and calcium carbonate (both since 2018) for gastrointestinal reflux disease.

On 02 Nov 2020 (Day 54), the subject presented to the emergency room and was subsequently hospitalized because of a cerebrovascular accident. Relevant tests were unknown. It was unknown whether a COVID-19 test was performed during the hospital stay. The subject remained hospitalized at the time of this report and the discharge information was not available.

The cerebrovascular accident was ongoing at the time of the last available report.

In the opinion of the investigator, there was no reasonable possibility that the cerebrovascular accident was related to the study intervention, concomitant medications, or clinical trial procedures. Pfizer concurred with the investigator's causality assessment.

The narrative comment for subject #102110211190 (a healthy 66-year-old woman with no pertinent medical history) reveals she suffered a cerebrovascular accident (stroke) 32 days after her second Pfizer dose. She remained hospitalized with no discharge date at the time of the report. Both the trial investigator and Pfizer declared: "no reasonable possibility" the stroke was related to the vaccine or trial procedures.

Cerebrovascular accidents were listed as an Adverse Events of Special Interest in Pfizer's own post-marketing safety documents (later discussed in this chapter) yet causality was dismissed without investigation.

## The Missing Third Death

In my fourth *TrialSite News*[702] investigative report (published in July 2022), I exposed what is, in my opinion, by far the most damning discovery to emerge from the entire court-ordered release of Pfizer documents: the missing third death not included in the pivotal *New England Journal of Medicine* paper by Polack et al.[703] (published December 10, 2020, one day before the FDA's emergency authorization). The data cutoff date for the interim analysis in the paper is October 9, 2020.

The paper stated: "Two BNT162b2 recipients died (one from arterio-sclerosis, one from cardiac arrest)" from the vaccine trial arm.

These two deaths included: subject #11621327 (a 60-year-old male who received his first (and only) dose of BNT162b2 on September 10. 2020.

**Compound: PF-07302048; Protocol: C4591001**
**Reason(s) for Narrative: Death**
**Unique Subject ID: C4591001 1162 11621327; Country: USA**
**Vaccine Group (as Administered): BNT162b2 (30 µg)**
**Date of First Dose: 10SEP2020; Date of Last Dose: 10SEP2020**

He was found dead at home three days later during a police welfare check. The medical examiner attributed the death to progression of atherosclerotic disease (with no autopsy performed), both the trial investigator and Pfizer ruled it unrelated to the vaccine.

The authors also included a later fatal event, explicitly reporting the death of subject # 10071101, a 56-year-old female who received two doses of BNT162b2 on the following dates: July 30 and August 20, 2020.

**Compound: PF-07302048; Protocol: C4591001**
**Reason(s) for Narrative: Death**
**Unique Subject ID: C4591001 1007 10071101; Country: USA**
**Vaccine Group (as Administered): BNT162b2 (30 µg)**
**Date of First Dose: 30JUL2020; Date of Last Dose: 20AUG2020**

She died two months later from cardiac arrest on October 21, 2020. The narrative comment reads: "In the opinion of the investigator, there was no reasonable possibility that the cardiac arrest was related to the study intervention of clinical trial procedures, as the death occurred 2 months after receiving Dose 2. Pfizer concurred with the investigator's causality assessment."

However, there was also a third death that I found, which was shockingly left out of the *NEJM* paper. The death of subject #11521497 (a 72-year-old male) who received his first (and last dose) on October 7, 2020 was admitted to hospital on October 26 after he had "fainted in the middle of the night" and was confirmed dead by his sister on November 11, 2020.

**Narrative Comment**

Subject C4591001 1152 11521497, a 72-year-old white male with a pertinent medical history of type 2 diabetes mellitus (since 2010) and hypertension (since 2018), received Dose 1 on 07 Oct 2020. The subject reported syncope on 26 Oct 2020, 19 days after receiving Dose 1.

Concomitant medications reported within 2 weeks prior to the onset of syncope included metformin (since 2013) for diabetes, ibuprofen (since 2015) for osteoarthritis, lisinopril (since 2018) for hypertension, and doxazosin (since 2019) for benign prostatic hypertrophy.

The subject missed Visit 2 on 28 Oct 2020 (Day 22). On 06 Nov 2020 (Day 31), it was reported that the subject was admitted to the hospital on 26 Oct 2020 (Day 20) since he fainted in the middle of the night. The subject was transferred to the intensive care unit. Family medical history relevant to the syncope was unknown. The subject tested negative for COVID-19 at the hospital. On an unspecified date, the syncope resolved and the subject was discharged from the hospital.

The subject was discontinued from the study intervention on 06 Nov 2020 and remains in the study to be evaluated for safety, immunogenicity, and efficacy.

During the follow-up, the site contacted the subject's sister, who confirmed that the subject died on 11 Nov 2020. The cause of death was reported as unknown. It was not reported if an autopsy was performed. A death certificate might be available at a later date.

In the opinion of the investigator, there was no reasonable possibility that the syncope was related to the study intervention, concomitant medications, or clinical trial procedures. Pfizer concurred with the investigator's causality assessment. Per Pfizer, the syncope was most likely coincidental and associated with underlying clinical conditions.

**PFIZER CONFIDENTIAL SDTM Creation: 17NOV2020 (10:49) Source Data: dm, vs, mh, ex, ae, cm, ds Output File: ./nda2_unblinded/C4591001_SNAP_2MPD2_Safety_Narratives/profile Date of Generation: 20NOV2020 (21:12)**

The third vaccinated death would have been known to Pfizer and the paper's authors before publication, yet it was not even recorded as a death in Pfizer's own files, instead it was somehow classified as "Safety-Related Subject Withdrawal."

Could this be the reason this death got omitted? If so, how many other deaths slipped under the radar because they were similarly misclassified?

**Compound: PF-07302048; Protocol: C4591001**
**Reason(s) for Narrative: Safety-Related Subject Withdrawal**
**Unique Subject ID: C4591001 1152 11521497; Country: USA**
**Vaccine Group (as Administered): BNT162b2 (30 µg)**
**Date of First Dose: 07OCT2020; Date of Last Dose: 07OCT2020**

Some might argue the third death was omitted because it occurred after the October 9 cutoff. However, the authors included the October 21 cardiac-arrest death of Subject #10071101, also a post-cutoff event. This inconsistency in applying the data cutoff has led independent analysts to question whether the reporting criteria were applied uniformly. Whether this represents different interpretations of what constitutes reportable post-cutoff data, the misclassification of subject #11521497's death as "Safety-Related Subject Withdrawal," or selective disclosure, remains a matter of ongoing scrutiny and debate.

**Compound: PF-07302048; Protocol: C4591001** **Page 4 of 149**
**Reason(s) for Narrative: Death**
**Unique Subject ID: C4591001 1007 10071101; Country: USA**
**Vaccine Group (as Administered): BNT162b2 (30 µg)**
**Date of First Dose: 30JUL2020; Date of Last Dose: 20AUG2020**

**Study Vaccination(s)**

| Vaccination Number | Vaccine | Vaccination Date (Study Day) | Time of Vaccination |
|---|---|---|---|
| 1 | BNT162b2 | 30JUL2020 (1) | 13:11 |
| 2 | BNT162b2 | 20AUG2020 (22) | 11:45 |

**Adverse Events**

| AE Number | MedDRA SOC | MedDRA Preferred Term | Investigator Text | Start Date (Study Day) | Start Time | Stop Date (Study Day) | Stop Time | Duration (Days) | Toxicity Grade | Action to Subject | SAE |
|---|---|---|---|---|---|---|---|---|---|---|---|
| 1 | CARD | Cardiac arrest | Cardiac Arrest | 18OCT2020 (81) | | 21OCT2020 (84) | | 4 | 4 | W | Y |

**Adverse Events**

| AE Number | AE Still Present? | AE Related To: | Prior Vaccination Number | Relative Day From Prior Vaccination | Narrative Event |
|---|---|---|---|---|---|
| 1 | Fatal (21OCT2020) | NOT RELATED/OTHER: Heart attack. Occurred 2 months after last receipt of study agent | 2 | 60 | Y |

As a direct consequence: the single publication that convinced regulators and the world the vaccine was safe reported only "two deaths" in the vaccine arm instead of three, artificially cutting the disclosed vaccine-recipient mortality figure by 50% at the most critical moment. Coupled with the paper's claim of only four "related" serious adverse events while Pfizer's internal records list dozens of post-cutoff heart attacks, strokes, pulmonary embolisms and other grave conditions, all uniformly dismissed as unrelated. These findings demonstrate that the safety data presented in the RN article was knowingly and materially incomplete compared with what Pfizer held at the time of publication.

## The Smoking Gun: FDA's October 2020 Slide

During the FDA's Vaccines and Related Biological Products Advisory Committee (VRBPAC) meeting on October 22, 2020, a startling slide on vaccine safety grabbed my attention, prompting me to write a report for *TrialSite News*[704] entitled, "The FDA's 'smoking gun' presentation slide from October 2020." It lay bare the undeniable truth: the regulator knew about the harms of the experimental mRNA shots before authorization.

On August 23, 2021, the U.S. Food and Drug Administration (FDA) granted approval[705] (or licensure) to the first ever COVID-19 mRNA gene therapy product by Pfizer/BioNTech, which from the onset was misbranded as a "vaccine."

The Acting FDA Commissioner Janet Woodcock, M.D., said at the time: "The FDA's approval of this vaccine is a milestone as we continue to battle the COVID-19 pandemic. While this and other vaccines have met the FDA's rigorous, scientific standards for emergency use authorization, as the first FDA-approved COVID-19 vaccine, the public can be very confident that this vaccine meets the high standards for safety, effectiveness, and manufacturing quality the FDA requires of an approved product." The very next day, the U.S. Defense Secretary, Lloyd Austin, issued a memorandum mandating the COVID-19 vaccine for all military service members.

Woodcock's claim that the Pfizer/BioNTech mRNA vaccine met "the FDA's rigorous, scientific standards for Emergency Use Authorization," granted on December 11, 2020, is paradoxical considering the less stringent nature of the EUA process. For instance, in times of a public health emergency or crisis, investigational medical countermeasures can be authorized under an Emergency Use Authorization (EUA) mechanism without complete clinical trial data. In addition, the FDA can grant an EUA of an investigational vaccine on the vague notion that it may be effective and that its known, potential benefits outweigh the known, potential risks.

In the lead-up to the EUA, a public meeting[706] of the FDA's Vaccines and Related Biological Products Advisory Committee (VRBPAC) was convened on October 22, 2020, to deliberate on the "development, authorization, and/or licensure of vaccines intended to prevent COVID-19."

Ironically, Phase III COVID-19 vaccine trials were never designed[707] to prevent transmission of COVID-19 or measure reductions in serious outcomes, like hospitalizations and death. This critical aspect was completely overlooked in the FDA's deliberations. From the start of the COVID-19 vaccine rollout, government officials, public health authorities, and mainstream media engaged in a concerted effort to disseminate misinformation by claiming that COVID-19 vaccines "stop the spread," despite them never being designed to prevent transmission.

At the October 22 VRBPAC meeting, Dr. Peter Marks, then the FDA Chief of the Center for Biologics Evaluation and Research, chose to remain silent on that issue. However, four years later, during the February 15, 2024, congressional hearing[708] of the Select Subcommittee on the Coronavirus Pandemic, Dr. Marks confessed when queried by Rep. Michael Cloud about whether the "COVID-19 vaccines stop transmission," he acknowledged, "it does not absolutely prevent transmission."

Another striking anomaly emerged during the 9-hour meeting: the brief glimpse of a bombshell FDA vaccine safety slide that seemed to go unnoticed. This damning slide, which flashed for just a moment, was part of Steven Anderson's presentation, the FDA's Director of the Office of Biostatistics and Pharmacovigilance (OBPV), on the Center of Biologics Evaluation and Research (CBER)'s plans for monitoring COVID-19 vaccine safety and effectiveness.

At the 2:33:40 mark in the proceedings, the "FDA Safety Surveillance of COVID-19 Vaccines" slide flashed on screen for a second. This single slide contained the FDA's own working list of the most severe adverse events they expected the vaccines to cause: Guillain-Barré syndrome, acute disseminated encephalomyelitis, myocarditis/pericarditis, thrombocytopenia, anaphylaxis, stroke, convulsions, and death.

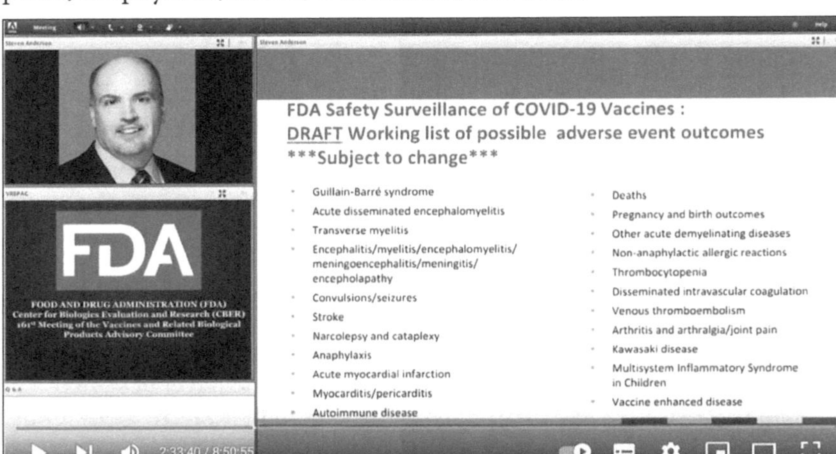


Source: Public meeting[709] of FDA's Vaccines and Related Biological Products Advisory Committee (VRBPAC) on October 22, 2020

The only reference made to the slide is when Anderson states, "Tom [Tom Shimabukuro] has a list of possible adverse outcomes of interest. I won't dwell on this.." And dwell he did not. The slide's brief flicker on screen underscored that the Director of the Office of Biostatistics and Pharmacovigilance at the FDA had zero intention of unpacking this inconvenient slide, opting instead to brush it aside entirely.

The fact that this extensive list of possible adverse events (AEs) "*subject to change*," was already in the FDA's crosshairs some two months prior to the EUA green light is a damning revelation. Equally troubling is the deliberate exclusion of the qualifier "serious" before "adverse event," given that every item on the list qualifies as such. Moreover, none of these prospective serious adverse events, apart from anaphylaxis, found their way into the initial package inserts for the investigational products.

The public disclosure of the myocarditis (inflammation of the heart muscle) and pericarditis (inflammation of the heart's outer lining) risk to young adolescent males did not emerge until April 2021,[710] several months after the mRNA shots had already been rolled out. Even more alarming is the FDA's decision to extend authorization of these experimental injections to individuals aged 12 through 15, a mere month later, on May 10, 2021, despite this known risk, as well as the agency's own presentation slide flagging "myocarditis/pericarditis" as far back as October 2020.

## Maddie de Garay: The Adolescent Trial's Hidden Victim

1,131 children aged 12–15-years-old were enrolled in Pfizer's adolescent clinical trial of their mRNA-based Covid shot. Maddie de Garay was a trial participant and aged twelve at the time. In December 2021, I had the opportunity of interviewing Stephanie de Garay, Maddie's mother for *TrialSite News*.[711] She shared her daughter's heart-breaking story of life-altering vaccine injuries, such as paralysis, seizures, severe vision impairment, tinnitus, mobility issues, blood in her urine, and needing a feeding tube.

Within 24 hours of receiving the second dose in early January 2021, Maddie experienced "zapping pain up and down her spine with severe abdominal pain...her toes and fingers turned white and were ice cold.." Maddie later cried out "Mum, it feels like my heart is being ripped out of my chest!"

After receiving a call back from Pfizer's adolescent trial hotline, Maddie's parents were told to send their daughter to the same hospital where the trial was being run, Cincinnati Children's Hospital. Even though it was obvious to Maddie's parents that she was suffering from adverse effects to the vaccine, the hospital ran tests for a suspected appendicitis and sent her home after having confirmation that there were no signs of a ruptured appendix. None of the tests that they should have done early on were carried out, Stephanie explained.

Between January-April 2021, Maddie went to the ER nine times. "It got to the point where we were not welcome anymore."

The de Garays asked Dr. Robert W. Frenck, principal investigator of Pfizer's adolescent trial and an infectious disease doctor at Cincinnati Children's hospital, whether he reported Maddie's case to VAERS. He said, "No, we report directly to Pfizer, the sponsor, and they report to the FDA."

When pressed on what symptoms were reported to Pfizer, he responded: "all of them" but avoided answering any further when Maddie's parents asked him for the specific list. From looking at Pfizer's EUA submission to the FDA, Maddie's case was shockingly downplayed as "functional abdominal pain, which is not even touching everything that's happened to her," Stephanie shared.

The following is an excerpt from the interview:

Stephanie de Garay: She [Maddie] had her MRI of her spine, that was March [2021], the middle of March. Ironically, it was the day before the data cut-off for the trial. And they had moved up her MRI. And she was in the hospital then. She was discharged the data cut off day for the trial for the 12- to 15-year-olds.

Sonia Elijah: Do you think that is significant?

Stephanie de Garay: I think it's kind of coincidental. They moved up her MRI it was scheduled for later.

Sonia Elijah: So, they discharged her the same day. Do you think they would classify her then as recovered, the fact that she was discharged, so she's not in the serious case category?

Stephanie de Garay: So, they put it as "functional abdominal pain." Basically, a stomach-ache and never mentioned that she couldn't walk. And then it said, they were still investigating.

Sonia Elijah: When you're saying, this is what they said, if you could clarify- this is on Pfizer's report of her?

Stephanie de Garay: Yeah

Sonia Elijah: Right, which you're able to see online?

Stephanie de Garay: Yes

Sonia Elijah: So, they've classified Maddie as just having, and you've described a whole array of symptoms, but they have just classified her as having functional abdominal pain, which is essentially a stomach-ache.

Stephanie de Garay: Right and neuralgia, which is the pins and needles or the numbness.

Sonia Elijah: How would they explain the seizures, the neurological?

Stephanie de Garay: They didn't. None of that was in there. And the seizures got really bad after that.

Later in May, Pfizer's principal investigator, Dr. Frenck, told Stephanie that the hospital doctors had informed him that nothing that Maddie was experiencing was "related to the vaccine."

The same month, the FDA extended EUA of the Pfizer/BioNTech's Covid shot to 12-15-year-olds and the pivotal report,[712] "Safety, Immunogenicity, and Efficacy of the BNT162b2 COVID-19 Vaccine in Adolescents" was published in *The New England Journal of Medicine.*

It was the primary publication reporting results from Pfizer-BioNTech's Phase III clinical trial, evaluating their mRNA COVID-19 shot, specifically in adolescents aged 12–15 years. It should be noted that Dr. Frenck was the lead author and would have been responsible for writing the results of the study which stated: "There were no vaccine-related serious adverse events."

## Post-Marketing Signals They Ignored

The FDA's "DRAFT working list of possible adverse event outcomes" that flashed on screen for mere seconds in October 2020, has proved to be chillingly prophetic. The true horror, however, is how rapidly the list grew once the injections were rolled out.

My 2021 analysis[713] of Pfizer's own post-marketing document,[714] "Cumulative Analysis of Post-Authorization Adverse Event Reports of PF-07302048 (BNT162B2) received through 28 February 2021," finalized on April 30, 2021 and quietly delivered to the FDA, recorded 42,086 case reports containing 158,893 adverse events in the first ninety days alone. Among them were 1,223 fatalities. Attached was an eight-page appendix titled "List of Adverse Events of Special Interest," a catalogue of conditions ranging from myocarditis and anaphylaxis to stroke, miscarriage, and acute kidney injury. Every serious outcome the FDA had privately flagged six months earlier was already appearing in real-world data, in volume, and within weeks of authorization.

This document only became publicly available thanks to a Freedom of Information Act (FOIA) release with the request filed on August 27, 2021, to access all the Pfizer documentation that the FDA relied on to approve Pfizer-BioNTech COVID-19 vaccine for individuals 16 years of age and older on August 23. It took the FDA though three months to release the first 91 redacted pages, on November 20.

The FOIA request was issued by a group of over 30 scientists and academics (Public Health and Medical Professionals for Transparency, PHMPT) who filed a civil action lawsuit[715] against the agency because they failed to fully comply with the request, since less than one percent of the documentation was released and with the FDA taking the position that all the data would be shared by 2076. Subsequently, the governmental agency had the audacity to push the date back even further to 2096. This was due to their disclosure of the existence of thousands of additional pages, totaling 451,000 versus the originally stated 320,000 pages.

It is interesting to note that Pfizer's post-marketing document represents an amended analysis provided by the company, a response to their failings associated with the incomplete submittal of a safety data package to the FDA, which the agency commented on.

A reference is made to the FDA's March 9, 2021 request to Pfizer "We are most interested in a cumulative analysis of post-authorization safety data to support your future BLA submission. Please submit an integrated analysis of your cumulative post-authorization safety data, including U.S. and foreign post-authorization experience, in your upcoming BLA submission. Please include a cumulative analysis of the Important Identified Risks, Important Potential Risks, and areas of Important Missing Information identified in your Pharmacovigilance Plan, as well as adverse events of special interest and vaccine administration errors (whether or not associated with an adverse event). Please also include distribution data and an analysis of the most common adverse events. In addition, please submit your updated Pharmacovigilance Plan with your BLA submission."

## The Many Unknowns

In the short three-month period in which the data was "reported spontaneously to Pfizer," 42,086 cases were recorded with 158,893 events.

According to the data, one can interpret that the average person (case) would have suffered from just under four symptoms (events). Particularly troubling, the FDA opted to protect Pfizer's interests by redacting the total number of doses to (b) (4), hindering the ability to calculate the incidence rates and provide a meaningful analysis of the data. Another deeply concerning fact centers on important limitations cited by Pfizer: "the magnitude of underreporting is unknown."

In relation to this topic, investigators leading a prominent Harvard study[716] conducted from 2007-2010, discovered that "less than 0.3% of all adverse drug events and 1-13% of serious events are reported to the FDA." Assuming this math is correct, we can conclude that the 42,086 cases represent a staggeringly underreported amount.

Other significant "unknowns" peppered throughout Pfizer's analysis are:

- 2990 cases where the gender is unknown
- 6876 cases where the age is unknown
- 9440 cases where the outcomes are unknown

Another anomaly that stands out is that for case outcomes, Pfizer has chosen to include those recovering from adverse events in the same category with those recovered, under the label, "Recovered/Recovering." This move alone seems questionable.

## The Large Numbers of Spontaneous Adverse Event Reports

Alarmingly, the analysis makes note of the fact that there has been such a large volume of adverse events, classified as "serious cases" in that short period of time, that Pfizer has had to take on more full-time employees and make significant technology changes to cope with the processing of the voluminous reports while also meeting regulatory reporting timelines. As recorded in the document:

"Due to the large numbers of spontaneous adverse event reports received for the product, the MAH has prioritized the processing of serious cases, to meet expedited regulatory reporting timelines and ensure these reports are available for signal detection and evaluation activity." The report went on to state how Pfizer has dealt with these large numbers of adverse event reports. "Pfizer has also taken multiple actions to help alleviate the large increase of adverse event reports. This includes significant technology enhancements, and process and workflow solutions, as well as increasing the number of data entry and case processing colleagues. To date, Pfizer has onboarded additional (b4) full-time employees (FTEs)..." (*b4 is a redacted term)

## The 1228 Deaths in the First Three Months

Within Pfizer's self-generated document, a serious red flag surfaces: 1228 people were recorded to have died within three months after taking the vaccine, while no record accounts for the gender of the study participants who died. This data, which has significant safety implications, was known to Pfizer by the end of February 2021, yet on April 12, Dr. Mace Rothenberg, Pfizer's former Chief Medical Officer, when talking to the Washington Journal about the development of the Pfizer vaccine said "I can tell you that no corners were cut" and "there have been no deaths that have occurred directly as a result of the vaccine alone."

Those defending the safety of the Pfizer vaccine have raised the argument that "correlation does not imply causation, in which two events occurring together does not establish a cause-and-effect relationship."

Page 10 of the Pfizer analysis presents an important identified risk of anaphylaxis with nine reported fatalities. Four out of the nine occurred on the same day the individuals were vaccinated. Pfizer emphasized that these individuals had underlying medical conditions, but for all four of them to die on the same day that they received the vaccine, suggests potential vaccinal death causality.

In Table 7 of pages 16-17, 1403 cases of Cardiovascular AESIs (Adverse Event of Specific Interest) were reported and segmented by the following: arrhythmia; cardiac failure; cardiac failure acute; cardiogenic shock; coronary artery disease; myocardial infarction; postural orthostatic tachycardia syndrome; stress cardiomyopathy; tachycardia.

The relevant event onset latency ranged from less than 24 hours to 21 days. This means that relevant events occurred from any time less than 24 hours up to 21 days of receiving the vaccine, with a median of less than 24 hours. 136 relevant event outcomes were fatal. Therefore, 50 percent of these relevant outcomes (including deaths) occurred less than 24 hours after receiving the vaccine. A temporal pattern that independent safety analysts have characterized as warranting investigation for potential causal relationship.

However, Pfizer concludes: "This cumulative case review does not raise any new safety issues. Surveillance will continue."

## Women Were More Affected & The Missing Information

Across the board, in every category of AESI (adverse events of special interest), women were generally three times more adversely affected than men. However, nowhere was this as pronounced as in the case of anaphylaxis (a potentially life-threatening allergic reaction), where women were over eight times more affected.

Out of the 1002 anaphylaxis cases reported meeting the Brighton Collaboration level of 1-4 (level 1 being the highest level of diagnostic certainty of anaphylaxis) 876 females were affected compared to 106 males. Women were also significantly more affected by cardiovascular events; 1076 females were reported as cases compared to 291 males. The statistically significant data reveals the real possibility of gender-specific vaccine safety risks. Yet nowhere in Pfizer's analysis does the company comment on this data, but instead confidently reasserts, "the cumulative case review does not raise any new safety issues."

Also noteworthy, the data associated with the "Use in pregnancy and lactation" were somehow excluded in the original analysis submitted to the FDA. In the amended version, 413 adverse cases are reported with 84 classified as serious.

Pregnancy outcomes for the 270 pregnancies were reported as spontaneous abortion (23), outcome pending (5), premature birth with neonatal death, spontaneous abortion with intrauterine death (2 each), spontaneous abortion with neonatal death, and normal outcome (1 each).

It is alarming that Pfizer makes the assertion that "there were no safety signals that emerged from the review of these cases of use in pregnancy and while breastfeeding." The data contained in the heavily redacted document appears to contradict this upbeat assessment.

In pediatric individuals < 12 years of age, which was originally missing from Pfizer's analysis, 34 cases were reported with 24 categorized as serious. The fact young children were administered the Pfizer vaccine raises concern since emergency use authorization was not awarded to the company to administer to the pediatric population at that time. Moreover, the age range raised considerable alarm given its "from 2 months to 9 years." The report lacks data on how many children in total were administered the vaccine, hence, there is no way of calculating incidence rates to extrapolate a meaningful analysis.

A thorough review of this one report suggests that the FDA and Pfizer have appeared to conceal the full extent of the Pfizer-BioNTech vaccine side effects from the public—throwing informed consent out the window.

It's a travesty that months later, the FDA dragged its feet and released this important safety document based on adverse event case reports under FOIA law. Case reports play an important role in pharmacovigilance. The recognition of the link between thalidomide given to mothers and malformations in their babies was triggered by a case report.

## Pfizer's Pregnancy and Lactation Cumulative Review

In April 2023, I was among the first to uncover[717] and publicize[718] another damning Pfizer document that had been withheld by the FDA: the Pregnancy and Lactation Cumulative Review.[719] This critical document was signed off on April 20, 2021, just as global health authorities began aggressively promoting COVID-19 shots for pregnant and lactating women.

The report is a cumulative review and summary of relevant (pregnancy and lactating) cases reported in Pfizer's pharmacovigilance (safety) databases from the time of drug development through to February 28, 2021. It contains disturbing data.

673 individual case reports were identified in total: 458 cases involved vaccine exposure during pregnancy (mother/fetus) and 215 cases involved exposure during breast feeding. Out of the 458 pregnancy cases, 248 (more than half) reported adverse events, see screenshot below.

> Among the remaining 248 cases, the most commonly reported AEs were product use issue (83), off-label use (81), pain (including but not limited to vaccination site pain/pain/pain in extremity)(101), headache (57), abortion spontaneous (51), fatigue (43), pyrexia (26), chills (24), myalgia (23), nausea (22), arthralgia (16), dizziness (15), malaise (12), lymphadenopathy (11) and asthenia (11).

Of the 458 cases involving vaccine exposure during pregnancy, 51 events were reported for spontaneous abortion (miscarriage), abortion (1 event) and abortion missed (1 event).

BNT162b2
Cumulative Review from Pharmacovigilance Database

- There were 53 reports of spontaneous abortion (51)/ abortion (1)/ abortion missed (1) following BNT162b2 vaccination. Of these reports, 4 cases were COVID-19 positive (including suspected), and 13 cases had relevant medical history of endometriosis (1), abortion spontaneous (10), polycystic ovaries (1), menstruation irregular (1). These cases were therefore excluded from the review. One patient had a medical history of COVID-19 (unknown if ongoing) and was excluded from the review. The remaining 39 cases are summarized in Table 1.

According to Pfizer, 53 reports of spontaneous abortion were noted but four cases were excluded from the review because of COVID-19 (included suspected) and 13 cases were further excluded because of the women's medical history. There was one patient who had a medical history of COVID-19 and was also excluded. This should leave 35 remaining cases but Pfizer erroneously writes, "the remaining 39 cases are summarized.." Of the "39" cases that were reviewed, 38 were actually listed. Another reporting error, perhaps?

What immediately stands out (where gestational age was known) that all the pregnant women in those cases experienced a miscarriage in their first trimester.

A further six disturbing cases out of the 458, involved babies being exposed to the vaccine "via transplacental route," leading to premature delivery. Their cases are described in the following screenshot.

- AER 2021166927 Baby report of fetal tachycardia noted 1 week after the neonate's mother received the second dose of the vaccine. The baby was delivered at 35 weeks and 3 days of gestation due to non-reassuring status during monitoring post vaccination. The baby was hospitalized for 5 days. The clinical outcome of fetal tachycardia was unknown.
- AER 2021015910 Maternal report of a 29-year old female who was pregnant when receiving BNT162B2. She had spontaneous rupture of membranes at 36 weeks of gestation, one day after her 2nd dose of vaccine. Unspecified therapeutic measures were taken as a result of premature rupture of membranes and the mother was recovering.
- AER 2021191405 Baby case of a fetus of unspecified gender who received BNT162B2 transplacentally. The patient's mother received vaccination during the second trimester (13-28 weeks) and experienced premature labor. A live infant was delivered but passed away a day later. Cause of death was cited as extreme prematurity with severe respiratory distress and pneumothorax.
- AER 2021182609 Maternal report (AER 2021193635 associated Baby report) of a 32-year-old female patient received BNT162B2 during the second-trimester (13-28 weeks) and experienced preterm premature rupture of membranes, premature baby/Premature delivery. Outcome of preterm premature rupture of membranes and premature delivery was recovered with sequelae. Concomitant medications included acetylsalicylic acid and dalteparin sodium.
- AER 2021155967 Baby report: A neonate patient's mother (mother was reported as 37-year-old) received BNT162B2 during 13-28 weeks of gestation and experienced foetal exposure during pregnancy, premature baby less than 26 weeks, respiratory distress and pneumothorax. Cause of death for the neonate was premature baby less than 26 weeks and severe respiratory distress and pneumothorax.
- AER 2021203938 Baby report: Patient's 33-year old mother had preterm delivery at 24 weeks and 2 days via emergency caesarean section. The fetus experienced maternal exposure during pregnancy via transplacental route on an unspecified date.

CONFIDENTIAL
Page 3

FDA-CBER-2021-5683-0779747

In two of the premature delivery cases, the babies died because of severe respiratory distress and pneumothorax. Both the mothers received the Pfizer-BioNTech mRNA vaccine in their second trimester. In another shocking case, a baby developed fetal tachycardia (heart rate over 160 beats per minute) where "the clinical outcome of the fetal tachycardia was unknown."

This bombshell real-world evidence was known back in early 2021 by the FDA and Pfizer/BioNTech. Just before the big push to get pregnant women vaccinated, it showed significant safety risks to the fetus due to indirect (transplacental) exposure of the Pfizer-BioNTech mRNA vaccine, with spontaneous abortion (miscarriage) being one of the known outcomes.

In regard to the lactation cases: 41 (~20%) of the 215 cases reported adverse events in infants indirectly exposed to the vaccine via the trans-mammary route (through breast milk). The extensive list of adverse events reported in breast feeding infants, range from facial paralysis, lymphadenopathy and blurred vision.

A study by Hanna et al.,[720] published in JAMA Pediatrics in September 2022, revealed that researchers found trace amounts of the COVID-19 vaccine mRNA in the breast milk of lactating women, as soon as one hour after vaccination. They went on to state, "We speculate that, following the vaccine administration, lipid nanoparticles containing the vaccine mRNA are carried to mammary glands via hematogenous and/or lymphatic routes."

However, this vitally important information was already known for some time by Pfizer/BioNTech, since it was observed in real-world data from their own review and signed off by the FDA on April 20, 2021, where 3 days later the CDC began recommending[721] it for pregnant women.

## The V-Safe Text Data Hidden By the CDC

Returning to the October 2020 FDA meeting, another key speaker was Dr. Tom Shimabukuro from the CDC's COVID-19 Vaccine Task Force (referred to later by Anderson), who addressed the group on the CDC post-authorization/post-licensure safety monitoring. This included the use of Vaccine Adverse Event Reporting System (VAERS), Vaccine Safety Data link (VSD) and the launch of the new V-safe program.

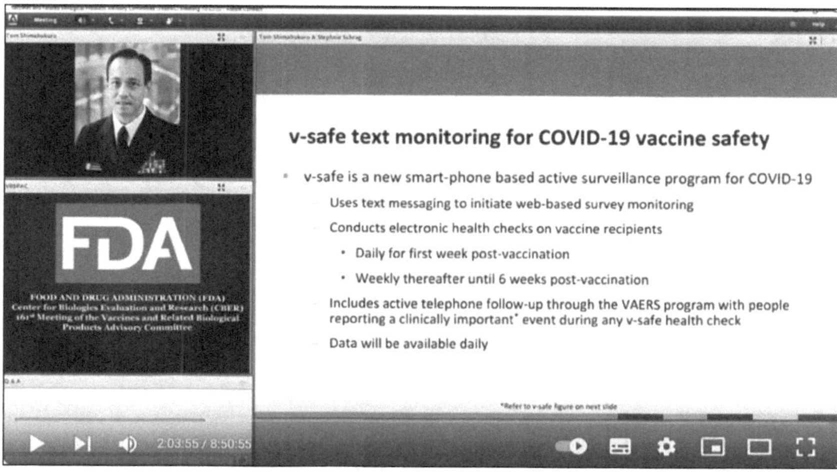


Dr. Shimabukuro discussed how the CDC's pivotal V-safe,[722] a smartphone-based active surveillance program, would use text messaging to initiate web-based survey monitoring after COVID-19 vaccination. He made a point of stating how the "data will be available daily."

Approximately 10 million people signed-up and submitted health reports after COVID-19 vaccination, none of the data was made available daily- in fact, it was never released at all. The ICAN's[723] legal team sued the CDC twice to obtain the data, which led to a court-order requiring the release of it. It took until February this year for ICAN to receive the first production of the V-safe free text data.

In an interview with Del Bigtree,[724] Aaron Siri, legal counsel of the ICAN legal team said: "A federal judge in an incredible 29-page decision has now issued an order requiring the CDC to make every single one of those 7.8 million free text entries available to the public over the next twelve months. Every month they have to produce a few hundred thousand of them...It will be an incredible opportunity to actually see what was being told to the CDC by the public...I think this is going to be the death blow to this cover-up. It is clear that they've been hiding something and now the world is about to see what people wrote after getting the vaccine."

Out of the 10,108,273 users, roughly a third were impacted by adverse health from the period January 2020-January 2022.

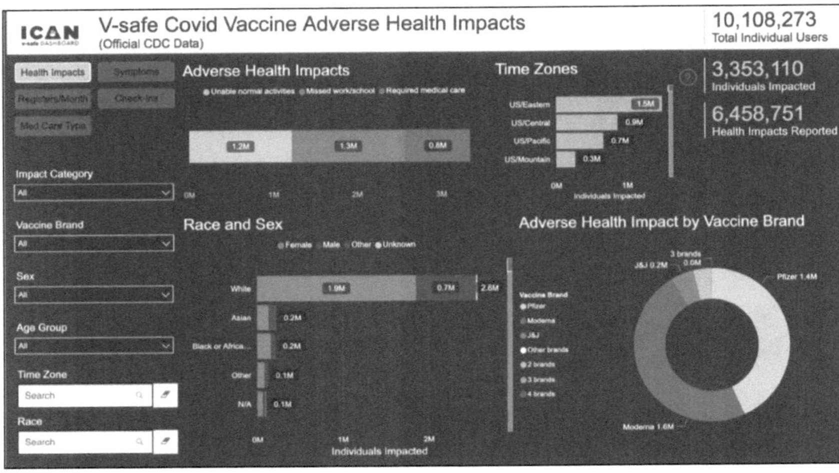


Screenshot showing breakdown of CDC data sourced by ICAN[725]

During the February 15, 2024, congressional hearing[726] of the Select Subcommittee on the Coronavirus Pandemic, Chairman Dr. Brad Wenstrup asked Dr. Peter Marks the following question: "As of February 2024, Vaccine Adverse Event Reporting System (VAERS) reports for COVID-19 vaccines total significantly higher than all other vaccines combined since 1990. This is a surprising figure. Dr. Marks, was the government prepared for such an avalanche of reports to VAERS?"

Marks responded: "We tried to be prepared for that, but the avalanche of reports was tremendous. It, again, required re-tasking people on the fly...We had to usually staff up and had many meetings working to increase our ability to go through these reports."

Then he went on to openly admit: "I fully agree with you that we probably have not done a good enough job of communicating sometimes the actual numbers of deaths versus what's in VAERS."

## The Child Deaths Found in the Pfizer/BioNTech's Safety Reports

While the FDA and CDC allegedly attempted to manage the "avalanche of reports" flooding VAERS and V-safe, across the Atlantic, their European counterpart, the European Medicines Agency (EMA), was engaging in a similar form of regulatory inaction and restricted transparency around the data: by quietly endorsing Pfizer/BioNTech's confidential Periodic Safety

Update Reports (PSURs), which contained equally concerning volumes of adverse events.

According to the EMAS's definition: "PSURs are pharmacovigilance[727] documents intended to provide an evaluation of the risk-benefit balance of a medicinal product at defined time points after its authorization. The objective of the PSUR is to present a comprehensive and critical analysis of the risk-benefit balance of the product, taking into account new or emerging safety information in the context of cumulative information on risk and benefits."

In 2023, I was asked by Children's Health Defence, Europe to analyze these reports which were only made public thanks to the persistent efforts by a group of European doctors known as PSUR4doctors. The group repeatedly filed Freedom of Information Act (FOIA) requests to secure the release of thousands of pages of PSUR safety data for all the COVID shots. PSURs contain worldwide data, including adverse event reports from the United States and other regions. In the case of the Pfizer/BioNTech shots, it is the MAH (Marketing Authorization Holder), BioNTech, who is legally required to submit PSURs (which cover 6-month periods) to the EMA. The Agency assesses these reports to determine whether any new risks are identified or if the risk-benefit balance has changed. All available PSURs can be accessed from Dr. Silvia Behrendt's Substack[728] and the German blog, tkp.[729]

Below is a summary of key findings (with screenshots from source documents) based on my original investigation[730] analyzing PSUR#3, covering the six-month period of December 2021 through to June 2022, for the Pfizer/BioNTech shot.

For 5–11-Year-Olds:

- Adverse Events: 9,605 individual cases (1.9% of 507,683 total cases), a 683% increase from 1,227 cases in PSUR #2 (covering the second half of 2021). The U.S., Australia, Philippines, and Germany reported the most cases.
- Seriousness and Outcomes: 17% of 22,457 AEs were serious, 40% had "unknown" outcomes, and 14.5% were "not resolved."
- Deaths: 20 fatal cases reported.

Two deaths (ages 6 and 7) were reported linked to myocarditis and cardio-respiratory arrest post-vaccination (dose 1 or 2). The 6-year-old boy's death was dismissed as "natural causes," despite myocarditis onset 7 days post-dose 1, with a pending autopsy.

> – In one case, the reporter concluded that the death "had nothing to do" with the administration of BNT162b2 and was due to natural causes:
>
> o MC case; age: 6 years; gender: male; fatal PTs: Myocarditis, Cardio-respiratory arrest, COVID-19, occurred 7 days after the 1st dose of BNT162b2; medical history: rhinitis allergic, autoimmune thyroiditis), type I diabetes mellitus); autopsy: performed, results are pending.

Two other death cases were dismissed with "death" as the only reported event and a further two, due to underlying conditions (autopsies not performed or unknown). In six cases, causality could not be ruled out due to temporal proximity, though no autopsy/lab data confirmed vaccine linkage. There were no confounding factors identified in 15 other cases.

For the 12–17-Year-Olds:

- Adverse Events: 21,945 cases (4.3% of total cases), a 20% increase from 18,451 in PSUR #2. Germany, Philippines, and Australia led in reports.
- Seriousness and Outcomes: 32% of 61,071 AEs were serious, 33% had "unknown" outcomes, and 20% were "not resolved."
- Deaths: 62 fatal cases reported, three times higher than the younger group.

There were three deaths (all age 13) linked to myocarditis; two lacked autopsy data, one cited "adverse event following immunization."

Fatal myocarditis cases in subjects aged 12-15 years (2 cases, medically confirmed; 1 case non-medically confirmed):

- A 13-year-old male subject from ███, ███████:
  - Medical history: None.
  - Co-suspect medications: None.
  - PTs with fatal outcome: Cardiac failure, Myocarditis.
  - Time to onset (myocarditis): 69 days after dose 2.
  - Causes of death: Cardiac failure; Myocarditis.
  - Autopsy: Not reported if autopsy was performed.
- A 13-year-old male subject from ██:
  - Medical history: Abdominal pain, Chest pain.
  - Co-suspect medications: None.
  - PTs with fatal outcome: Anuria, Asthenia, Cardiac arrest, Compartment syndrome, Enterovirus infection, Malaise, Multi-organ disorder, Multiple organ dysfunction syndrome, Myocarditis, Pulseless electrical activity, Renal failure, Rhinovirus infection, Ventricular tachycardia.

PRAC PSUR assessment report
EMA/PRAC/849/2023

Page 131/272

  - Time to onset (myocarditis): 5 days after dose 2.
  - Causes of death: Asthenia; Cardiac arrest; Compartment syndrome; Enterovirus infection; Malaise; Multi-organ disorder; Myocarditis; Pulseless electrical activity; Renal failure; Rhinovirus infection; Ventricular tachycardia.
  - Autopsy: Not reported if autopsy was performed.
- A 13-year-old female subject from █████:
  - Medical history: None.
  - Co-suspect medications: None.
  - PTs with fatal outcome: Myocarditis.
  - Time to onset (myocarditis): 6 days after dose 1.
  - Causes of death: Myocarditis.
  - Autopsy: Adverse event following immunisation.

The other 15 fatal cases lacked sufficient detail ("death" only), two were accidents, six involved underlying conditions (e.g., a 16-year-old girl with pulmonary embolism and cardiac arrest 2 days post-dose 3, autopsy performed but results not provided), and 20 where causality could not be excluded due to temporal links, though unconfirmed by lab/autopsy data. No confounding factors were noted in 39 cases. 19 cases were dismissed due to "limited information," reflecting Pfizer/BioNTech's failure to investigate further.

## 161 Child Deaths In A Year

Following my original report, I went on to further investigate[731] the disturbing cases of child deaths. An extract from that article reads: "As of June 2022, 161 fatal pediatric cases were recorded from the reporting interval of PSUR #1 through to PSUR#3. Even though this technically covered an 18-month period, regulators like the EMA and FDA first authorized the Pfizer/BioNTech vaccine for 12-15-year-olds at the end of May 2021 and for 5-11-year-olds, from October that year. This means that these pediatric deaths would have occurred in just 12 months."

Notably, in the EMA's Pharmacovigilance Risk Assessment Committee (PRAC) assessment report for PSUR #3 (December 2021 through to June 2022), the 82 pediatric fatal cases were later revised down to 79, due to three of the cases being allegedly non-fatal (see snapshot below showing the rapporteur assessment comment).

MAH's conclusion

There is no information in the review of these 82 paediatric fatal cases that identifies BNT162b2 as a contributor to the reported deaths. Fatal cases will continue to be monitored via routine pharmacovigilance.

*Rapporteur assessment comment:*

Of the 82 cases retrieved 3 cases were non-fatal cases, resulting in 79 cases:

- 18 cases are considered unlikely related to Comirnaty exposure;
- 4 cases unclassified;
- 57 cases unassessable.

Overall, MAH's conclusion is endorsed that based on the provided data no causal association of Comirnaty with the reported deaths can be concluded. No new important information could be identified concerning the reported deaths. The MAH should closely monitor any new cases, patterns, or trends of reporting fatal outcome through routine pharmacovigilance.

**Issue solved**

BioNTech, the MAH's (Marketing Authorization Holder) dismissive conclusion: "no information in the review of these 82 pediatric fatal cases that identifies BNT162b2 as a contributor to the reported deaths" is revealing. It proves that BioNTech did not properly review these fatal cases, because if they had done, they would have also known that 3 out of the 82 cases were apparently non-fatal, just like the EMA's rapporteur.

Notably, in the EMA's Rapporteur comment box, common phrases and terms describing these fatal cases can be read throughout the assessment report, such as, "unlikely related to Comirnaty exposure," "unclassified" and "unassessable."

What is particularly disturbing is the EMA's endorsement of the MAH's conclusion and their signing off with "issue solved."

EuroMOMO,[732] which graphs pooled weekly total number of deaths in the data provided by EuroMOMO partner countries, showed cumulative excess deaths in children aged 0-14 years in Europe, from week 1, 2019- week 22, 2023. A significant increase can be observed, just around the time the EMA approved the Pfizer-BioNTech COVID-19 vaccine for children aged 12-15 years of age.

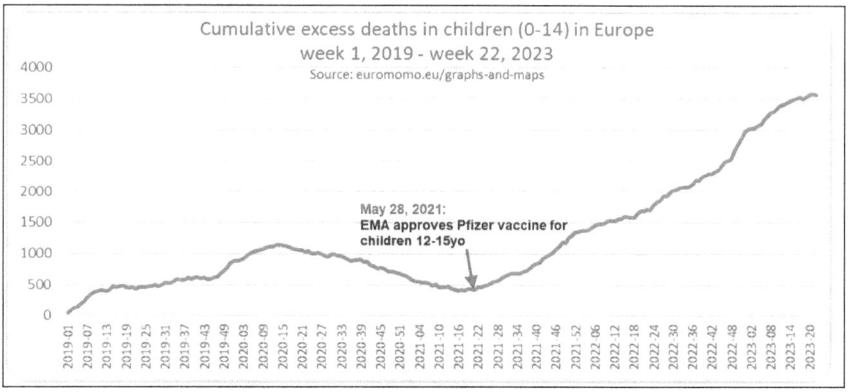
Cumulative excess deaths in children (0-14) in Europe
week 1, 2019 - week 22, 2023
Source: euromomo.eu/graphs-and-maps
May 28, 2021:
EMA approves Pfizer vaccine for children 12-15yo

Image source: @P_McCulloughMD[733]

## The FDA's "Proper Investigation" into Child Deaths

In September 2025, the U.S. Food and Drug Administration (FDA) Commissioner Dr. Marty Makary announced in a CNN interview:[734] "We're reviewing the autopsy reports" as part of the FDA's "proper investigation" into child deaths following COVID vaccination.

Two months later, a leaked internal memo[735] by Dr. Vinay Prasad (FDA vaccine division director) claiming "at least 10 children have died after and because of receiving COVID-19 vaccination" was obtained by *The Washington Post.*[736]

Notably, my analysis of the Periodic Safety Update Reports (PSURs) revealed that autopsies were frequently not performed, not reported, or results were unavailable for many pediatric cases. This lack of critical data is particularly egregious given that these deaths involved young children.

Tragically, the FDA's investigation into child deaths following COVID vaccination, arrives five years too late for the many families who lost a child. And why wasn't a thorough investigation launched from the start?

Perhaps the most revealing insight into that question comes from Dr. Eric Rubin, Editor-in-Chief of the *New England Journal of Medicine* and a member of the FDA's Vaccines and Related Biological Products Advisory Committee. During the October 26, 2021, VRBPAC meeting[737] discussing authorization of the Pfizer-BioNTech COVID-19 vaccine for children aged 5–11, he stated: "We're never going to learn about how safe the vaccine is unless we start giving it. That's just the way it goes. That's how we found out about rare complications of other vaccines like the rotavirus vaccine. And I do think we should vote to approve it."

## What the EMA's Eudravigilance Revealed

While the EMA quietly endorsed Pfizer's cursory dismissal of dozens of child deaths in the official PSURs, an even darker picture was emerging in their own spontaneous reporting database, EudraVigilance, where the sheer volume of harm reports dwarfed anything seen in the past two decades. It took an independent senior data analyst, Wouter Aukema from The Netherlands, to finally expose what the agency appeared to bury.

EudraVigilance, is the EMA's central pharmacovigilance database and data-processing system for collecting and analyzing reports of suspected adverse reactions to medicines (including vaccines). Its highly cumbersome and opaque interface makes it very difficult to assess the true risks of a pharmaceutical product or vaccine. That is until Wouter Aukema decided to do something about it. He teamed up with a software expert to develop a tool where they were able to download all 15 million case safety reports over the past 20 years, for 6000 medicinal drug products and substances (within and outside of Europe) including the COVID-19 shots.

In my interview[738] with Aukema, he was able to showcase through his Tableau dashboard,[739] the true horrors of the safety data buried within the European Medicines Agency's EudraVigilance case safety reporting system, like never before.

Aukema demonstrated the many problems with the system and explained: "If I would want to understand the history of all side effects for this particular drug, I need to repeat this action 16 times for the Covid shots, due to an EMA restriction of a maximum 250,000 row download. If I want to go back to 2018, I need to do that seven times for one drug. Mind you, seven times, 6,000 different drugs and substances. That's 42,000 times that I need to click on buttons, download files. This is undoable. Nobody can do this."

However, thanks to Aukema and his colleague's unique tool, the public can see for the first time the true harms caused by the COVID-19 shots. With color coded visual graphs and diagrams, the damning data is presented for the first time in a truly transparent way, in stark contrast to the EMA's nebulous system.

Aukema's dashboard of data showcased a staggering threefold increase in case safety reports for the COVID-19 vaccines (at the start of the rollout) compared to all the other drug products and substances, over the past 20 years. The blue graph line represents the number of case safety reports for the COVID-19 vaccines. The orange graph line is for the other 6000 drug products and substances.

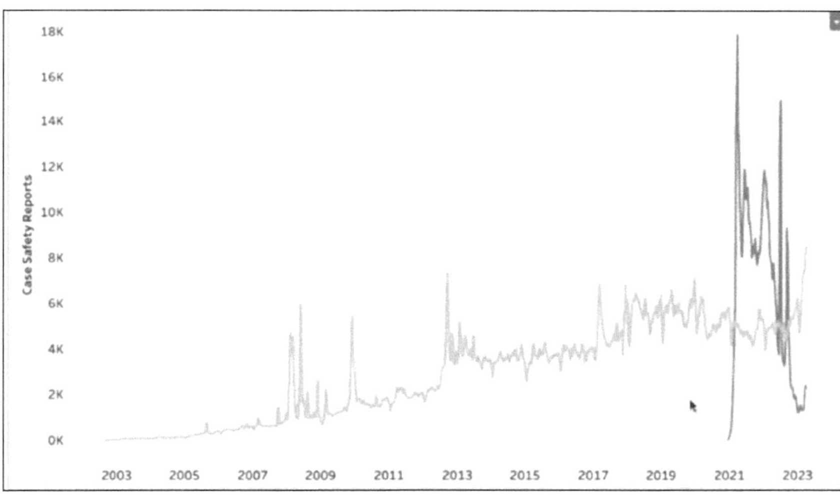


Aukema went on to reveal: "What is the most reported side effect reported for all the COVID vaccines? I was flabbergasted by this. It is COVID itself. But I thought the COVID vaccines were going to prevent COVID."

The diagram below depicts the reaction, "COVID-19" as the largest blue bubble.

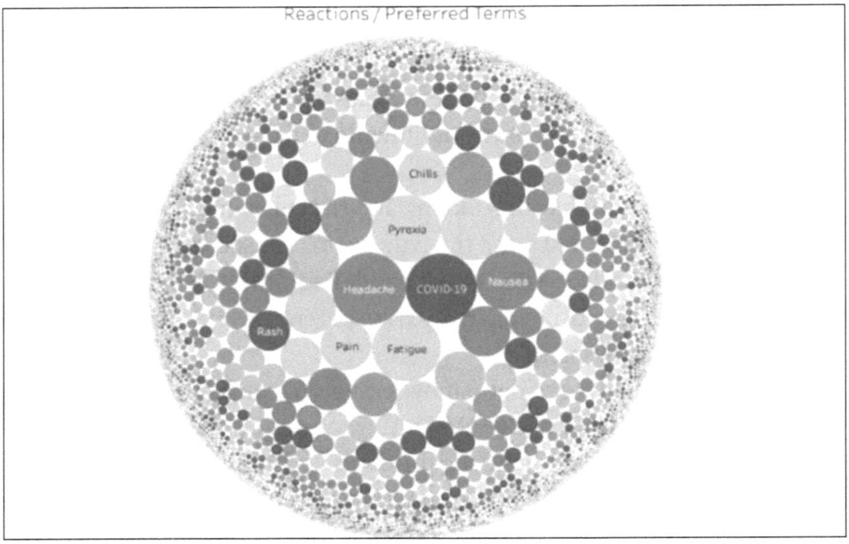


Aukema disclosed more bombshell findings from the data, this time for all other drugs. The sudden explosion starting from January 2023 onwards of case safety reports for two specific drugs.

1. Keytruda,[740] a cancer drug mainly used in adults for cancers that are advanced, have spread or returned, are not responding to other treatments or cannot be removed by surgery.
2. Inflectra,[741] an anti-inflammatory medicine to treat diseases such as rheumatoid arthritis, Crohn's disease, ulcerative colitis and psoriasis. It is usually used when other medicines or treatments have failed.

What could have caused such a sudden demand (hence an increase in reporting of side effects) for a cancer drug and a medicine for chronic inflammation from the start of January 2023? Could there be a link between the increase in use for these drugs to treat certain side effects of the Covid shots?

During the interview, Aukema highlighted another critical finding: Myocardial Infarction (heart attack) was one of the top reported cardiac disorders following Covid vaccination. The data expert made a point of stating how pericarditis and myocarditis were listed as known side effects in the packaging inserts of the Covid vaccines but myocardial infarction was surprisingly absent.

• • •

Based on the investigations documented in this chapter, it can be argued that regulatory agencies had substantial early warning signals yet did not act with the urgency the data appeared to warrant. Some observers have characterized this pattern as regulatory capture[742], noting that agencies including the FDA and EMA receive significant funding from the pharmaceutical industry they regulate, a structural conflict highlighted by public health advocates for decades. Whether these funding relationships influenced decision-making, or whether regulators genuinely assessed the benefit-risk balance differently than independent analysts, remains a subject of intense debate. What is documented here is the timeline: warnings flagged, data submitted, and harms reported. However, regulators seemingly turned a blind eye and in doing so protected the narrative instead of the people. Juvenal's ancient question: "Who will guard the guards themselves?" has rarely felt more urgent, as these same regulatory structures remain in place today.

The next chapter examines the censoring of harms: deplatformed scientists erased from professional networks, grieving families shadow-banned for sharing their children's injuries, peer-reviewed studies retracted under pressure or relegated to obscurity by institutional gatekeepers. What began as the suppression of lockdown skeptics evolved into a comprehensive effort to silence anyone, expert or injured, who dared document the human cost of the "safe and effective" mantra.

CHAPTER FIFTEEN

# CENSORING HARMS

*"When you tear out a man's tongue,*
*you are not proving him a liar, you're only telling the*
*world that you fear what he might say."*

~George R. R. Martin's *A Song of Ice and Fire series,*
spoken by Tyrion Lannister in
*A Clash of Kings*

The true purpose of censorship is to control the narrative. Since 3/11, governments, public health authorities, mainstream media, Big Tech platforms, scientific journals, and fact-checking organizations have relentlessly enforced a single, unchallengeable mantra: the Covid shots are "safe and effective."[743]

This chapter spotlights the victims of this vast censorship-industrial complex: the vaccine-injured who dared to speak, and the eminent scientists, health advocates, journalists, and frontline medical professionals who challenged the official line. It examines the systematic suppression of inconvenient science: the retraction, withdrawal, or burial of peer-reviewed studies that revealed harms from the Covid shots. It also uncovers the deliberate withholding of data, from the untraceable and retroactive alteration of serious adverse event reports in the EMA's EudraVigilance database to the UK Health Security Agency's ongoing refusal to release anonymized record-level data linking vaccination dates to deaths.

This machinery of censorship was not born with the Covid shots. The same tactics: smear campaigns, deplatforming, shadow-banning, and institutional pressure, were deployed against scientists and doctors who questioned blanket lockdowns, school closures, or one-size-fits-all restrictions, including the authors of the Great Barrington Declaration. What began as the silencing of lockdown dissent seamlessly evolved into the systematic marginalization of anyone raising legitimate concerns about the Covid shots.

The evidence reveals a scorched battlefield of narrative warfare, where truth, and those who seek it, are always the first casualties.

## Censoring Dissenting Scientists

In my July 2021 interview[744] with Dr. Robert Malone, first featured in chapter 9, he was one of the scientists who spoke out early about the potential health risks associated with COVID-19 mRNA shots. The following is a segment summary from that conversation, with a particular focus on the censorship he described experiencing as a direct result of his public statements.

In the interview, Malone described what he saw as a coordinated, multi-institutional system of censorship that had been deployed against scientists and others who raised evidence-based concerns about the safety of the COVID-19 genetic shots. He recounted his own dramatic experience of being completely erased from LinkedIn, where he had maintained a professional profile for over fifteen years, including valuable documentation and photographs from his work inside the WHO during the Ebola outbreak.

"It wasn't that they just closed my account; I no longer existed," he said. "You couldn't find 'RW Malone MD' on LinkedIn anymore… poof, gone."

The justification notice he received from LinkedIn cited three main reasons: his discussion of scientific literature on the spike protein's biological activity and potential toxicity; his sharing of a mainstream Wall Street Journal editorial excerpt highlighting vaccine risks; and his comments about the problem of censorship itself. Malone highlighted the irony, noting, "I got censored, in part, for talking about censorship." He stressed that the top-cited reason was his post exposing the chairman of Reuters' board also sitting on Pfizer's board [James C. Smith]. "That is the first, the top post that they cite as the reason for ghosting me," he explained. The deletion occurred within approximately 48 hours of that revelation, and the notice itself contained typos and misspellings, leading him to infer it had been "hastily composed by a person rather than generated automatically."

Malone linked this personal deplatforming to a broader mechanism: the Trusted News Initiative, led by the BBC and involving major tech platforms (Google, Microsoft, Meta/Facebook, and others) along with legacy media. He stated that these organizations had agreed to restrict acceptable discourse to only those "truths" endorsed by official public health bodies such as the CDC and WHO, effectively suppressing scientific speech that deviated from those positions, even when grounded in peer-reviewed publications.

He attributed the rise of this censorship apparatus to two primary forces. First, widespread fear during the height of the crisis had caused institutions and individuals to tolerate or participate in actions they would normally reject: "Fear drives groups of people to do things in moments of stress that they wouldn't otherwise do—to cross lines and agree to stuff they wouldn't in a normal situation." Second, and more disturbingly, he raised the possibility that powerful actors had deliberately exploited the atmosphere of fear: "Are there people exploiting this window for their own purposes, whether financial, political, or power-related?"

Malone framed the situation as a profound distortion of normal scientific and political behavior. He warned that the suppression of open debate, even uncomfortable or dissenting debate, represented a serious departure from free inquiry and informed consent. In his view, the environment was not the result of isolated overreactions, but the visible outcome of a deliberate, cross-institutional effort to enforce a single approved narrative about the vaccines, where questioning official claims, citing evidence, or even discussing the existence of censorship itself could result in swift and total digital erasure.

Notably, my interview with Malone, originally posted on YouTube on July 6, 2021, was promptly removed from the platform shortly after its upload, reflecting the very censorship dynamics Malone was describing. It remained unavailable for nearly three years until it was resurrected and reinstated on YouTube in May 2024. Dr. Robert Malone's media appearance on *The Joe Rogan Experience*[745] was also removed within hours in January 2022. He was also suspended from Twitter in December 2021but reinstated a year later after Elon Musk's acquisition of the social media platform, now X.

Another distinguished scientist, Dr. Peter McCullough, a physician, and one of the most published cardiologists in history with over 1000 publications to his name, encountered censorship when his former employer, Baylor Scott & White Health, obtained a restraining order[746] against him in July 2021. The order prohibited him from continuing to reference his institutional affiliations while discussing vaccine safety concerns publicly. His media appearances, including those highlighting myocarditis risks associated with the COVID-19 shots, most notably on *The Joe Rogan*

*Experience*,[747] were subsequently labeled by medical authorities as promoting "debunked conspiracy theories." The retraction of several of his scientific papers on related topics will be addressed later in this chapter.

Dr. Martin Kulldorff, a world-renowned epidemiologist, Harvard Medical School professor since 2003 specializing in vaccine safety surveillance and co-author of the Great Barrington Declaration, which advocated focused protection of the vulnerable instead of universal lockdowns (discussed in chapter 4), faced widespread censorship and professional repercussions for challenging official COVID-19 vaccine policies.

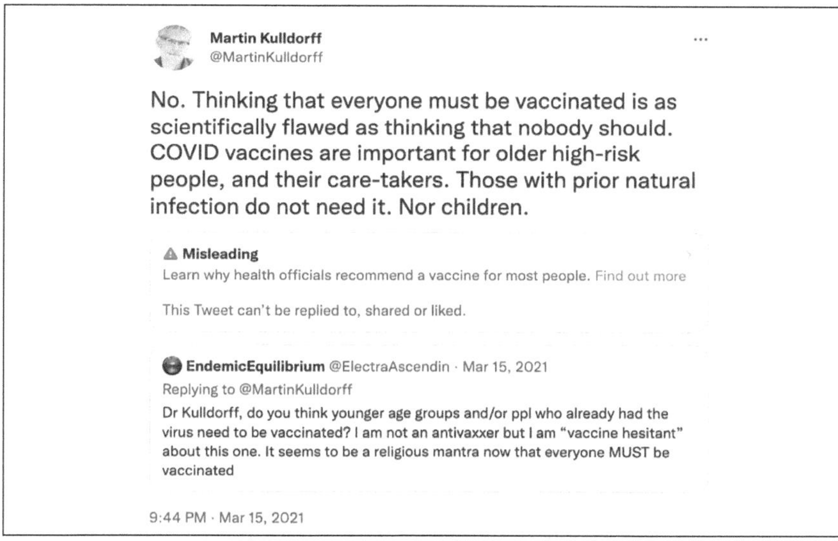


Source: Public.News[748]

Kulldorff publicly argued that individuals with natural immunity did not require vaccination. A view grounded in established immunological principles. At the encouragement of the U.S. government (as revealed through the Twitter Files, which is explored in chapter 16) he was censored across major platforms: Twitter (now X), LinkedIn, Facebook, and YouTube repeatedly removed or suppressed his posts for contradicting CDC guidance on natural immunity and vaccination.

In November 2021, Mass General Brigham terminated his position for refusing the COVID-19 shot despite his documented natural immunity. This was followed by his dismissal from Harvard Medical School in March 2024, effectively ending a distinguished 20-year academic career.

In a *City Journal* article[749] titled "Harvard Tramples the Truth," he wrote: "I am no longer a professor of medicine at Harvard. The Harvard motto is Veritas, Latin for truth. But, as I discovered, truth can get you fired. This is my story—a story of a Harvard biostatistician and infectious-disease epidemiologist, clinging to the truth as the world lost its way during the Covid pandemic."

Dr. Jay Bhattacharya, emeritus professor at Stanford School of Medicine, rose to prominence in 2020 as co-author of the Great Barrington Declaration. In response, then-director of the NIH Francis Collins labelled him one of the "three fringe epidemiologists" in an email to Anthony Fauci (exhibited in chapter 4). Consequently, he was shadow-banned and placed on Twitter's "Trends Blacklist" in 2020, preventing his tweets from trending or gaining visibility.

In December 2022, upon release of the Twitter Files, he took to X (formerly Twitter): "Still trying to process my emotions on learning that Twitter blacklisted me. The thought that will keep me up tonight: censorship of scientific discussion permitted policies like school closures & a generation of children were hurt."

In 2025, Bhattacharya was appointed director of the NIH after being nominated by President Trump. Not bad, for a "fringe epidemiologist."

In the UK, Professor Sunetra Gupta, a theoretical epidemiologist at Oxford University and the third author of the Great Barrington Declaration, endured a brutal smear campaign. This involved baseless accusations portraying her as a "charlatan" funded by libertarian interests, alongside defamatory attacks on her credentials. In her witness statement[750] to the UK COVID-19 Inquiry, she detailed being vilified as a right-wing extremist, bombarded with abuse, and confronted by orchestrated institutional and media efforts to stifle discussions on alternative pandemic approaches.

## Censoring The Injured

The suppression did not stop with the experts. When ordinary families began speaking out about injuries to their children, the same digital guillotine fell.

Chapter 14 featured my 2021 interview with Stephanie de Garay, whose daughter Maddie suffered catastrophic, life-altering injuries shortly after receiving her second dose of Pfizer's mRNA Covid shot as a participant in the company's adolescent clinical trial in the United States. She was aged

12 at the time. In the interview, Stephanie described the severe censorship her family encountered when they courageously went public with Maddie's story. Below is a key excerpt from our conversation.

Sonia Elijah: I read that Maddie's TikTok account got shut down. She got locked out.

Stephanie de Garay: Two of them.

Sonia Elijah: So, would you not consider that as censorship?

Stephanie de Garay: I guess, I mean they don't give you a reason. They just shut it down. She's never had one shut down ever! So, when she was younger, she had one and we shared one, you know, because then I can monitor it. I still have access to it. But she never had one shut down ever before because she's pretty conservative and she wasn't even posting controversial things. She's on there with her NG [feeding] tube and she's done some joking ones. I mean, because that's how she copes. She just keeps opening new accounts.

Sonia Elijah: And they shut it down when she opens new ones?

Stephanie de Garay: She has one that hasn't been shut down yet.

Sonia Elijah: What about Facebook?

Stephanie de Garay: Facebook? I have been very careful because I knew what could happen so I don't post a lot. Like I just posted my story on Maddie's. So, what I did notice is that if I would post links to articles, I would literally get zero responses. I'm like, something's not right. You know, nobody's even responding to this. It's things like that, you can't post because they'll just push it down. Nobody will see it. But if you post without, like if I posted a story about Maddie and I don't use certain words. I've learned how to play the system. Just like a lot of other people.

Sonia Elijah: You're selective with the words that you choose?

Stephanie de Garay: I'm selective with the words and the pictures and I don't use links because links get blocked.

Sonia Elijah: I've heard that a lot of the Facebook accounts set up as support groups for COVID vaccine injured victims have been shut down.

Stephanie de Garay: Yeah. I mean, there's rules when you join them, like you can't use this word, this word, this word. They'll get notifications, they'll be flagged. And, when I've joined some of these groups, it'll give you the warning: "This group talks about misinformation. Do you still want to join?" I'm like, yeah. There's a group for parents of kids and the name-you wouldn't be able to find it if you search for it. We literally are using the other groups that are for adults, and we invite people to it. Because there's already people in there that shouldn't be in there. It's a lot different when it's parents, like that's what people don't get. If it is you, when you're talking about you, you know what I mean? Versus your child. It's just different. And you're less likely to be open. You're just scared because it's okay to screw up with yourself. It's not okay to screw up with your kid. Yes, that's one thing that has been difficult. A lot of parents are not speaking out. They're afraid.

In December 2022, I went on to interview[751] Heather Hudson from Florida, the mother of a severely mRNA vaccine injured young man, Cody. She spoke openly about his catastrophic injuries following the Pfizer/BioNTech Covid shot given to him in 2021: pulmonary embolisms (blood clots in the lungs) and neuropathy left him hospitalized. She spoke how his condition, vaccine-induced antiphospholipid syndrome (APS), which causes a rare autoimmune disorder where the body attacks proteins involved in blood clotting, leading to hypercoagulability (excessive clotting), is related to the lipid nanoparticles found in the Pfizer-BioNTech Covid shot, particularly the modified phospholipids.

His case is described as one of the most severe APS instances known, with catastrophic APS (CAPS) features, which has ravaged his brain, all four limbs and his lungs.

The family has received no compensation from federal programs like CICP (Countermeasures Injury Compensation Program), which has a one percent approval rate and backlog. Heather has relentlessly advocated for expedited Medicare/Medicaid for the vaccine-injured. She has even authored proposed legislation in Florida, entitled "Cody's Law,"[752] to ensure medical care for vaccine-injured, addressing abandonment.

Heather has repeatedly documented heavy suppression on Facebook, where her posts about Cody's injury, vaccine adverse events, medical gaslighting, and Cody's Law receive little to no engagement. She describes her account as "completely suppressed" since 2021, with content related to vaccine injuries treated as "dirty words."

In a 2025 open letter[753] to Mark Zuckerberg (Co-founder and CEO of Meta Platforms, formerly Facebook), she accused the platform of censoring vaccine injury cases, preventing warnings from reaching others, and contributing to crimes against humanity by silencing affected families.

Turning to the UK, in February 2024, then Prime Minister Rishi Sunak faced an intense grilling by a vaccine-injured man, John Watt, live on GB News's People's Forum.[754] The previously healthy Scot was left with life-altering injuries from postural orthostatic tachycardia syndrome (POTS) after his third Covid vaccine. His tragic but far from isolated story was highlighted in the documentary, "Safe and Effective: A Second Opinion."[755]

Watt, who is also a leading figure in the Scottish Vaccine Injury Group, seized the opportunity during the People's Forum to question Sunak on why the vaccine-injured have been "left to rot." He urged Sunak to look him "in the eye and do the right thing." His "look me in the eye" line did not go unnoticed, alluding to the fear-mongering advertising campaign used by the UK government (highlighted in chapter 3).

Watt's highly emotive speech also shone a light on how the vaccine-injured have been silenced by the mainstream and social media. "We are silenced, Rishi. On social media and everything. We are silenced! We are the most silenced people in this country!"

The morning after Watt's questioning of Sunak on GB News, Kevin McGuire, editor of the Daily Mirror newspaper, went on Good Morning Britain and dismissively stated about Watt: "Did you watch the bit where that anti-vaxxer went on and on and on at Sunak.."

Egregiously, injuries and deaths caused by the experimental COVID shots, were systematically dismissed, with anyone sounding the alarm bells branded as "anti-vaxx."

The BBC, leader of the Trusted News Initiative, set up on March 16, 2020, just five days after the WHO declared COVID-19 a global pandemic, to counter "disinformation," collaborated with Facebook to take down the accounts of COVID vaccine-injured groups, by drawing attention to the fact that certain "anti-vaxx" groups used **carrot emojis**[756] to circumvent Big Tech censors.

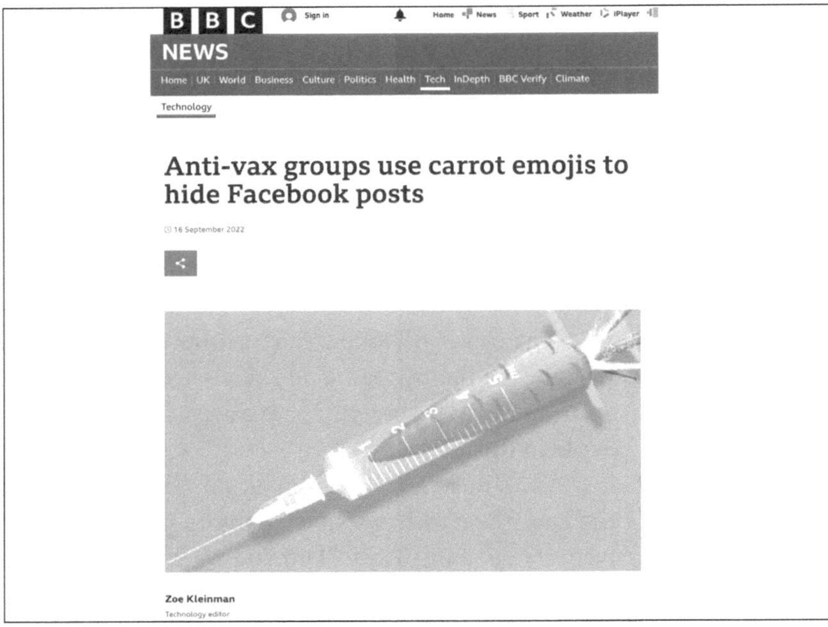


The next chapter further explores the systematic coordination between major technology corporations, prominent media organizations, and government entities in their initiatives to address "misinformation."

## Censoring The Science

In early June 2024, a revelatory study was published in *BMJ Public Health* [757]by a group of researchers (Mostert et al.) from Vrije Universiteit, Amsterdam. The group's findings were shared in the mainstream media with *The Telegraph* daring to write:[758] "Covid vaccines may have helped fuel rise in excess deaths."

The researchers from The Netherlands analyzed all-cause mortality reports abstracted from 47 countries using the "Our World in Data" database. Only countries that had all-cause mortality reports available for all three consecutive years (2020–2022) were included. To calculate the baseline of expected deaths, a Karlinsky and Kobak's estimate model was used. This model uses historical death data in a country from 2015 until 2019 and accounts for seasonal variation and year-to-year trends in mortality.

The alarming results revealed: "The total number of excess deaths in 47 countries of the Western World was 3,098,456 from 1 January 2020 until

31 December 2022. In 2020, the year of the COVID-19 pandemic onset and implementation of containment measures, records present 1,033,122 excess deaths. In 2021, the year in which both containment measures and COVID-19 vaccines were used to address virus spread and infection, the highest number of excess deaths was reported: 1,256,942 excess deaths. In 2022, when most containment measures were lifted and COVID-19 vaccines were continued, preliminary data present 808,392 excess deaths."

The authors went on to state: "During 2021, when not only containment measures but also COVID-19 vaccines were used to tackle virus spread and infection, the highest number of excess deaths was recorded: 1,256,942 excess deaths. Scientific consensus regarding the effectiveness of non-pharmaceutical interventions in reducing viral transmission is currently lacking. During 2022, when most mitigation measures were negated and COVID-19 vaccines were sustained, preliminary available data count 808,392 excess deaths."

The researchers importantly pointed out: "Although COVID-19 vaccines were provided to guard civilians from suffering morbidity and mortality by the COVID-19 virus, suspected adverse events have been documented as well. Both medical professionals and citizens have reported serious injuries and deaths following vaccination to various official databases in the Western World."

Their study is one of the few to examine excess deaths[759] on a global level; a disturbing phenomenon that has virtually been ignored by governments and the mainstream media. Also, it is one of the few to dare point to the massive elephant in the room: the experimental COVID-19 shots that allegedly "saved over 20 million lives,"[760] a claim based on mathematical modeling.

The authors spot lit studies documenting suspected adverse events following vaccination. For instance, the Fraiman et al. study[761] which presented a secondary analysis of the placebo-controlled, phase III randomized clinical trials of mRNA COVID-19 vaccines. The results showed that the Pfizer trial had a 36% higher risk of serious adverse events in the vaccine group. The Moderna trial had a 6% higher risk of serious adverse events among vaccine recipients.

They pointed to a study comparing adverse event reports to VAERS and EudraVigilance following mRNA COVID-19 vaccines versus influenza vaccines. A higher risk of serious adverse reactions was observed for COVID-19 vaccines in comparison to influenza vaccines. These reactions included cardiovascular diseases, coagulation, hemorrhages, gastrointestinal events and thromboses.

In addition, they referred to an important study which revealed that excess deaths were only seen in Germany "from April 2021 onward." The German authors went on to state: "These findings indicate that something must have happened in spring 2021 that led to a sudden and sustained increase in mortality."

What could have happened in the Spring of 2021? Perhaps it was the world's unprecedented rollout of experimental gene-based injections?

Mostert et al. saliently concluded: "Excess mortality has remained high in the Western World for three consecutive years, despite the implementation of COVID-19 containment measures and COVID-19 vaccines. This is unprecedented and raises serious concerns. During the pandemic, it was emphasized by politicians and the media on a daily basis that every COVID-19 death mattered and every life deserved protection through containment measures and COVID-19 vaccines. In the aftermath of the pandemic, the same morale should apply. Every death needs to be acknowledged and accounted for, irrespective of its origin."

Shortly afterwards, the integrity of the peer-reviewed, Mostert et al.[762] study on excess deaths, came under simultaneous attack from both the organization affiliated with the Dutch authors, Princess Máxima Center,[763] and the journal which published it.

On June 11th, the wildfire-like news coverage of the scientific paper was abruptly stamped out by the Princess Máxima Center (the Pediatric Oncology institution affiliated with the authors) issuing a statement, "distancing itself" from the publication. Their statement can be read in full:

> 11-06-2024
>
> The Princess Máxima Center distances itself from the publication "Excess mortality across countries in the Western World since the COVID-19 pandemic: 'Our World in Data' estimates of January 2020 to December 2022".
>
> Serious questions have arisen regarding the publication "Excess mortality across countries in the Western World since the COVID-19 pandemic: 'Our World in Data' estimates of January 2020 to December 2022". Therefore, we will further investigate the scientific quality of this study. The Princess Máxima Center

> deeply regrets that this publication may give the impression that the importance of vaccinations is being questioned.
>
> Originally, the idea was to look at the effect of COVID measures on, among other things, the mortality rate of children with cancer in low-income countries. During the course of the study, the focus shifted and diverted in a direction that we felt was too far from our expertise: pediatric oncology. We are not experts in epidemiology, nor do we want to give that impression. The Máxima Center therefore emphatically distances itself from this publication. We should have been more alert to the formation and results of this publication and will further investigate the way it was created. If it turns out that carelessness was involved in the realization of this publication, it will of course be withdrawn.
>
> We, as the Princess Máxima Center, want to emphasize that we strongly support vaccination, and that this publication should certainly not be read as an argument against vaccination. The study in no way demonstrates a link between vaccinations and excess mortality; that is explicitly not the researchers' finding. We therefore regret that this impression has been created.

This prompted *BMJ Public Health* to respond with an "expression of concern"[764] a few days later, on June 14. Their full statement can be read in full:

> "The integrity team and editors are investigating issues raised regarding the quality and messaging of this work. The Princess Máxima Centre, which is listed as the affiliation of three of the four authors, is also investigating the scientific quality of this study. The integrity team has contacted the institution regarding their investigation.
>
> Readers should also be alerted to misreporting and misunderstanding of the work. It has been claimed that the work implies a direct causal link between COVID-19 vaccination and mortality. This study does not establish any such link. The researchers looked only at trends in excess mortality over time, not its causes. The research does not support the claim that vaccines are a major contributory factor to excess deaths since the start of the pandemic. Vaccines have, in fact, been instrumental in reducing the severe illness and death associated with COVID-19 infection.

Update January 2025: *BMJ* are awaiting the result of an institutional investigation into the conduct of the work, which was due to be finalized by the end of 2024. At present, the institution can offer no update on when the information will be sent to *BMJ*."

The backlash triggered by the peer-reviewed paper does not come as a surprise. This is because the Mostert et al. study is not the only scientific paper to be censored because it dared question the safety of the Covid shots. Post 3/11, numerous peer-reviewed papers have been either retracted, withdrawn, had an "expression of concern" or "under investigation" notice slapped on them.

Take for instance, the peer-reviewed paper by Walach et al.,[765] "The Safety of COVID-19 Vaccinations- We should Rethink the Policy." The main finding of the paper showed: "For three deaths prevented by vaccination we have to accept two inflicted by vaccination." Following its June 24, 2021 publication in Vaccines, several of the editors of the journal resigned in protest.

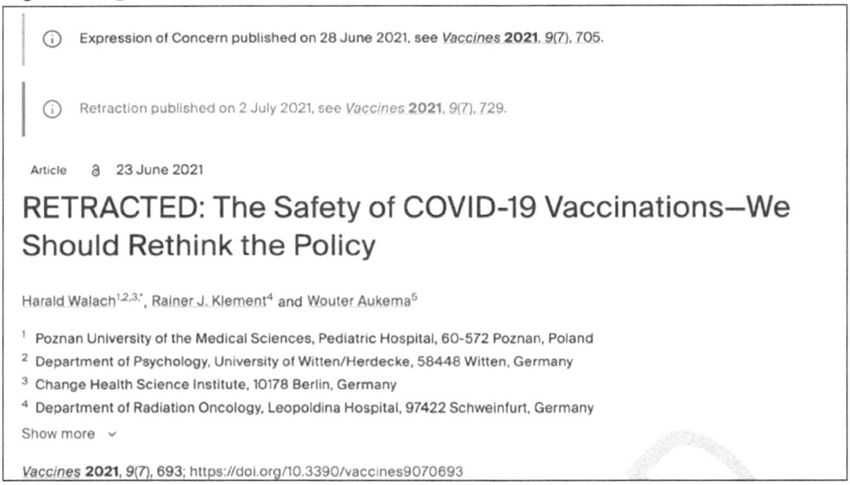
Expression of Concern published on 28 June 2021, see *Vaccines* **2021**, 9(7), 705.

Retraction published on 2 July 2021, see *Vaccines* **2021**, 9(7), 729.

Article 23 June 2021

RETRACTED: The Safety of COVID-19 Vaccinations—We Should Rethink the Policy

Harald Walach[1,2,3,*], Rainer J. Klement[4] and Wouter Aukema[5]

[1] Poznan University of the Medical Sciences, Pediatric Hospital, 60-572 Poznan, Poland
[2] Department of Psychology, University of Witten/Herdecke, 58448 Witten, Germany
[3] Change Health Science Institute, 10178 Berlin, Germany
[4] Department of Radiation Oncology, Leopoldina Hospital, 97422 Schweinfurt, Germany
Show more

*Vaccines* **2021**, 9(7), 693; https://doi.org/10.3390/vaccines9070693

Earlier in 2024, there was the retraction of "COVID-19 mRNA Vaccines: Lessons Learned from the Registrational Trials and Global Vaccination Campaign" by Mead et al.[766] (including authors, Dr. Jessica Rose Ph.D. and Dr. Peter McCullough MD, MPH) from *Cureus*.

"Based on the research presented in this narrative review, the global COVID-19 vaccination campaign should be regarded as a grave medical error" the authors stated in the paper.

Cureus

Publishing Beyond Open Access

▸ Cureus. 2024 Feb 26;16(2):r137. doi: 10.7759/cureus.r137

**Retraction: COVID-19 mRNA Vaccines: Lessons Learned from the Registrational Trials and Global Vaccination Campaign**

M Nathaniel Mead [1,✉], Stephanie Seneff [2], Russ Wolfinger [3], Jessica Rose [4], Kris Denhaerynck [5], Steve Kirsch [6], Peter A McCullough [7,8]

Editors: Alexander Muacevic, John R Adler

▸ Author information ▸ Article notes ▸ Copyright and License information

PMCID: PMC10897748 PMID: 38414517

Dr. Peter McCullough, is no stranger to censorship, as referenced earlier in this chapter, along with Dr. Jessica Rose, an immunologist and computational biologist. Their peer-reviewed October 2021 seminal paper: "A Report on Myocarditis Adverse Events in the U.S. Vaccine Adverse Events Reporting System (VAERS) in Association with COVID-19 Injectable Biological Products," which showed a staggering 19 times the expected number of myocarditis cases in the vaccination volunteers over background myocarditis rates for the 12-15-year-old age group, was withdrawn[767] from *Elsevier*, the same week the FDA voted on whether to offer the experimental Pfizer/BioNTech mRNA shot to 5-11 year olds.

Provided to the PMC COVID-19 Collection by

Elsevier

▸ Curr Probl Cardiol. 2021 Oct 1:101011. Online ahead of print. doi: 10.1016/j.cpcardiol.2021.101011

**WITHDRAWN: A Report on Myocarditis Adverse Events in the U.S. Vaccine Adverse Events Reporting System (VAERS) in Association with COVID-19 Injectable Biological Products**

Jessica Rose [a,∗], Peter A McCullough [b]

▸ Author information ▸ Copyright and License information

PMCID: PMC8483988 PMID: 34601006

In my 2021 interview[768] with Dr. McCullough, he stated: "*Elsevier* is illegally attempting to censor this paper- right at the moment when it's needed the most, when the vaccine manufacturer is going to the U.S. FDA and seeking approval for emergency authorization use for children aged 5-11."

Later in July 2023, a paper by Hulscher et al.,[769] "A Systematic Review of Autopsy Findings in Deaths after COVID-19 Vaccination" (including

Dr. Peter McCullough and Dr. Harvey Risch Professor Emeritus of Epidemiology at the Yale School of Public Health and Yale School of Medicine among the co-authors ) was first removed and then later officially withdrawn from *The Lancet's* preprint server. The paper's damning findings showed: "A total of 240 deaths (73.9%) were independently adjudicated as directly due to or significantly contributed to by COVID-19 vaccination."

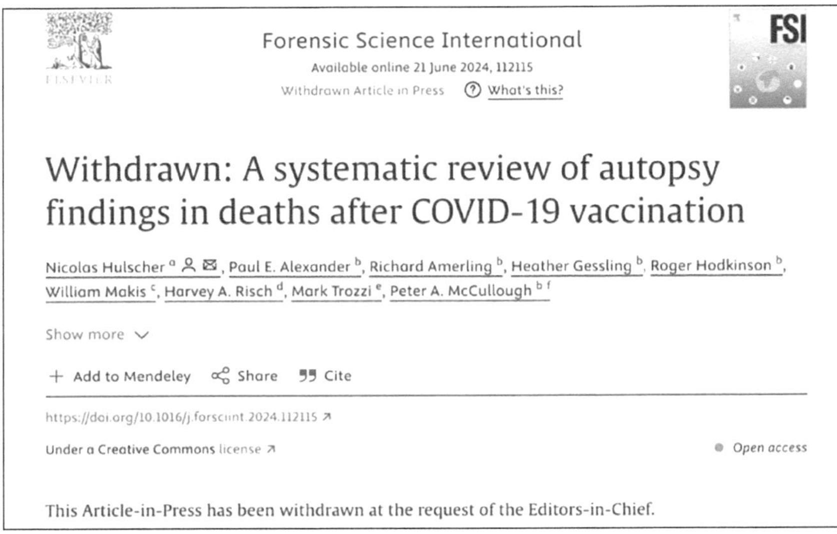
Forensic Science International
Available online 21 June 2024, 112115
Withdrawn Article in Press What's this?

FSI

Withdrawn: A systematic review of autopsy findings in deaths after COVID-19 vaccination

Nicolas Hulscher[a], Paul E. Alexander[b], Richard Amerling[b], Heather Gessling[b], Roger Hodkinson[b], William Makis[c], Harvey A. Risch[d], Mark Trozzi[e], Peter A. McCullough[b f]

Show more

+ Add to Mendeley Share Cite

https://doi.org/10.1016/j.forsciint.2024.112115

Under a Creative Commons license Open access

This Article-in-Press has been withdrawn at the request of the Editors-in-Chief.

Dr. McCullough offered me this comment: "This act of medical censorship occurred after the paper met all the criteria for listing on *The Lancet* PrePrint Server and appears to be triggered by very heavy worldwide interest and rapid downloading of the paper. This speaks to the importance of our findings as the largest summary of autopsies after COVID-19 vaccination. *Elsevier* and *The Lancet* are trying to suppress critical scientific observations on COVID-19 vaccine safety. Their actions are reprehensible."

Furthermore, an investigation[770] by journalist, Rebekah Barnett revealed that politics and financial interests, not scientific concerns, led to the retraction of a 2021 peer-reviewed study that found the spike protein from SARS-CoV-2 and the mRNA vaccine impair critical DNA repair mechanisms, could lead to cancer.

In late 2025, I interviewed[771] a group of scientists: Dr. Jessica Rose, Dr. David Speicher, and Kevin McKernan, scientists whose research on the Pfizer and Moderna COVID-19 mRNA shots has revealed massive DNA contamination exceeding regulatory limits. Chapter 12 addressed the DNA contamination scandal in detail.

These scientists' fight for truth has not stopped at the lab; it has escalated into a war against a coordinated censorship machine, complete with fabricated claims, and conflicted reviewers.

The story traces back to April 2023, when McKernan, a genomics pioneer and founder of Medicinal Genomics, first uncovered DNA fragments in vaccine vials through independent testing. This sparked an October 2023 preprint, later expanded with David Speicher and Maria Gutschi's contributions using properly sourced Canadian vials. Their analysis was damning: fluorometry revealed DNA levels soaring up to 600 times the 10 nanograms per dose safety threshold.

"Fluorometry binds any double-stranded DNA... including plasmid sequences and E. coli remnants," McKernan explained. Regulators, however, lean on qPCR, which targets narrow regions like the kanamycin resistance gene, potentially masking the true extent. "They're looking at a region that's 100 times lower than the spike DNA," he added, noting Australia's TGA as the only agency claiming independent replication, while the FDA and Health Canada blindly trust Pfizer's word.

Speicher highlighted the risks: this isn't harmless "naked" DNA with a 10-minute half-life; it's shielded by lipid nanoparticles (LNPs), potentially ferrying SV40 promoter sequences, known nuclear localizers, straight into cells, raising alarms about integration, immune disruption, and even cancer pathways.

"Cells that are dividing don't have a nucleus... these LNPs go to dividing cells," McKernan warned.

By September 2025, their peer-reviewed paper: "Quantification of Residual Plasmid DNA in SV40 Promoter Enhancer Sequences in Pfizer-BioNTech and Moderna modRNA COVID-19 Vaccines from Ontario, Canada" was published in *Autoimmunity*.[772] They tackled critiques head-on, using RNase A to eliminate RNA crosstalk: "The signal comes down... but it's still way over the limit."

The publication should have been a triumph but within 11 days, an investigation loomed, ignited by PubPeer complaints, an anonymous post-publication peer-review platform, dubbed "PubSmear" by the group.

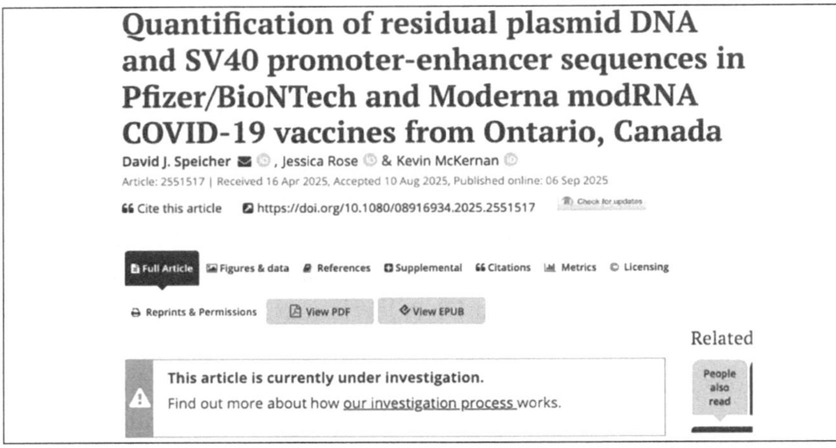
**Quantification of residual plasmid DNA and SV40 promoter-enhancer sequences in Pfizer/BioNTech and Moderna modRNA COVID-19 vaccines from Ontario, Canada**

David J. Speicher, Jessica Rose & Kevin McKernan

Article: 2551517 | Received 16 Apr 2025, Accepted 10 Aug 2025, Published online: 06 Sep 2025

Cite this article https://doi.org/10.1080/08916934.2025.2551517 Check for updates

Full Article Figures & data References Supplemental Citations Metrics Licensing

Reprints & Permissions View PDF View EPUB

Related

**This article is currently under investigation.**
Find out more about how our investigation process works.

People also read

"We got the first email in our inbox letting us know that the paper was under investigation because of some PubPeer commenter…but the comment was fabricated in the first place," Rose explained.

"PubSmear," is a cog in a machine funded by the Arnold Foundation, which was set up by John and Laura Arnold. John Arnold, a former senior Enron trader, received an $8 million bonus (the largest in Enron history) and left unscathed with no criminal charges or accusations of wrongdoing related to Enron's accounting fraud. The same foundation also funds Retraction Watch.

"It's a network aiming to retract papers against certain narratives... some brag about $5,000 bounties," she said. The smears included outright lies: pseudonymous user Kevin Patrick (alias Actinopolyspora bicolorensis, which is one of his alleged 20 usernames) fabricated a quote from a referenced Klinman et al. paper to dogpile (mob-attack) the investigation.

McKernan noted the asymmetry of the fight: "We have to disclose all of our conflicts but all the people attacking us do not. We have to disclose our methods, we have to pay $3,000 to get our thing in there... they flood anonymously without repercussions…And then all of our rebuttals to their work are kept captive by the journal while they are out in public and flaming the paper and getting it put into this sort of investigational purgatory."

According to the scientists, Retraction Watch escalated the scandal, unintentionally leaking a review from one of the peer-reviewers of their paper, whose metadata revealed it came from Rolf Marschalek, who is co-author of the Kaiser et al. paper downplaying DNA contamination (Marschalek's methods overlook small DNA fragments below 150 base pairs, which the Speicher et al. paper critiqued). "They lose all the DNA below 150... ours looks at everything," Speicher countered.

McKernan noted that Marschalek has received research funding from DFG (German Research Foundation) which supported the foundational work on BioNTech's mRNA vaccine platform. "This is a huge conflict. He shouldn't have reviewed us," McKernan said. He went on to assert that despite two other reviewers approving (with modifications the team made), Marschalek falsely claimed rejection, a lie affirmed by the editor. "This echoes his hit-and-run against Brigitte König's MDPI paper:[773] lob complaints, dodge rebuttals, flee to preprints" explained McKernan.

Expression of Concern published on 25 June 2025, see *Methods Protoc.* **2025**, *8*(4), 68.

Commentary 7 May 2024

**Methodological Considerations Regarding the Quantification of DNA Impurities in the COVID-19 mRNA Vaccine Comirnaty®**

Brigitte König[1,2] and Jürgen O. Kirchner[3,*]

The suppression tactics appear to go even further. On January 3, 2026, *Oncotarget* published a systematic review by cancer researchers Dr. Wafik El-Deiry (Brown University) and Charlotte Kuperwasser (Tufts University). They systematically analyzed 69 previously published studies and case reports (from 2020–2025) across 27 countries, identifying 333 instances where cancer was newly diagnosed, recurred, or rapidly progressed (sometimes described as "hyperprogression" or "turbo cancers") shortly after COVID-19 vaccination (often within days to weeks, especially after boosters). The paper flagged temporal links: tumors near injection sites, flare-ups of dormant cancers, virus reactivations like human herpesvirus 8, urging mechanistic probes without claiming causation.

Mere days later, *Oncotarget's* site crashed under a cyberattack, showing "bad gateway" errors, possibly a DDoS flood. The journal reported it to the FBI and alleged ties to PubPeer. The anonymous peer-review platform flatly denied[774] involvement: "No officer, employee or volunteer... has any involvement whatsoever."

El-Deiry, who is also Editor-in-Chief of *Oncotarget*, decried it as "censorship... keeping important information about COVID vaccines and cancer signals from reaching the scientific community."

He wrote on X:[775] "Freedom of the Press is protected under the First Amendment of the US Constitution. But: Censorship is alive and well in the U.S. and has come into medicine in a big, awful way. The future is bleak if weaponized censorship in medicine continues to suppress any narratives that stand up to pharma, that expose inconvenient or suppressed truth."

As McKernan, Speicher and Rose face "PubSmear" onslaughts, El-Deiry's ordeal suggests a pattern: vaccine-critical papers draw digital sabotage.

McKernan tied it together: "PubSmear has anonymous attackers... funded by the same sources as Retraction Watch." Speicher noted selective outrage: PubPeer ignores real fraud, like the hidden data for seniors[776] in Pfizer's mRNA flu jab trial in the *e*. These scientists aren't backing down. "We haven't committed fraud... we're presenting what we find," Rose asserted.

Speicher also criticized how PubPeer rips papers apart anonymously; Retraction Watch flags and shames them publicly and it is all U.S. taxpayer-deductible. Essentially, U.S. taxes subsidize this censorship network targeting inconvenient science.

It is not hard to conclude that the scientific papers highlighting the risks of harm associated with the COVID-19 shots along with the scientists who spoke up against these harms, suffered the same fate as those demonstrating ivermectin and hydroxychloroquine as effective early treatments for the virus and advocating for its use, as discussed in chapter 10.

This pattern of selective scrutiny and swift suppression has led some critics to suggest a coordinated effort to protect a dominant narrative: one promoting experimental gene-based injections as the primary solution while systematically sidelining safer, cheaper, and readily available options that could have challenged the necessity of mass vaccination.

## Censoring The Data

Back in 2023, I wrote about how governments and mainstream media had imposed a "veil of silence"[777] on the issue of excess deaths, particularly after the rollout of COVID-19 shots in mid-2021, in stark contrast with their earlier obsession with daily COVID-19 death tallies.

It centered on a pivotal UK House of Commons 30-minute adjourned debate[778] on October 20, 2023, secured by then-independent MP Andrew Bridgen (after 20 prior rejections). The debate focused on the ongoing issue of excess deaths, with the chamber nearly empty in contrast to an enthusiastic public gallery.

Notably, the BBC inserted live captions throughout Bridgen's debate to fact-check and undermine him in real-time.

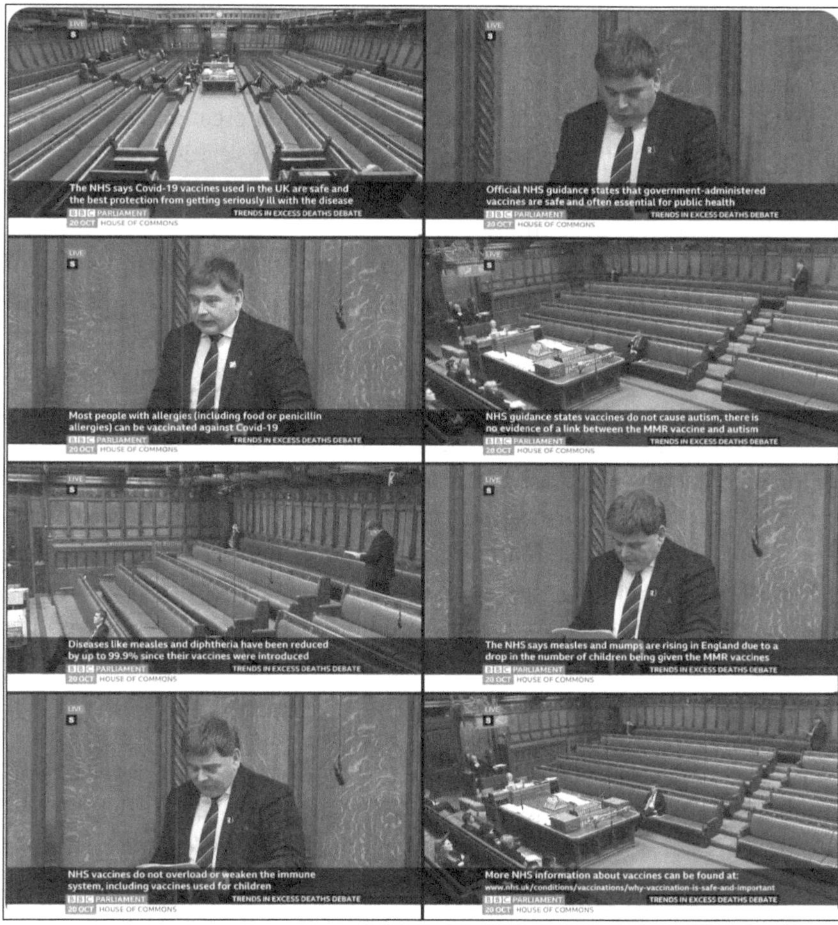
The NHS says Covid-19 vaccines used in the UK are safe and the best protection from getting seriously ill with the disease
BBC PARLIAMENT
TRENDS IN EXCESS DEATHS DEBATE
20 OCT HOUSE OF COMMONS
Official NHS guidance states that government-administered vaccines are safe and often essential for public health
Most people with allergies (including food or penicillin allergies) can be vaccinated against Covid-19
NHS guidance states vaccines do not cause autism, there is no evidence of a link between the MMR vaccine and autism
Diseases like measles and diphtheria have been reduced by up to 99.9% since their vaccines were introduced
The NHS says measles and mumps are rising in England due to a drop in the number of children being given the MMR vaccines
NHS vaccines do not overload or weaken the immune system, including vaccines used for children
More NHS information about vaccines can be found at:
www.nhs.uk/conditions/vaccinations/why-vaccination-is-safe-and-important

Source: @robinmonotti[779]

The BBC issued a statement[780] on November 3, 2023, admitting the captions were disproportionate and created an incorrect impression of editorial bias: "We have reviewed our use of on-screen captions during an Adjournment Debate at the House of Commons called 'Trends in Excess Deaths'. There were concerns that the captions, which outlined the NHS guidance on vaccines for COVID-19 and other diseases, showed bias against Andrew Bridgen MP who was making a speech that challenged the Government's position on the safety and efficacy of the COVID-19 vaccines. It is normal practice to provide accurate information and context to these debates on screen and in this case it was an important aspect of our coverage due to the nature of the assertions being made in relation to public health. However, we accept that there was a lack of consistency in our use of these captions and that the number posted during the speech was not proportionate, nor always relevant, which created the incorrect impression that there was an editorial approach in relation to the views expressed. We apologize for this and are reviewing the way we use captions during such proceedings."

Bridgen highlighted that the UK has recorded more excess deaths since July 2021 than during the whole of 2020. Unlike the pandemic period, these deaths are not mainly among the elderly but are disproportionately affecting people in the prime of life and occurring across all age groups. He criticized the Office for National Statistics (ONS) for including 2021 deaths in the baseline for expected deaths, arguing that this treats an abnormal year as normal and artificially minimizes the reported excess.

It is worth highlighting here, my early 2022 interview[781] with Prof. Norman Fenton, a British mathematician and computer scientist, serving as Professor Emeritus of Risk Information Management at Queen Mary University of London, who has authored hundreds of peer-reviewed papers and several books. He revealed how the ONS had been manipulating the data on deaths involving COVID-19 by vaccination status.

Fenton co-authored a paper[782] with Prof. Martin Neil (Queen Mary University of London), Dr. Clare Craig (diagnostic pathologist) and Joel Smalley, analyzing an ONS report:[783] "Deaths involving COVID-19 by vaccination status, England: deaths occurring between 2 January and 24 September 2021."

Their paper concluded that the ONS was guilty of "systematic mis categorization of vaccine status" and that the COVID-19 vaccines did not reduce all-cause mortality but rather produced genuine spikes in all-cause mortality shortly after vaccination.

Turning back to Bridgen's parliamentary speech, where he pointed out a serious failure in death registration: deaths referred to coroners face long delays, sometimes years, before formal registration, particularly affecting younger age groups, meaning the true death toll for 2021 and beyond remains uncertain.

Bridgen noted unexplained rises in deaths among adolescents and children, including the ONS's refusal to release statistically significant data on excess deaths in young males in late 2021 during a judicial review.

He cited high excess deaths in heavily vaccinated countries such as Ireland, Malta, Portugal and the Netherlands, and presented Australia, where COVID-19 circulation was negligible before Omicron, as a near-ideal control group, showing sharp increases in cardiac emergencies among younger adults that coincided precisely with vaccine rollout.

Bridgen highlighted how Dr. Clare Craig was the first to point out the sharp rise in ambulance calls for cardiac arrests in England following the vaccine rollout. He stated: "Ambulance data for England provides another clue. Ambulance calls for life-threatening emergencies were running at a steady 2,000 calls per day until the vaccine rollout. From then they rose to 2,500 daily, and calls have stayed at that level since."

He also referenced studies from Israel and Australia linking cardiac issues to vaccination timing rather than COVID-19 infection.

Bridgen raised concerns about the Pfizer clinical trial, where more deaths occurred in the vaccine arm than the placebo arm (21 versus 17, including four cardiac arrests versus one), with suggestive delays in reporting vaccine-group deaths.

Crucially, he went on to share how the product manufactured for trial participants differed substantially from the version rolled out to the public, and regulators waived the requirement to compare safety and efficacy data between the two processes. Mass production introduced risks of bacterial DNA contamination far exceeding permitted leve, with lipid nanoparticles potentially delivering this material into human cells and organs. This scandal was discussed in detail in chapter 12.

In closing, Bridgen stated: "The experimental COVID-19 vaccines are not safe and are not effective. Despite there being only limited interest in the Chamber from colleagues, I am very grateful to those who have attended. We can see from the Public Gallery that there is considerable public interest. I implore all Members of the House, those who are present and those who are not, to support calls for a three-hour debate on this important issue. Mr. Deputy Speaker, this might be the first debate on excess deaths in our Parliament, indeed, it might be the first debate on excess deaths in the world but, very sadly, I promise you it will not be the last."

• • •

Six months later, on April 18, 2024, Bridgen managed to secure a landmark two-hour House of Commons debate[784] on excess deaths and their link to the mRNA Covid shots. This specific address to parliament by Bridgen was referred to earlier in chapter 5.

Describing it as "the greatest medical scandal in living memory," he opened the debate stating: "I've been called an anti-vaxxer as if I rejected these vaccines based on some ideology. I want to say clearly and unequivocally that I am not. I am in fact double vaccinated and vaccine harmed."

He accused bodies like the Office for National Statistics (ONS) and the UK Health Security Agency (UKHSA) of opacity and manipulation. He highlighted the ONS' halt in data releases (on August 25, 2023, the ONS announced[785] that it would no longer update its "Deaths by vaccination status, England" series, marking the end of its regular publications) and its methodological shift in calculating excess deaths that erased roughly 20,000 excess deaths in 2023. The UKHSA's refusal to release anonymized record-level data on deaths by vaccination status was also heavily criticized by Bridgen.

This leads to the next explosive scandal. In late 2025, the UK's Health Security Agency (UKHSA) was exposed for its outright refusal to release critical data that could reveal a potential link between COVID-19 shots and the UK's alarming surge in excess deaths. This has not been a simple case of bureaucratic foot-dragging but can be described as a deliberate data blackout.

*The Telegraph*[786] revealed in a damning exposé, how the UKHSA officials invoked the "distress or anger" of bereaved families as their shield, arguing that any hint of correlation in the data might shatter the emotional well-being of those left behind.

According to *The Telegraph*: "Last year, a cross-party group expressed alarm about 'growing public and professional concerns' over the UK's rates of excess deaths[787] since 2020. In a letter to UKHSA and Department for Health, the MPs and peers said that potentially critical data, which map the date of people's Covid vaccine doses to the date of their deaths, had been released to pharmaceutical companies but not put into the public domain.

They argued that the data should be released 'on the same anonymized basis that it was shared with the pharmaceutical groups, and there seems to be no credible reason why that should not be done immediately.'

UsForThem, a campaign group, requested that UKHSA release the data under freedom of information laws. But the agency refused, making a number of different arguments including that publishing the data 'could lead to misinformation' that would 'have an adverse impact on vaccine uptake' in the public.

UKHSA also claimed there would be a risk of individuals being identified, despite the request being made for an anonymized dataset. After a two-year battle, the Information Commissioner ruled in the UKHSA's favor, backing its refusal to publish the data."

Gareth Eve whose wife, Lisa Shaw died from the Astra-Zeneca Covid jab, took to social media to express his opinion on the UKHSA's refusal to disclose the data under the guise that it will risk "damaging the well-being and mental health of families and friends of people who died."

He wrote on X:[788] "As someone who lost his amazing wife to a Covid jab As a Dad of a little boy who lost his Mammy at the age of 6 I can assure you, my heart and my mental health is already very much broken."

UsForThem was not the only party seeking this crucial data through Freedom of Information requests. As early as 2022, diagnostic pathologist and statistician Dr. Clare Craig submitted a series of FOI requests to UKHSA and ONS seeking detailed data on deaths following COVID-19 vaccination.

On August 4, 2023 she made a specific request for anonymized individual-level NIMS records of adults over 20 who died after December 2020 (age at first dose, vaccination dates, and barbarized date of death). Barbarized data is used primarily in the UK to protect privacy and prevent the identification of individuals in aggregated datasets.

UKHSA refused disclosure. After the Information Commissioner upheld the refusal in June 2024, Dr. Craig appealed to the First-tier Tribunal against both the Information Commissioner and UKHSA. The tribunal dismissed her appeal on October 14, 2025.

Dr. Craig kindly gave me permission to review the First-tier Tribunal's 27-page decision. Several anomalies stood out to me. Firstly, the UKHSA repeatedly changed its legal grounds. When Dr. Clare Craig made her request in August 2023, the UKHSA originally said "no" under section 40(2) FOIA (personal data exemption). Even with barbarized death dates, the UKHSA argued that the combination of age at first dose, exact vaccination dates, and approximate death date could still allow some individuals to be re-identified. So, the UKHSA treated the requested data as third-party personal data and refused it outright. Later, probably in preparation for the tribunal they downplayed section 40(2) and relied mainly on section

38 FOIA (Health and Safety). Section 38(1) says information is exempt if its disclosure would or would likely to: a] endanger the physical or mental health of any individual b] endanger the safety of any individual.

This exemption is not absolute but is subject to the public-interest balance test. The UKHSA also shifted to other arguments: sections: 12 (Cost), 4 (Vexatious or repeated requests), 36 (Prejudice to effective conduct of public affairs), 41 (Actionable breach of confidence). They ultimately succeeded with the broad "health and safety" exemption (s.38) based on speculative risks of harassment or violence.

- Releasing these records (even barnardized) could lead to bereaved families being identified and harassed.
- It could fuel anti-vaccine campaigns that incite threats or violence against doctors, scientists, or public-health staff.
- It could cause serious distress to relatives who discover their loved one's details are being discussed online.
- Misinformation/misinterpretation of the data could itself damage public confidence and therefore harm mental health on a wider scale.

In short, the UKHSA started with "this is personal data, full stop," which later became "well, maybe it can be anonymized, but releasing it anyway would endanger people's health or safety." Then they threw in every possible additional exemption (cost, vexatious, damage public confidence, and legal confidentiality) to make absolutely sure at least one would stick.

When asked for comment, Dr. Craig wrote: "There is more than enough evidence that the vaccine products caused death. The majority were covid deaths in the first two weeks after injection and in the period after the third mRNA dose. Non-covid deaths also rose and these did not come in waves. However, the ONS stopped publishing their data when the problem became undeniable. I hope this story about hiding the data wakes people up to the failure of our institutions to respect the truth over their own agendas."

• • •

The previous chapter detailed my first interview with senior data patterns & forensics analyst, Wouter Aukema, whose groundbreaking work: using enhanced software to download 15 million case safety report files from the EMA's EudraVigilance[789] and transform them into user-friendly Tableau dashboards.[790] These tools allow the public to navigate through data points on thousands of medicinal products, including COVID-19 shots, offering a holistic view that the official EMA website lacks, which is limited to individual product searches.

Shockingly, the data revealed a three-fold increase in these reports for the Covid vaccines (at the start of the rollout) compared to all other drug products and vaccines, over the past 20 years. A surge Aukema attributed in part to the massive scale of vaccinations, though he noted comparable usage rates for general medications across populations.

In the second interview[791] with Aukema, several months later, he dropped another bombshell: "And what is disturbing Sonia is that if you repeatedly download all that data, then I can investigate how many records were added every week. And I can investigate how many got lost or ended up deleted/missing. 40% of serious case safety reports end up missing." This was from the period of October 2021 through to November 2022. What appeared at first to be mass deletions of serious case safety reports turned out to be something even more calculated. Later revelations in this chapter detail the systematic process that made the original versions vanish forever, replaced without a trace.

In addition, case safety reports were also retroactively modified, after their data lock point (DLP). Aukema went on to share, "I think it is a crime that they are hiding the data from us so that we cannot find the truth."

In the third revealing interview,[792] the Dutch ethical hacker and data analyst opened up about the unexpected pressures he has encountered for making public data more accessible. A key feature of Aukema's platform is the "case locator" dashboard, designed to help individuals verify the accuracy of their submitted adverse event reports.

Drawing from personal experience, Aukema recounted filing a report for a family member who developed acute pancreatitis following an mRNA COVID shot. A hospital specialist had linked it to the jab, citing similar cases among other patients. However, upon checking the EMA database using his tool, Aukema discovered the report had been miscategorized: the hospitalization was downplayed as "other" rather than marked as serious. When he confronted the Dutch pharmacovigilance authority Lareb, they admitted the error but initially blamed him, promising a correction.

This incident underscored the tool's value, as dozens of users contacted Aukema to report similar discrepancies in their cases, ranging from omitted side effects to misattributed reporters. Issues that could diminish the weight of reports from healthcare professionals in pharmacovigilance assessments. While Aukema refrained from speculating on whether such errors have led to missed safety signals, emphasizing his non-medical background, he stressed the dashboards' role in empowering patients, doctors, and families to ensure data integrity.

The interview took place at the "Back to the Future"[793] conference in the Netherlands, where Aukema was slated to speak. However, just days prior, he stumbled upon a startling email from the EMA in his spam folder, demanding the immediate deletion of what they deemed "non-public information" from his Tableau dashboards. The agency cited privacy risks, claiming that unique worldwide case identifiers and country of residence data could indirectly lead to patient identification, despite the absence of names, birth dates, or addresses in the datasets Aukema handles. "I have no access to patients' birth dates or names," he insisted. "Even if that data was available, I would never have downloaded it. My objective is to gather insights on patterns, not to find people."

He expressed shock at the letter, viewing it as a form of legal pressure and censorship, especially given the EMA's proclaimed commitment to data transparency. "My initial reaction is I'm being censored," he shared. (Later, it came to light that similar EMA letters were sent to French researchers Emma Darles and Pavan Vincent.)

This isn't the first time Aukema has faced pushback. In a 2022 interview on Dutch YouTube channel Blackbox,[794] he highlighted the mysterious disappearance of 40% of serious adverse event cases from the EudraVigilance system over time. The EMA's press office responded by accusing him of "misleading allegations" without clarifying what he got wrong or engaging in dialogue. "They didn't correct me," Aukema said. "They just accused me."

He pointed out apparent double standards, contrasting Europe's stringent privacy stance with the U.S. VAERS system, which openly shares state-level details and full case narratives without similar concerns. In response, Aukema spent hours redacting his conference presentation to comply, removing sensitive elements while planning to inform the audience about the EMA's intervention.

The EMA's insistence that country of origin data could indirectly identify patients seems inconsistent, particularly when Aukema's dashboards require a case identifier, accessible only to the reporter, to be useful. When asked what he believes the EMA's true fears are, Aukema hesitated to speculate beyond the stated privacy concerns but expressed a willingness to engage in open dialogue. "I'm more than happy to have a debate with them," he said. noting that his redacted presentation demonstrates his goodwill. Yet, the timing and tone of the EMA's demands suggest an attempt to silence a researcher whose work has exposed uncomfortable truths: not just about the COVID shots but also other medicinal products.

After further discussions with Aukema, he revealed a disturbing practice affecting approximately 40% of serious (including fatal) COVID-19 vaccine adverse-event reports. Whenever a case narrative is updated, even for the most trivial edit, such as inserting a comma, the system generates an entirely new case ID number and a new receipt date. The previous version of the report, with its original identifier and timestamp, is permanently overwritten and becomes untraceable. There is no audit trail, no version history, and no way to retrieve the original entry. Aukema described it as "a floating duck."

On the surface everything appears normal, but the critical reference points are in constant motion, making it impossible to track changes or hold anyone accountable for what has been altered or suppressed. He suspects that this selective updating of original reports is not accidental. In his view, the manipulation originates from the pharmaceutical companies themselves and from national pharmacovigilance authorities, including Lareb in the Netherlands and, by extension, equivalent bodies such as the MHRA (Yellow Card scheme) in the United Kingdom, whose databases feed into the European system.

In short, not only are serious and fatal cases being under-reported or retrospectively downgraded; in a large proportion of instances, the original evidence that they were ever reported in the first place is being deliberately and irreversibly destroyed.

Turning back to the UKHSA's blank refusal to release critical data, which could expose the link between excess deaths and the Covid shots. Perhaps, this link could be found in Aukema's damning data sets, which include case safety reports from the UK for the Covid shots. Each individual case safety report (ICSR) in EudraVigilance includes (when reported): date of vaccination, date of onset of the adverse reaction, and the date of death (if fatal). If a large, tightly clustered peak of fatal reports were visible in the first 0–14 days and especially if that peak exceeded the reporting bias and background mortality expected in the vaccinated population, it would represent a very strong safety signal requiring urgent investigation.

The timing of the EMA's demands have led some observers to suspect that the agency's stated privacy concerns may conceal deeper institutional fears about what comprehensive data analysis could uncover. Independent analysts including Aukema have raised questions about whether regulatory resistance to data transparency reflects coordination among agencies facing potential liability exposure, allegations the EMA has not directly addressed. Whether this represents legitimate privacy protection, bureaucratic caution, or what critics characterize as systematic suppression of inconvenient evidence remains a matter of ongoing dispute and investigation.

• • •

In March 2024, the American comedian and political commentator, Bill Maher on *Real Time with Bill Maher*,[795] delivered a poignant takedown of pandemic policies and the COVID "experts" who got it wrong. He reflected on how many suppressed or ridiculed views have since been vindicated.

Maher said. "I get it that we didn't know what exactly was happening at the beginning of COVID and some mistakes were inevitable. But four years on, I'm tired of hearing: 'Well we didn't know.' No, we didn't but some people guessed better than others and the people who got it wrong don't seem to want to acknowledge that now… Yes, some very bad ideas were embraced as the conventional wisdom ideas that haven't aged well. And a lot of the dissent, dissenting opinions that were suppressed and ridiculed at the time have proven to be correct."

The question is no longer whether censorship occurred, but how deeply it was orchestrated. The final chapter reveals the systematic collaboration between governments, non-governmental organizations (NGOs), technology giants, media organizations, and public health authorities that made this silence possible.

CHAPTER SIXTEEN

# "FOR YOUR SAFETY"

*"Governments and the private sector should assign a greater priority to developing methods to combat mis- and disinformation prior to the next pandemic response. Governments will need to partner with traditional and social media companies to research and develop nimble approaches to countering misinformation ...For their part, media companies should commit to ensuring that authoritative messages are prioritized and that false messages are suppressed including through the use of technology."*

~Recommendations from Event 201,
a global pandemic exercise,
October 18, 2019[796]

The phrase "For your safety" has become the justification for almost every new layer of control. What started as temporary emergency measures during a declared pandemic has hardened into permanent infrastructure.

This final chapter looks at how the biodefense-industrial complex in lockstep with the machinery of censorship, did not emerge spontaneously in the aftermath of 3/11. Its roots stretch back two decades through a recurring pattern: crisis, fear, and expanded powers. However, it took a major disruptive event, like 3/11, for the apparatus to be fully scaled and globalized: culminating in binding pandemic-preparedness agreements; public-private partnerships coordinating suppression; governments applying pressure; NGOs supplying ideological cover, military-grade psyops "inoculating" against dissent, and the accelerating descent into digital authoritarianism now underway across the West.

## The "Amerithrax" Template

The beginning of this final chapter draws heavily on the investigative groundwork laid in my earlier reports: "Mpox, Project BioShield, Everyone's Dark Winter?"[797] and the follow-up piece "Cashing in on a very 'Dark Winter.'"[798]

Those investigations highlighted the enduring biosecurity framework built around Project BioShield, the role of longtime biodefense expert, Dr. Robert Kadlec, across multiple eras, the suspicious circumstances of the 2001 anthrax-letter attacks officially dubbed as "Amerithrax" by the FBI, and Emergent BioSolutions' opportunistic rise as the sole supplier of the anthrax vaccine BioThrax and the primary supplier of ACAM2000 (a smallpox vaccine later used for mpox). Here, these threads are woven together to reveal how the "Amerithrax" crisis established a template that was later refined and redeployed for 3/11.

The 2001 "Amerithrax" attacks, erupted shortly after 9/11, killing five people and sickening many others. The attacks involved weaponized anthrax spores mailed to media outlets and politicians, sparking fears of bioterrorism and justifying a massive expansion of U.S. biodefense spending. They also established a powerful precedent for how a bioterror crisis could be exploited to entrench a single company as the indispensable supplier of a critical medical countermeasure.

The FBI's close to nine-year investigation[799] ultimately pinned[800] the (Ames-strain) Anthrax attacks on senior biodefense researcher Bruce E. Ivins[801] working at the United States Army Medical Research Institute of Infectious Diseases (USAMRIID) at Fort Detrick, Maryland. Ivins died by suicide in 2008 before charges could be filed. However, serious doubts[802] persist over the FBI's investigation. The Ames strain database at Iowa State University was destroyed on FBI orders. According to the late Francis A. Boyle, Professor of International Law, who drafted the Biological Weapons Anti-Terrorism Act of 1989, which passed into law, he stated:[803] "FBI's decision to order the destruction of the Ames strain database was an obstruction of justice, a federal crime…That collection should have been preserved and protected as evidence. That's the DNA, the fingerprints right there."

Earlier security lapses[804] at Fort Detrick raised questions about internal access and narrative control. Notably, the same USAMRIID labs at Fort Detrick were temporarily shut down[805] after failing CDC inspections due to safety concerns in the summer of 2019 and they have cooperated with the Institute of Medical Virology of Wuhan University, "since the 1980s."[806]

In the aftermath of the "Amerithrax" attacks, Emergent BioSolutions, formerly BioPort, solidified its position as the sole U.S. producer of BioThrax, the anthrax vaccine. Having acquired the failing Michigan Biological Products Institute facility in 1998 for well below market value,[807] BioPort secured a $45 million DoD contract (a mere 11 days after the sale was finalized) that guaranteed payments even if the vaccine failed to achieve full licensing. This structure shielded the company from market risk while capitalizing on post-9/11 biodefense panic.

Serendipitously for Emergent BioSolutions, this occurred the same year when the mandatory Anthrax Vaccine Immunization Program (AVIP)[808] was set up under the Clinton Administration in 1998.

The "Amerithrax" attacks directly catalyzed the creation of Project BioShield Act of 2004.[809] This Act, which passed through Congress under the Bush administration, authorized billions in public funding ($5.6 billion later expanded to over $60 billion) to stockpile medical countermeasures (including vaccines, drugs, and diagnostics) against chemical, biological, radiological, and nuclear (CBRN) threats.

It was also under Dr. Anthony Fauci's leadership at the National Institute of Allergy and Infectious Diseases (NIAID) and directly in response to the post-9/11 Anthrax attacks, that the institute "markedly expanded, intensified and accelerated its ongoing research programs in biodefense."

During his keynote address at the 12th annual Joseph B. Brennan Lecture on October 17, 2002, in Georgetown University's ICC Auditorium, Fauci described the post-2001 shift: "Events of 2001 have had an impact not only on the nation but on the biomedical field, which is now concerned with emerging diseases and defense," as reported in The Hoya's article "Fauci Addresses Bioterrorism Threats."[810] He added that "eighteen cases and five deaths associated with anthrax has led to a total transformation in what the biomedical community would have to deal with. The anthrax scare has resulted in a situation unprecedented...and would be a new challenge for American medicine."

A key element of Project BioShield is that it allowed the stockpiling and distribution of vaccines that had not been tested for safety or efficacy in humans, "due to ethical concerns." This is because the agents could not have been tested in humans without also exposing them to the threat. Instead, animal testing was used to establish efficacy.

Project BioShield created the legal framework for Emergency Use Authorizations, liability immunity later expanded via the PREP Act, and accelerated procurement. These were precisely the mechanisms repurposed in 2020 to fast-track the experimental mRNA products while shielding manufacturers from responsibility, as detailed in earlier chapters.

A central figure in this trajectory, one who played a pivotal role across both eras, is Dr. Robert Kadlec.[811] A former U.S. Air Force colonel, physician and biodefense expert, who has spent decades at the intersection of national security, pandemic preparedness, and lucrative pharmaceutical contracts.

On June 22-23, 2001, a simulation exercise code-named "Dark Winter"[812] at Andrews Air Force Base was conducted, depicting a smallpox bioterror attack on the U.S., which eerily preceded the anthrax attacks by mere months. It was introduced via mock news briefings reporting confirmed smallpox cases, initially in Oklahoma, with rapid spread to other states. One of the key findings from the exercise was that "should a contagious bioweapon pathogen be used, containing the spread of disease will present significant ethical, political, cultural, operational, and legal challenges."

Dark Winter was a collaborative effort led by the John Hopkins Center for Civilian Biodefense Strategies, the ANSER Institute for Homeland Security, and the Oklahoma City National Memorial Institute for the Prevention Terrorism. Those who were present included several Congressmen, a former CIA director (James Woolsey), Dr. Tara O'Toole (then Director of John Hopkins Center for Civilian Biodefense Strategies and since 2014 has held leadership roles at the CIA hedge fund, In-Q-Tel) and CIA's former deputy director for Science and Technology (Ruth David) and selected members of the press.

Notably, in a video,[813] which appears to be archival footage from the 2001 exercise mock news briefing, Robert Kadlec states: "it could be a very dark winter for America" (referring to a vaccine shortage leading to uncontrolled spread and high casualties).

Retired U.S. Airforce Colonel Randall Larsen, who had recruited Kadlec to teach at the National War College in the mid-1990s and collaborated with him on biodefense studies, was a key co-designer of Dark Winter alongside Dr. Tara O'Toole and Tom Inglesby, the Center's current director.

Larson and Kadlec's joint work focused on the need for enhanced U.S. preparedness against bioweapons, including stockpiling vaccines and antibiotics, ideas that directly informed the scenarios in Dark Winter.

The pattern repeated in 2019 with "Crimson Contagion,"[814] an exercise directly overseen by Kadlec during his tenure as Assistant Secretary for Preparedness and Response (ASPR). This nationwide simulation from January to August 2019 that modeled a severe influenza pandemic originating in China, uncannily mirroring COVID-19's trajectory. The exercise exposed catastrophic gaps: PPE shortages, ventilator chaos, supply-chain breakdowns, and interagency dysfunction. Yet, despite damning internal reports warning of "cascading"[815] failures, little was done to address them before 3/11 hit months later.

Kadlec's engagement extended beyond exercises; on July 11, 2019, he participated as a federal representative in a Blue Ribbon Study Panel on Biodefense workshop in New York City titled, "A Manhattan Project for Biodefense,"[816] discussing federal/military biodefense research needs and requirements for a major national R&D push against biological threats.

It drew an explicit analogy to the WWII Manhattan Project's[817] massive, public-private mobilization to develop the atomic bomb. The event called for a similarly bold national R&D effort to rally federal agencies, military, academia, and industry in accelerating innovations (e.g., universal vaccines, diagnostics, medical countermeasures) against pandemics, bioterrorism, and engineered threats. Kadlec, on the federal/military panel, endorsed it, declaring it was time to "go big or go home"[818] on biodefense to comprehensively address these risks.

Just weeks after Crimson Contagion concluded, on October 18, 2019, the same Johns Hopkins Center (Dark Winter's host) co-sponsored Event 201[819] with the World Economic Forum and Bill & Melinda Gates Foundation. This tabletop exercise simulated a novel zoonotic coronavirus outbreak, complete with global spread, economic collapse, and explicit calls for governments to partner with media and tech companies to suppress "mis- and disinformation."

Turning back to Kadlec's rise to power, following 9/11 and the Anthrax attacks (where he contributed[820] to the FBI's "botched" investigation), he joined the White House Homeland Security Council as biodefense director. From that position, he played a central role in drafting, advocating for, and helping create Project BioShield.

Kadlec, also played a key role in drafting the Pandemic and All-Hazards Preparedness Act (PAHPA). Introduced in 2006 and signed into law by President George W. Bush on December 19, 2006. BARDA (Biomedical Advanced Research and Development Authority) was also established the same month, as part of PAHPA, to oversee aspects of Project Bioshield. The act conveniently created the powerful Assistant Secretary for Preparedness and Response (ASPR) position at HHS, a role Kadlec himself would later occupy from 2017 to 2021, while expanding federal authority and funding for emergency responses to bioterrorism, pandemics, and natural disasters, often favoring biodefense contractors.

One of those biodefense contractors who was very much favored[821] was Emergent BioSolutions, which emerged as the sole U.S. supplier of the Anthrax vaccine (BioThrax) and the primary supplier of the Smallpox vaccine ACAM2000, which was later given FDA approval[822] for the prevention of Mpox in 2024, under Project BioShield's lucrative framework.

However, these countermeasures came with severe risks that were often downplayed or suppressed in the name of preparedness. BioThrax, Emergent's anthrax vaccine, was mandated for U.S. troops during the 1990s Gulf War era under the Anthrax Vaccine Immunization Program (AVIP), leading to widespread reports of debilitating illnesses that many veterans and researchers have linked[823] to Gulf War Syndrome: a constellation of chronic symptoms including fatigue, muscle/joint pain, neurological issues, and autoimmune disorders.

Dr. Meryl Nass, a physician, biological warfare epidemiologist and anthrax expert, has repeatedly highlighted[824] these adverse events, citing VAERS data, peer-reviewed studies, and congressional testimony showing elevated rates of serious reactions, including Guillain-Barré syndrome and deaths among service members.

Similarly, ACAM2000 for Smallpox and Mpox carries serious warnings[825] of myocarditis, pericarditis, encephalitis, and potentially fatal complications.

**WARNING: SERIOUS COMPLICATIONS**

**Myocarditis and pericarditis (suspect cases observed at a rate of 5.7 per 1000 primary vaccinees (95% CI: 1.9-13.3)), encephalitis, encephalomyelitis, encephalopathy, progressive vaccinia, generalized vaccinia, severe vaccinial skin infections, erythema multiforme major (including STEVENS-JOHNSON SYNDROME), eczema vaccinatum resulting in permanent sequelae or death, accidental eye infection (ocular vaccinia) which can cause ocular complications that may lead to blindness, and fetal death, have occurred following either primary vaccination or revaccination with ACAM2000 or other live vaccinia virus vaccines that were used historically. These risks are increased in certain individuals and may result in severe disability, permanent neurological sequelae and/or death [see Warnings and Precautions (5)].**

Alarmingly, the FDA-approved prescribing information for this product also states: "ACAM2000 contains live vaccinia virus that can be transmitted to persons who have close contact with the vaccine and the risks in contacts are the same as those for the vaccinee... Death has also been reported in unvaccinated contacts accidentally infected by individuals who have been vaccinated."

Despite these dangers, liability immunity under the PREP Act shielded Emergent from accountability.

Emergent BioSolutions' rise was no accident: in the revolving door of biodefense policy, Kadlec himself had deep ties[826] to the company. Between 2012 and 2015, while in the private sector, he served as a paid strategic adviser through his firm RPK Consulting, earning at least $360,000 (including a reported $120,000 annual retainer). He also co-founded a biodefense startup, East West Protection, with Emergent's founder and chairman Fuad El-Hibri, serving as managing director and part-owner until selling his stake for $20,000.

When Kadlec was nominated for ASPR in 2017 (the very position created by the PAHPA legislation he helped draft), he failed to disclose[827] these financial ties or the biodefense startup on his Senate ethics forms, simply answering "None" to potential conflicts. Confirmed nonetheless, he took charge of the Strategic National Stockpile in 2018 (away from the CDC, enabling centralized control over acquisitions) and promptly awarded Emergent billions in contracts: a 10-year, up to $2.8 billion deal for smallpox vaccine in 2019 (at double the previous per-dose price), extensions on anthrax vaccine worth hundreds of millions, and over $733 million in total ASPR payments during his tenure.

This favoritism culminated in the COVID-19 response. In June 2020, Kadlec's office handed Emergent a $628 million task order[828] under Operation Warp Speed for "fill-finish" manufacturing of Johnson & Johnson and AstraZeneca's Covid vaccines at its Baltimore Bayview plant. What followed was disaster:[829] systemic contamination ruined ingredients for up to 400 million doses (with congressional probes revealing deliberate concealment from FDA inspectors), wasting taxpayer funds on a massive scale. Emergent executives cashed in millions in stock sales before the scandals broke, yet the company pocketed billions overall. Congressional investigations in 2021–2022 exposed Kadlec's undisclosed consulting and apparent cronyism.

Here, a parallel can easily be drawn with Moderna. A company with no approved products prior to 2020, which received billions in BARDA funding and massive advance-purchase commitments through Operation Warp Speed, transforming it overnight into a pharmaceutical giant (as discussed in chapter 9). Similarly, BioNTech, founded in 2008, had no products approved prior to 3/11, yet the COVID-19 crisis catapulted it to global prominence through its Pfizer partnership and the rapid authorization of the first mRNA vaccine.

Evidently, the "Amerithrax" template was never discarded. It was simply refined and redeployed for the mRNA era, where crisis once again guaranteed monopoly profits and narrative control, all, of course, under the guise of national security.

However, the most insidious evolution of this machinery was not merely bolstering the biodefense-industrial complex through insider enrichment and countermeasure stockpiling: it was the deliberate construction of tools to silence dissent, framed as combatting "mis- and disinformation." In the pages that follow, I will trace how the recommendations from Event 201 and similar exercises became the blueprint for a coordinated censorship apparatus, where governments, tech giants, and biosecurity experts worked in lockstep to decide what the public could see, say, and believe, all inevitably, "for your safety."

## The Trusted News Initiative: "Ministry of Truth"

The global pandemic exercise of Event 201 and its clarion call: urging governments and media/tech companies to "develop methods to combat mis- and disinformation" and "suppress false messages" through technology, became operational reality in the Trusted News Initiative (TNI).

Initially formed by the BBC in July 2019 to counter election disinformation, and rapidly expanded on March 27, 2020, to "tackle harmful Coronavirus disinformation,"[830] TNI united legacy media (BBC, Reuters, Associated Press, Financial Times, and the Washington Post) with tech giants (Google, Meta, Microsoft) in a formal alliance that coordinated suppression of content deviating from official narratives, turning Event 201's rehearsal into a global censorship cartel.

The TNI's expansion was not a spontaneous response to a crisis. It was launched roughly two weeks after the World Health Organization's pandemic declaration, before the public could even begin to question the emerging narrative. It brought together an unprecedented coalition: the world's dominant technology platforms, alongside legacy media giants. Partners explicitly agreed to restrict discourse to only those "truths" endorsed by official bodies such as the CDC, WHO, and national health agencies. Any deviation (even when supported by peer-reviewed evidence, emerging data, or credentialed expertise) was to be flagged, demoted, labeled as misinformation, or erased entirely.

The TNI described itself as an "early warning system" to identify and combat "harmful disinformation." In practice, it operated as a real-time, cross-platform censorship network. Perfectly in-line with Event 201's call for "nimble approaches to countering misinformation."

Post 3/11, the TNI coordinated and amplified the suppression of several key areas of legitimate scientific debate. The laboratory-origin hypothesis (lab-leak theory), dismissed as a conspiracy theory (outlined in chapter 1). Arguments for natural immunity as superior or equivalent to vaccination, a position later vindicated but initially branded dangerous (discussed in chapter 15).

In addition, early treatment protocols such as ivermectin and hydroxychloroquine, were systematically blacklisted despite emerging clinical evidence (detailed in chapter 10). The Great Barrington Declaration itself, co-authored by Drs. Martin Kulldorff, Jay Bhattacharya, and Sunetra Gupta, which advocated focused protection over universal lockdowns (outlined in chapters 4 and 15), was smeared as dangerous and fringe. Its signatories censored and vilified by the very public-private apparatus Event 201 had rehearsed.

Turning back to my July 2021 interview with Dr. Robert Malone, he described the TNI's effect in stark terms: "The Trusted News Initiative… agreed to restrict acceptable discourse to only those 'truths' endorsed by official public health bodies such as the CDC and WHO, effectively suppressing scientific speech that deviated from those positions, even when grounded in peer-reviewed publications."

This was not reactive moderation. It was proactive narrative enforcement. The TNI's expansion predated widespread vaccine rollout, the first major waves of adverse event reporting, and even the full implementation of lockdowns in many countries. It was infrastructure built in anticipation of dissent, exactly as the Event 201 exercise had recommended just months earlier.

The initiative did not merely respond to misinformation; it defined what constituted misinformation, then mobilized the combined power of global media and technology to enforce that definition. The consequences were far-reaching. As explored in chapter 15, the TNI collaborated directly with Facebook to identify and dismantle accounts of COVID vaccine-injured groups, even highlighting their use of carrot emojis as a circumvention tactic. The same network helped shadow-ban Kulldorff's posts on natural immunity, contributed to the removal of Malone's Joe Rogan appearance within hours, and facilitated the broader epistemic quarantine of anyone challenging the "safe and effective" mantra.

The Trusted News Initiative was criticized as an Orwellian "Ministry of Truth" in congressional testimony and antitrust lawsuits. During the July 20, 2023, hearing [831]of the U.S. House Judiciary Committee's Select Subcommittee on the Weaponization of the Federal Government, Rep. Jim Jordan (R-OH), Chairman, declared in his opening statement: "This is the Ministry of Truth… the government working with Big Tech to silence Americans."

Rep. Thomas Massie (R-KY) described coordinated efforts as "a Ministry of Truth operation… the government and these organizations [including TNI partners] deciding what is true and what is not."

Witness Michael Shellenberger (Twitter Files journalist) testified: "The Trusted News Initiative is part of a broader censorship cartel… it functions like a Ministry of Truth."

In a July 2023 interview[832] with David Rubin of "The Rubin Report", Robert F. Kennedy Jr. (now the 26th United States Secretary of Health and Human Services) explained: "The Trusted News Initiative was a conspiracy that was initiated by the BBC where they called together all of the legacy news sites… they married them to the social media sites… and they all made an agreement with each other that they would censor certain kinds of information. For example, any information about COVID that departed from government orthodoxies."

A month prior, Children's Health Defense (CHD) led by Kennedy at the time, joined by plaintiffs: TrialSite News (TSN), Creative Destruction Media (CD Media), Erin Elizabeth Finn, Jim Hoft (Gateway Pundit) and other individuals focused on health, politics, and COVID-19 reporting, filed an anti-trust lawsuit[833] against TNI members: The Washington Post, The Associated Press, Reuters, and BBC News. The complaint explicitly referenced the TNI as a "coordinated censorship apparatus" functioning like a "de facto Ministry of Truth" that suppressed competition in the U.S. online news market, particularly for COVID-19 and political news.

In September 2022, I interviewed[834] Daniel O'Connor, an entrepreneur with extensive expertise in drug development and clinical trials and founder of TrialSite News (TSN). O'Connor announced that TSN and five other groups would be going after the Trusted News Initiative by filing an anti-trust lawsuit. He shared: "These large media entities are using censorship to thwart competition. There's been an explosion of new media sites and this is concerning to Big Media as they're losing market share. Our damages have been the revenue that we were generating from YouTube. As soon as they started censoring us for illicit reasons, over truthful facts-they would give us strikes then shadow ban us, so our revenues would go down 80-90%."

O'Connor went on to state: "I think the broader problem is that if the government has established a narrative and within that narrative, there are definitive truths that represent still an unfolding science, then is it right to classify any other interpretation as misinformation, then ask social networks to tag, flag and deal with those messages? If the government is proactively monitoring the American public and then reaching into the social networks and proactively having them define what is misinformation - you're getting into some questionable legal territory."

At the time of this book's publication the case remains pending with the Department of Justice filing a Statement of Interest[835] in July 2025 supporting the antitrust claims.

## Governments Exert Pressure While Spying on Their Citizens

After 3/11, governments did not merely request moderation, they demanded it. Backed by explicit threats of regulatory consequences. In the United States, the declassified "Twitter Files"[836] released between 2022 and 2023, along with the landmark Missouri v. Biden[837] lawsuit, later known as Murthy v. Missouri, revealed a sustained multi-agency campaign of coercion that went far beyond polite suggestions.

Shortly after Elon Musk's acquisition of Twitter on October 27, 2022, he released internal documents, known as the "Twitter Files" to journalists Matt Taibbi, Bari Weiss, Lee Fang, Michael Shellenberger, David Zweig,

Alex Berenson, and Paul D. Thacker, exposing how federal agencies routinely flagged content for removal or suppression.

The files showed White House officials, including former Press Secretary Jen Psaki, directly pressuring Twitter to censor true posts about vaccine side effects, natural immunity, and lockdown harms. Government agencies, including DHS, CDC, FBI and Cybersecurity and Infrastructure Security Agency (CISA), used specialized reporting mechanisms, such as Facebook's "Content Request System,"[838] to flag social media content for potential throttling, suppression, or removal, often under the umbrella of countering "mis-, dis-, and malinformation."

The files demonstrated that platforms complied not out of independent policy, but out of fear of antitrust action, Section 230 reform, or other regulatory retaliation.

The most consequential legal challenge was Missouri v. Biden, mentioned earlier. It was filed in May 2022 by the Attorneys General of Missouri and Louisiana, alleging that the Biden administration violated the First Amendment by coercing social media companies to suppress protected speech. The case expanded to include private plaintiffs, including Dr. Martin Kulldorff, Dr. Jay Bhattacharya, Dr. Aaron Kheriaty, and Jill Hines, co-authors and advocates of the Great Barrington Declaration.

Key revelations from discovery[839] showed White House officials repeatedly berating Facebook and Twitter executives for not doing enough to censor vaccine-related content. Emails revealed direct pressure:[840] "We are gravely concerned that your service is one of the top drivers of vaccine hesitancy - period."

In July 2021, President Biden publicly accused platforms like Facebook of "killing people"[841] by allowing vaccine misinformation to spread. White House Communications Director Kate Bedingfield followed up by saying platforms "should be held accountable"[842] and that the administration was "reviewing" Section 230 protections, which shield platforms from liability for user content.

Jenin Younes, Litigation Counsel for the New Civil Liberties Alliance, represented the private plaintiffs. In our 2022 interview,[843] she explained the core violation: "Members of the Biden Administration had made statements to tech companies saying that if they didn't censor people more, they would face consequences in the form of regulatory or other legal action. When a lot of people think that this is private companies doing the censorship on their own, but when the government is using private companies or telling private companies what to do to censor people, that's a First Amendment violation."

Younes highlighted the chilling breadth of the suppression: "The views were very much within the realm of legitimate scientific discourse. Masks maybe don't work that well, do children really need the vaccine, should people be forced to get the vaccine at the threat of losing their jobs, those were the sort of tweets that led to their suspensions from Twitter."

Discovery in the case uncovered a massive, coordinated effort across agencies. Younes described it plainly: "There's clearly this massive, coordinated effort. They're constantly giving presentations about what to censor. This kind of topic should be censored."

This dynamic was laid bare even more starkly during congressional testimony on the Twitter Files and government weaponization. In the March 9, 2023 hearing[844] of the House Judiciary Committee on the Weaponization of the Federal Government, journalists Matt Taibbi[845] and Michael Shellenberger[846] testified on the Twitter Files revelations. Taibbi described the government's role as creating a "censorship-industrial complex," while Shellenberger detailed how federal agencies pressured platforms to suppress COVID-related dissent, including accurate information on vaccine side effects and origins. Shellenberger stated: "The Twitter Files show the government was directly involved in suppressing speech."

In a July 2023 hearing of the U.S. House Judiciary Committee's Select Subcommittee on the Weaponization of the Federal Government. Rep. Nancy Mace (R-SC) confronted Vijaya Gadde, Twitter's former Head of Legal, Policy, and Trust & Safety:

Rep. Mace: "Why do you think you or anyone else had the medical expertise to censor a doctor's expert opinion? Did the U.S. government ever contact you or anyone at Twitter to censor or moderate certain Tweets? Yes or no?"

Mr. Gadde: "We receive legal demands to remove content from the platform from the U.S. government and governments all around the world..."

Rep. Mace: "Thank God for Elon Musk for allowing to show us and the world that Twitter was basically a subsidiary of the FBI, censoring real medical voices with real expertise that put real Americans' lives in danger because they didn't have that information."

The exchange crystallized the reality: unelected platform executives, under direct government pressure, were overriding the expertise of licensed physicians and researchers, often with life-or-death consequences.

The report, "The Censorship-Industrial Complex"[847] (May 1, 2024, by House Judiciary Republicans) is perhaps the most comprehensive in detailing the Biden White House coercion of Facebook/Meta, YouTube/Google, and Amazon to censor COVID-19-related content, including true information, satire, and criticism, via emails implying regulatory threats.

Some key individuals cited in the emails include: Andew Slavitt, Senior Advisor to the White House COVID-19 Response Team (January to June 2021). Sir Nick Clegg (former Deputy Prime Minister of the United Kingdom), President of Global Affairs at Meta (formerly Facebook) from 2018 until early 2025. Robert Flaherty, Assistant to the President and Director of Digital Strategy at the White House during the Biden administration (2021–2023). Dr. Vivek H. Murthy, U.S. Surgeon General during the Biden administration, who took over as lead petitioner after the change in administration and appeal to the Supreme Court, in the Missouri v. Biden case. The following list highlights these key emails and internal communications taken from the report:

March 2, 2021 (Slavitt to Amazon VP): Criticized "high levels of propaganda/misinformation" in vaccine book searches; stated CDC warnings insufficient, prompting "Do Not Promote" policy for anti-vax books (Page 7, The Amazon Files).

March 15, 2021 (Slavitt to Facebook): "Internally we have been considering our options on what to do about it" re: perceived lack of transparency on hesitancy data (Page 18, The Facebook Files).

April 18, 2021 (Slavitt to Clegg/Facebook): "Outraged" over satirical meme comparing vaccines to asbestos; demanded removal as it "inhibits confidence" (Page 29, The Facebook Files).

April 21, 2021 (Flaherty to Facebook): "Not for nothing, but last time we did this dance, it ended in an insurrection" re: Tucker Carlson video (Page 26, The Facebook Files).

April 27, 2021 (Draft Meta to Zuckerberg/Sandberg): White House demanded removal of "vaccine discouraging humorous meme" despite it being "humorous/satirical and arguably true" (Page 33, The Facebook Files)

July 14, 2021 (Internal Meta to Clegg): Censored lab-leak theory "Because we were under pressure from the [Biden] administration... We shouldn't have done it" (Page 13, The Facebook Files).

July 21, 2021 (Internal Meta to Clegg): White House/Surgeon General wanted removal of "true information about side effects," "negative opinions," and "satirical content suggesting vaccine isn't safe" (Page 43, The Facebook Files).

August 2, 2021 (Internal Meta): Brainstormed "additional policy levers... to be more aggressive against misinformation" due to "continued criticism from the [Biden] administration" (Page 46, The Facebook Files)

August 10, 2021 (Internal Meta to Clegg): Scoped four changes to censor vaccine content per Surgeon General's (Dr. Vivek H. Murthy) request (Page 48, The Facebook Files).

Returning to the Murthy v. Missouri case, in July 2023, Judge Terry A. Doughty issued a preliminary injunction blocking several federal agencies from communicating with social media companies to suppress content except for illegal activity. The 155-page ruling[848] described a massive campaign of censorship and called it "Orwellian." The Fifth Circuit largely affirmed the injunction in September 2023 but narrowed it slightly.

However, on June 26, 2024, a 6-3 Supreme Court ruling,[849] the Court reversed the Fifth Circuit and vacated the injunction. The Court held that plaintiffs lacked standing, as they failed to prove a direct causal link between government pressure and specific platform actions that harmed them. The decision did not address the merits of whether coercion violated the First Amendment. The dissent, written by Justice Alito and joined by Justices Thomas and Gorsuch, argued that the government's pressure was unprecedented and created a coercive environment that chilled speech. The ruling effectively ended the case without a merits decision on censorship or coercion.

This insidious form of government censorship was not isolated to the U.S.; it was repeated across the Atlantic. In the UK, the civil liberties group Big Brother Watch published a damning report[850] based on whistleblower accounts and FOIA disclosures entitled, "Ministry of Truth: The Secretive Government Units Spying on Your Speech" in January 2023.

It exposed five secretive Whitehall units: the Counter Disinformation Unit (CDU), Rapid Response Unit (RRU), 77th Brigade (a specialist unit of the British Army focused on information warfare), Government Information Cell, and Research, Information and Communications Unit (RICU), all involved in monitoring, flagging, and suppressing online speech under the guise of countering disinformation, especially during the COVID-19 pandemic.

These units secretly surveyed UK citizens and labeled lawful political dissent, policy criticism, and mainstream media scrutiny as "misinformation" or "vaccine hesitancy," including tweets from MPs. According to the report: "David Davis, the senior Conservative backbench MP and former Brexit Secretary, was mentioned in RRU analyses on multiple occasions, providing further evidence that even elected MPs were not outside the scope of the unit's monitoring. A weekly vaccine hesitancy report from July 2021 featured a tweet from Mr. Davis from June 30th of the same year which celebrated the government's decision to scrap mandatory COVID-19 certificates for large events. The MP argued that the passports were aimed at solving a 'non-existent problem of poor vaccine take-up.' It was still circulated in a 'vaccine hesitancy report,' although Mr. Davis made no reference to the vaccine's efficacy. Mr. Davis also appeared in a second report from 25th August 2021 after he tweeted a *The Telegraph* article covering findings suggesting that although COVID-19 vaccination had been very successful in cutting hospitalization and death, it may have had little impact on transmission of the Delta variant of the virus."

The report went on to flag how dissenting academics were also under the watchful eyes of these clandestine units. In September 2020, Oxford Professor Carl Heneghan penned a *Spectator* article[851] questioning the evidence base for the UK's "Rule of 6" social gathering limit during COVID-19, arguing it lacked scientific justification for balancing infection risks against social-distancing harms and calling for evidence-based policies to minimize overall harm. The government's Rapid Response Unit (RRU) flagged the piece for officials after noticing lockdown critics sharing it on social media.

| Re: Rule of six Carl Heneghan article - RRU flag | 14/9/2020 | Just wanted to flag that a Spectator article by Carl Heneghan and [redacted] from Oxford University's Centre for Evidence-Based Medicine is being shared in anti-lockdown circles, including by some of the main influencers in that space. They argue that there is no scientific basis for the 'rule of six' and that it is an overreaction.<br><br>Thanks, | CO/Internal | Media Monitoring | |
|---|---|---|---|---|---|

The Big Brother Watch report stated: "As this report has demonstrated, the growing existence of censorship and surveillance units should concern anyone who believes in the importance of rights, freedoms and also following due process, something that is integral to maintaining liberal democracy. Through bodies such as the CDU, RICU and the RRU, the Government is using unaccountable teams of civil servants to extra-judicially censor lawful expression online. Not only is this a violation of the right to freedom of expression but as evidence in this

report has shown, in order to perform these censorship functions, the units in question also have to engage in significant levels of surveillance."

The report also called for the immediate shutting down of the CDU and RRU, prohibiting AI mass censorship, banning state propaganda via fronts, and repealing Online Safety Bill elements that enable similar censorship.

At the time of this book's publication, only one of these "truth units" have been disbanded: the Rapid Response Unit (RRU). The Counter Disinformation Unit (CDU) was rebranded in late 2023 to the National Security and Online Information Team (NSOIT). It now operates under the Department for Science, Innovation and Technology (DSIT). The rest remain intact.

This level of involvement, particularly the use of the military, in domestic speech monitoring underscores how far governments went to suppress key dissenting voices under the pretext of "safety."

## The Ideological Engine: Center for Countering Digital Hate

Governments were not the only entities in proactively controlling the narrative, non-governmental organizations (NGOs) performed an integral role too. The British-American nonprofit, Center for Countering Digital Hate (CCDH), led by co-founder and CEO Imran Ahmed, stands out above the rest, in that it appears to have provided the intellectual and policy justification for mass suppression. Their website[852] states: "The Center for Countering Digital Hate delivers change by exposing hate and disinformation producers, galvanizing support from the public and advertisers for tech reform, shaping informed debates, and driving policy changes, and collaborating with civil society leaders for social media reform."

Their infamous 2021 "Disinformation Dozen"[853] report, naming "twelve leading online anti-vaxxers:" Robert F. Kennedy Jr., Dr. Joseph Mercola, Dr. Sherri Tenpenny, Dr. Rashid Buttar, Erin Elizabeth, Ben Tapper, Dr. Kelly Brogan, Dr. Christiane Northrup, Rizza Islam, Ty and Charlene Bollinger, Kevin Jenkins and Sayer Ji, as being responsible for the majority of online vaccine skepticism.

Turning back to the Censorship-Industrial Complex report referenced earlier, the screenshot below is taken from page 44. It shows a Facebook internal memo specifically discussing the CCDH's "Disinfo Dozen."

**Disinfo Dozen Status On Platform:**

1. We have been aware of the Disinfo Dozen back in March. We took very aggressive actions based on them, and other entities we flagged, by expanding the amount of Misindo that we remove and by giving the "Worst of the Worst" entities 48 hours to remove all violating misinformation or otherwise they would be removed. As a result of that, we removed known anti-vaxxers such as RFK Jr.'s IG Account.
2. This resulted in behavior modification by these actors -- RFK stopped posting anti-vax content on his FB page, and some other members of the Disinfo Dozen also stopped posting violating content.
3. We have continued to monitor these accounts and have found the following:
    a. 91 entities are tied to the Disinfo Dozen (however, the majority of these entities do not share anti-vax content and some post infrequently or stopped posting altogether).
    b. 23 of those entities have been removed.
    c. We are confirming additional entities (approx. 15) that may be removed under our "Single Use Multiple Account" and Recidivism policies (we are aiming to have these results by EOD).
    d. 11 of the 12 Disinfo Dozen members have had one entity removed by us. The 12th posts mainly about internet censorship now. We are watching his profile closely.

The memo's description in the report, reads: "The memo outlined the 'aggressive actions' that Facebook had taken to censor the Disinfo Dozen since March 2021, including by 'expanding the amount' of misinformation it removed and by giving the 'Worst of the Worst' Entities 48 hours to remove all violating misinformation or otherwise be removed" from the platform. The memo boasted that, consequently, Facebook removed "known anti-vaxxers" such as Robert F. Kennedy Jr.'s Instagram account, chilling the speech of many of these individuals.

Here, it is important to return to the July 20, 2023 hearing of the U.S. House Judiciary Committee's Select Subcommittee on the Weaponization of the Federal Government, where Robert F. Kennedy Jr gave his oral testimony.[854] The following is an excerpt where he specifically refers to being targeted as part of the "Disinformation Dozen."

"I was included in a group called the disinformation dozen. Facebook and others were asked to censor us, which they did. By the way, my post was taken down. My whole Instagram account with 900,000 people was taken down because of that. Oh, they knew. Facebook knew that the disinformation dozen claim, and what they said was disinformation came from this very shady group called The Center for Preventing Digital Hate in England that was funded by dark money that should be looked into. They claimed that 65 percent of the vaccine misinformation on the internet was generated by those 12 people. Facebook itself said that is impossible. That is false information. We know that not to be true. Yet, when the White House asked them to censor this disinformation dozen, including me, they did it anyway when they knew it to be untrue."

In November 2025, I interviewed Sayer Ji,[855] founder of GreenMedInfo and one of the twelve named in the "Disinformation Dozen." He described how Meta's own content policy chief, Monique Bickert, publicly called it "a faulty narrative without evidence," revealing a 1300-fold exaggeration of their actual influence: "Monique Bickert… made it very clear in a blog post that when they looked at the actual statistics… only 0.05% of the content associated with vaccines would link to our account. So that's a 1300-fold exaggeration from the actual statistics provided from Facebook… It was a lie of gargantuan proportions out the gates."

However, the report's falsehoods did not prevent its weaponization. President Biden publicly declared during a press conference that the Disinformation Dozen was "killing people"[856] with misinformation. Ji reflected on the alarming escalation: "The narrative that it [the Covid shots] was safe and effective and necessary was so weaponized that any dissent, any question of safety… was considered radical, dangerous, irresponsible, and actually eventually was defined as domestic terrorism through DHS."

Within months, Ji's platforms, built over more than a decade aggregating peer-reviewed natural health research, were systematically deplatformed across Facebook, Pinterest, Twitter (pre-X), and beyond. "It was eerie," he said, "like a coordinated blackout."

CCDH's influence extended far beyond the 2021 Disinformation Dozen report. Central to this was their development of the STAR Framework,[857] a policy proposal they explicitly describe as "a blueprint for policymakers to combat online harms and fortify democracy in the digital age."

STAR stands for Safety by Design (embedding harm prevention in platform architecture), Transparency (mandatory reporting and algorithm disclosures), Accountability (independent oversight and audits), and Responsibility (personal liability for executives and consequences like fines for non-compliance).

While CCDH presents STAR as a tool to address hate, disinformation, and child safety risks, critics argue it supplied the ideological blueprint for mass suppression by empowering regulators and governments to mandate widespread content removal or deplatforming under vague "harmful content" categories.

This framework directly informed CCDH's advocacy[858] for the UK's Online Safety Act (OSA), with Imran Ahmed as the first expert witness[859] in pre-legislative scrutiny, and their input on the EU's Digital Services Act (DSA) implementation. Both Acts empower regulators to demand removal of "harmful" content under threat of massive fines or service suspension. These laws are discussed in greater detail later in this chapter.

Disturbingly, leaked internal CCDH documents from 2024 exposed "Kill Musk's Twitter" as the organization's top annual priority. A campaign involving advertiser boycotts, regulatory pressure via DSA/OSA, and lobbying U.S. congressional offices. These documents were leaked to investigative journalists Paul Thacker and Matt Taibbi by an anonymous source and published on Thacker's *The Disinformation Chronicle.*[860]

| Month Priorities | Annual Priorities | Backburner |
|---|---|---|
| • | • Kill Musk's Twitter<br>• Advertising focus<br>• Trigger EU & UK regulatory action<br>• Progress towards change in USA and support for STAR | |

According to Taibbi and Thacker's article: "The Center for Countering Digital Hate is the anti-disinformation activist ally of Prime Minister Keir Starmer's Labour Party, and a messaging vehicle for Labour's neoliberal think tank, Labour Together. Both the CCDH and Labour Together were founded by Morgan McSweeney, a Svengali credited with piloting Starmer's rise to Downing Street, much as Karl Rove is credited with guiding George W. Bush to the White House."

In a dramatic turn, McSweeney resigned[861] as Starmer's chief of staff on February 8, 2026, taking "full responsibility" for advising the appointment of Peter Mandelson (despite his documented ties to Jeffrey Epstein) as UK ambassador to the U.S.. The exit, amid mounting political pressure and calls for accountability, marked the sudden unraveling of the once-dominant behind-the-scenes operator who had shaped Labour's path to power.

Just a few months prior, in December 2025, the U.S. State Department imposed visa sanctions[862] on CCDH's co-founder Imran Ahmed for alleged "organized efforts to coerce American platforms to censor." Ahmed secured a temporary restraining order through March 2026, but the episode highlighted growing U.S. backlash against foreign-influenced censorship advocacy.

## The Arbiters of "Truth"

While CCDH supplied the ideological blueprint for mass suppression, the ecosystem of fact-checking organizations became the operational gatekeepers of the pandemic narrative. Certified by the International Fact-Checking Network[863] (IFCN) and often partnered with platforms like Meta, Google, and Twitter, these groups wielded the power to label dissent as "misinformation," triggering algorithmic de-amplification, shadow-banning, or outright removal.

Major scandals exposed their bias, funding conflicts, and selective enforcement. PolitiFact[864] and its parent, the Poynter Institute,[865] "the world's most influential school for journalists", have received funds from[866] the Open Society Foundations, Bill & Melinda Gates Foundation, Google, Facebook, and the U.S. State Department. They repeatedly labeled accurate claims: natural immunity[867] superiority, lab-leak plausibility[868], and early vaccine injury reports,[869] as "false" or "misleading," only updating rulings under pressure after the claims were later vindicated.

The IFCN certification system, which grants fact-checkers privileged status on platforms, faced criticism for lacking transparency and allowing financial conflicts to influence rulings. Science Feedback (IFCN-certified) flagged peer-reviewed papers questioning vaccine safety or origins, contributing to coordinated backlash campaigns, editor resignations, and retractions, including studies such as Walach et al. in Vaccines and Hulscher et al. autopsy reviews, discussed in the previous chapter.

Full Fact in the UK, which is primarily funded by tech companies (Meta, Google) and charitable trusts (Nuffield Foundation, Health Foundation), rarely challenged official overstatements while swiftly labeling lockdown skepticism[870] and vaccine safety[871] concerns as misinformation.

In a notable case, Full Fact deemed a 2023 parliamentary speech by former Conservative MP Andrew Bridgen, highlighting concerns over COVID-19 vaccine safety and excess deaths as "misleading."[872] The previous chapter discussed Bridgen's speech in detail, including the BBC's zealous use of live "fact-checking" captions, which it later issued a correction and clarification statement "admitting the captions were disproportionate and created an incorrect impression of editorial bias."

Bridgen responded by accusing Full Fact of bias and political motivation, claiming the organization's funding and affiliations compromised its independence.

It is particularly telling that Full Fact's own website describes its advocacy role in shaping the UK's Online Safety Act (2023): "Throughout 2022 and 2023, Full Fact worked with MPs and Peers from across the political spectrum to improve the legislation. We helped to table amendments that would better protect us all from harmful health misinformation, to improve freedom of speech, and to end the ability of internet companies to make unaccountable decisions for UK internet users from offices on the other side of the world." They added: "Full Fact was instrumental in making sure that Ofcom's media literacy duties were updated[873] to include social media and search platforms." Interestingly, they noted how they had "also campaigned to include protections from health misinformation in the Online Safety Bill." But went on to lament: "We originally secured a commitment from the then government to address online health misinformation,[874] but they reneged on this promise."

The UK's Online Safety Act (OSA), (discussed later in this chapter) represents one of the most sweeping pieces of digital control legislation in the Western world. The fact that Full Fact pushed hard for "harmful health misinformation" to be included in the Act, speaks to their intent to institutionalize the suppression of vaccine harm reports, safety concerns, and dissenting medical perspectives under the banner of public protection.

In the U.S., Reuters Fact Check drew scrutiny over conflicts of interest: chairman James C. Smith sat on Pfizer's board during the pandemic, while Reuters fact-checks consistently defended vaccine safety and origins narratives.

Similarly, Logically AI, another IFCN-certified group, received contracts[875] from the U.S. Department of Defense and UK Home Office to monitor "misinformation," raising concerns about intelligence-linked influence over fact-checking.

NewsGuard, a rating system heavily promoted by Microsoft and integrated into Bing, Edge, and other Microsoft products, also drew controversy for its funding[876] from the U.S. State Department, Pentagon-linked entities, and Publicis Groupe[877] (a major Pfizer marketing partner). Critics accused NewsGuard of systematically downgrading COVID-skeptic and alternative health sites while giving high ratings to legacy media, creating a de facto "trust score" that influenced search visibility and ad revenue. Meta's third-party fact-checking program, reliant on IFCN partners, further amplified these groups' reach by granting them privileged moderation status on platforms.

Evidently, these organizations were not just neutral arbiters. They provided the "trusted" justification for platform actions that would otherwise appear as direct censorship. Fact-checkers did not merely debunk errors; they policed the boundaries of acceptable science and discourse, serving as the operational arm of the censorship-industrial complex that Event 201 had envisioned and the TNI activated after 3/11.

## NATO's Psyops: "Inoculating" Dissent

Strikingly, this machinery of censorship went far beyond reaction into pre-emption. In my September 2025 analysis,[878] I examined NATO's Strategic Communications Centre of Excellence (StratCom COE) and its 2021 report "Inoculation Theory and Misinformation"[879] by Dr. Jon Roozenbeek and Professor Sander van der Linden (Cambridge Social Decision-Making Lab).[880]

The report proposed a psychological "vaccine" against "anti-vax groups" and "climate deniers," using pre-emptive "prebunks" via games like Bad News and Go Viral!, funded[881] by the UK Cabinet Office and World Health Organization. Players role-play as fake-news creators, learning to spot "tactics" like emotional manipulation and conspiracy-mongering, then internalize aversion to dissenting narratives.

NATO has a long history of psychological operations (psyops). During the Cold War it conducted psyops to counter Soviet propaganda, including initiatives resembling Operation Mockingbird-style programs[882] in which disinformation campaigns were used to influence public perception and undermine communist narratives, often in collaboration with intelligence agencies such as the CIA.

Today, NATO's Strategic Communications Centre of Excellence[883] (StratCom COE), headquartered in Riga, Latvia, upholds this legacy under the guise of "strategic communications." Funded by sponsoring nations including the United States, the United Kingdom and Germany, with project-specific funding from NATO itself, StratCom COE conducts research, develops training, advances military doctrine and provides practical support to NATO decision-makers. Its remit explicitly covers Information Operations, Psychological Operations, Public Diplomacy and Military Public Affairs.

The centre also hosts the annual Riga StratCom Dialogue, where military brass regularly meet Silicon Valley executives.

The 2021 report, published under NATO's banner during the peak of the global COVID vaccine rollout, explores "the role that psychology and behavioural science can play in the mitigation of online misinformation."

Drawing on inoculation theory[884] (first developed in the 1960s by psychologist William McGuire amid fears of North Vietnamese "brainwashing" during the Vietnam War), the authors advocate exposing citizens to a weakened dose of misleading arguments paired with refutation, so they develop resistance. The authors warn against the "harmful consequences" of misinformation and identify its primary spreaders: "anti-vax groups" and "climate deniers."

An excerpt from the report states: "The spread of false and misleading information both online and offline poses a threat to the well-being of individuals, democratic institutions, and societies around the world. The harmful consequences of the spread of false and/or misleading information can be seen in the proliferation of anti-vax groups on Facebook, lack of confidence in the science of climate change, acts of vandalism committed on the basis of false conspiracy theories about COVID-19."

The inoculation model does not persuade with evidence; it conditions aversion. Roozenbeek and van der Linden critique specific examples of COVID vaccine concerns, such as a Chicago Tribune headline about a healthy doctor's death after vaccination, by arguing that while the headline facts may be correct, the "implicit message is misleading."

They similarly downplay the Johnson & Johnson vaccine's thrombosis with thrombocytopenia syndrome (TTS) risk, citing 38 confirmed cases out of 12.8 million doses (approximately 1 in 337,000) and framing it as a "minor risk" compared with everyday hazards such as car accidents. In reality, TTS proved serious enough for the vaccine to be withdrawn from the U.S. market in May 2023.

The authors dismiss traditional fact-checking as reactive and ineffective because of the "continued influence effect," whereby debunked myths linger in memory. Their solution is pre-emptive "prebunks" that build psychological resilience before exposure. They conclude that the most effective tools are "technique-based inoculation games and videos."

Bad News, launched in February 2018, lets players act as fake-news tycoons and learn to spot manipulation tactics. Go Viral!, launched in October 2020 specifically for the pandemic, trains users to "go viral" by spreading COVID-19 disinformation so they can later recognize and resist it. Both games were developed by Cambridge's Social Decision-Making Lab, the Dutch nonprofit DROG and design agency Gusmanson.

The funding sources for the report reveal clear vested interests. While the document disclaims official NATO endorsement, it was published under the organisation's banner and supported largely at UK taxpayers' expense. Key funders include the IRIS Coalition[885] (launched by the UK Government in June 2021 to address vaccine confidence and misinformation), the Economic and Social Research Council, Jigsaw (Google's former "regime change" unit)[886] and the EU Horizon 2020 JITSUVAX (Joint Initiative on Tailored Strategies for Vaccine Uptake) project on vaccine hesitancy.[887] It is noteworthy that Pfizer and BioNTech received substantial Horizon 2020 funding (€2.15 billion through advance purchase agreements) for the development and scaling of their Comirnaty mRNA vaccine.

The authors never address the central question: who decides what qualifies as "misinformation"? In practice, these games function as gamified propaganda. Players earn points for mimicking disinformation tactics, then learn to spot them, implicitly trusting the curators: NATO-linked academics, the UK Government and the WHO, while critical thinking is pathologised as a symptom of disease to be vaccinated against.

These NATO-backed efforts to psychologically inoculate the public against dissenting views went far beyond research papers and online games. NATO was actively involved in the United Kingdom's official approach to COVID-19 disinformation and vaccine policy.

On 30 July 2025 I submitted[888] a Freedom of Information Act request to the Department for Science, Innovation and Technology (DSIT), the very ministry now housing the rebranded Counter Disinformation Unit (CDU). I asked for all correspondence, minutes and documents relating to NATO's involvement in the formulation of the United Kingdom's "disinformation" and "misinformation" policy with regards to the COVID-19 shots. In its response dated 29 August 2025, DSIT confirmed that it holds NATO directives, guidance and communications on countering COVID-19 vaccine "disinformation" during the pandemic. However, the department refused to release a single document, email or record. It invoked Section 27 of the FOIA (information whose disclosure would prejudice relations between the United Kingdom and any other state or international organisation) and Section 40 (personal data).

The four reasons given for the blanket refusal were, in their own words: disclosure would damage the relationship of trust between the UK and

NATO; it would harm ongoing negotiations and cooperation with NATO and other international partners; the information could be "misinterpreted" by the public; releasing it risked NATO and partner nations refusing to share information with the UK in future.

This extraordinary reply is deeply revealing. The department responsible for policing "misinformation" has now placed on record that NATO helped direct British domestic policy on what the public was permitted to discuss about a novel medical intervention, then ensured the public would never see the evidence of that influence. Such secrecy only reinforces what the preceding pages have documented: what was presented as public-health policy was, in significant part, shaped by military-strategic communications objectives. The machinery of "inoculation" against dissent was never merely academic or domestic. It carried an unmistakable transatlantic and military footprint.

## The Rise of Digital Authoritarianism

As this book draws to a close, it arrives at the culmination of the architecture of control exposed throughout these pages: the rise of digital authoritarianism seen across the West. The pre-emptive psychological conditioning rehearsed in NATO's inoculation games, the narrative enforcement of the Trusted News Initiative (TNI), the ideological blueprint supplied by the Center for Countering Digital Hate (CCDH), and the operational gatekeeping by fact-checking organizations, all have found their ultimate legal expression in binding laws and global frameworks, where "safety" justifies surveillance, conditional rights, and the policing of thought itself.

My October 2025 article, "How the UK and Canada Are Leading the West's Descent into Digital Authoritarianism,"[889] framed the UK and Canada as frontrunners in implementing expansive digital surveillance.

The following is an adaptation of the report, which has been updated to include the EU's parallel measures.

Under the guise of safety and innovation, the UK and Canada are deploying invasive tools that undermine privacy, stifle free expression, and foster a culture of self-censorship. Both nations are exporting their digital control frameworks through the Five Eyes alliance, a covert intelligence-sharing network uniting the UK, Canada, U.S., Australia, and New Zealand, established during the Cold War. Simultaneously, their alignment with the United Nations' Agenda 2030,[890] particularly Sustainable

Development Goal (SDG) 16.9, which mandates universal legal identity by 2030, supports a global policy for digital IDs, such as the UK's proposed Brit Card and Canada's Digital Identity Program, which funnel personal data into centralized systems under the pretext of "efficiency and inclusion." By championing expansive digital regulations, such as the UK's Online Safety Act and Canada's pending Bill C-8, which prioritize state-defined "safety" over individual liberties, both nations are not just embracing digital authoritarianism, they're accelerating the West's descent into it.

The United Kingdom has long positioned itself as a global leader in surveillance. The British spy agency, Government Communications Headquarters (GCHQ), runs the formerly-secret mass surveillance program, code-named Tempora,[891] operational since 2011, which intercepts and stores vast amounts of global internet and phone traffic by tapping into transatlantic fiber-optic cables. Knowledge of its existence only came about in 2013, thanks to the bombshell documents leaked by the former National Security Agency (NSA) intelligence contractor and whistleblower, Edward Snowden. "It's not just a U.S. problem. The UK has a huge dog in this fight," Snowden told the *Guardian*[892] in a June 2013 report. "They [GCHQ] are worse than the U.S."

Following that, is the Investigatory Powers Act[893] (IPA) 2016, also dubbed the "Snooper's Charter," which mandates that internet service providers store users' browsing histories, emails, texts, and phone calls for up to a year. Government agencies, including police and intelligence services (like MI5, MI6, and GCHQ) can access this data without a warrant in many cases, enabling bulk collection of communications metadata. This has been criticized for enabling mass surveillance on a scale that invades everyday privacy.

Recent expansions under the Online Safety Act (OSA) further empower authorities to demand backdoors in encrypted apps like WhatsApp, potentially scanning private messages for vaguely defined "harmful" content. A move critics like Big Brother Watch,[894] a privacy advocacy group, decry as a gateway to mass surveillance. The OSA, which received Royal Assent on October 26, 2023, represents a sprawling piece of legislation by the UK government to regulate online content and "protect" users, particularly children, from "illegal and harmful material." Implemented in phases by Ofcom, the UK's communications watchdog, it imposes duties on a vast array of internet services, including social media, search engines, messaging apps, gaming platforms, and sites with user-generated content forcing compliance through risk assessments and hefty fines. By July 2025, the OSA was considered "fully in force" for most major provisions. This sweeping regime, aligned with global surveillance trends via Agenda 2030's push for digital control, threatens to entrench a state-sanctioned digital dragnet, prioritizing "safety" over fundamental freedoms.

Elon Musk's platform X has warned that the act risks "seriously infringing" on free speech, with the threat of fines up to £18 million or 10% of global annual turnover for non-compliance, encouraging platforms to censor legitimate content to avoid punishment. Musk took to X to express his personal view on the act's true purpose: "suppression of the people."

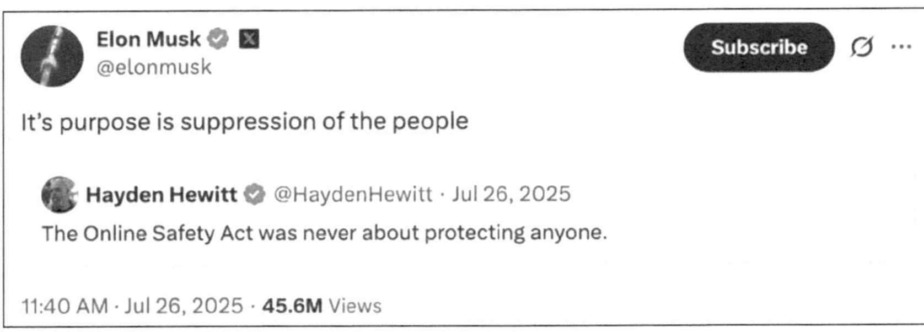
Elon Musk
@elonmusk
Subscribe
It's purpose is suppression of the people
Hayden Hewitt @HaydenHewitt · Jul 26, 2025
The Online Safety Act was never about protecting anyone.
11:40 AM · Jul 26, 2025 · 45.6M Views

In late September 2025, Imgur (an image-hosting platform popular for memes and shared media) made the decision to block[895] UK users rather than comply with the OSA's stringent regulations. Earlier in May, the video-sharing platform, BitChute, known for its emphasis on free speech, also blocked access for users in the UK. A statement[896] from BitChute reads: "To our valued users in the United Kingdom, after careful review and ongoing evaluation of the regulatory landscape in the United Kingdom, we regret to inform you that BitChute will be discontinuing its video sharing service for UK residents." This underscores the chilling effect such laws can have on digital freedom.

The act's stated purpose is to make the UK "the safest place in the world to be online."[897] However, critics argue it's a brazen power grab by the UK government to increase censorship and surveillance, all the while masquerading as a noble crusade to "protect" users.

Another pivotal development is the Data (Use and Access) Act 2025 (DUAA),[898] which received Royal Assent in June 2025. This wide-ranging legislation streamlines data protection rules to boost economic growth and public services but at the cost of privacy safeguards. It allows broader data sharing among government agencies and private entities, including for AI-driven analytics. For instance, it enables "smart data schemes" where personal information from banking, energy, and telecom sectors can be accessed more easily, seemingly for consumer benefits like personalized services but raising fears of unchecked profiling.

Cybersecurity enhancements further expand the UK's pervasive surveillance measures. The forthcoming Cyber Security and Resilience Bill,[899] announced in the July 2024 King's Speech and slated for introduction by year's end, expands the Network and Information Systems (NIS) Regulations to critical infrastructure, mandating real-time threat reporting and government access to systems.

This builds on existing tools like facial recognition technology, deployed extensively in public spaces. In 2025, trials in cities like London have integrated AI cameras that scan crowds in real-time, linking to national databases for instant identification, a capability that has moved from pilot to operational use in 2026,[900] evoking a biometric police state.

The *New York Times* reported:[901] "British authorities have also recently expanded oversight of online speech, tried weakening encryption and experimented with artificial intelligence to review asylum claims. The actions, which have accelerated under Prime Minister Keir Starmer with the goal of addressing societal problems, add up to one of the most sweeping embraces of digital surveillance and internet regulation by a Western democracy."

Compounding this, UK police arrest over 30 people a day for "offensive" tweets and online messages, per *The Times*,[902] often under vague laws, fueling justifiable fears of Orwell's thought police.

Yet, of all the UK's recent digital identity initiatives, none sparked greater public controversy than Prime Minister Starmer's proposed 'Brit-Card' digital ID scheme — initially presented as mandatory for proving the right to work, which critics warned could lead to increased tracking and surveillance risks.

First announced on September 4, as a tool to "tackle illegal immigration and strengthen border security," but rapidly the Brit Card's scope ballooned through function-creep to envelop everyday essentials like welfare, banking and public access. These IDs, stored on smartphones containing sensitive data like photos, names, dates of birth, nationalities, and residency status, are sold "as the front door to all kinds of everyday tasks,"[903] a vision championed by the Tony Blair Institute for Global Change and echoed by Work and Pensions Secretary Liz Kendall MP in her October 13 parliamentary speech.[904]

This digital shackle system has sparked fierce resistance across the UK. A scathing letter,[905] led by independent MP Rupert Lowe and endorsed by nearly 40 MPs from diverse parties, denounced the government's proposed mandatory "Brit Card" digital ID as "dangerous, intrusive, and profoundly un-British." Conservative MP David Davis issued a stark warning, declaring that such systems "are profoundly dangerous to the privacy and fundamental freedoms of the British people."[906]

By early October, an online petition opposing the proposal had garnered over 2.8 million signatures,[907] reflecting widespread public outcry. In response, on October 2nd, the government dismissed these objections, stating, "We will introduce a digital ID within this Parliament to address illegal migration, streamline access to government services, and improve efficiency. We will consult on details soon."

A parliamentary debate[908] on Digital ID took place on December 8, 2025, triggered by the public petition, revealing cross-party opposition. Facing sustained pressure, the government quietly U-turned[909] on the mandatory requirement for the digital ID in right-to-work checks in early 2026.

However, the broader GOV.UK One Login[910] digital identity infrastructure, (fully operational across over 50 government services since November 2024) continues its rollout under the same "efficiency and inclusion" rationale. The UK's GOV.UK Wallet (part of GOV.UK One Login), is currently in testing, with private trials for mobile driving licenses in late 2025 and wider rollout planned later in 2026, allowing citizens to store official documents on their phones for identity verification.

Across the Atlantic, Canada's surveillance surge under Prime Minister Mark Carney, former Bank of England head and World Economic Forum board member, mirrors the UK's dystopian trajectory. Carney, with his globalist agenda, has overseen a slew of bills that prioritize "security" over sovereignty. Take Bill C-2,[911] "An Act to amend the Customs Act", introduced June 17, 2025, which enables warrantless data access at borders and sharing with U.S. authorities via CLOUD Act (Clarifying Lawful Overseas Use of Data Act) pacts, essentially handing Canadian citizens' digital lives to foreign powers. Despite public backlash prompting proposed amendments in October, its core, enhanced monitoring of transactions and exports, remains ripe for abuse.

Complementing this, Bill C-8,[912] first introduced June 18, 2025, amends the Telecommunications Act to impose cybersecurity mandates on critical sectors like telecoms and finance. It empowers the government to issue secret orders compelling companies to install backdoors or weaken encryption, potentially compromising user security. These orders can mandate the cutoff of internet and telephone services to specified individuals without the need for a warrant or judicial oversight, under the vague premise of securing the system against "any threat."

Opposition to this bill has been fierce. In a parliamentary speech Canada's Conservative MP Matt Strauss decried the bill's sections 15.1 and 15.2 as granting "unprecedented, incredible power" to the government. He warned of a future where individuals could be digitally exiled, cut off from email, banking, and work without explanation or recourse, likening it to a "digital gulag."

The Canadian Constitution Foundation (CCF) and privacy advocates have echoed these concerns, arguing that the bill's ambiguous language and lack of due process violate fundamental Charter rights, including freedom of expression, liberty, and protection against unreasonable search and seizure.

Bill C-8 complements the Online Harms Act (Bill C-63),[913] first introduced in February 2024, which demanded platforms purge content like child exploitation and hate speech within 24 hours, risking censorship with vague "harmful" definitions. Inspired by the UK's OSA and EU's Digital Services Act (DSA), C-63 collapsed amid fierce backlash for its potential to enable censorship, infringe on free speech, and lack of due process. The CCF and Pierre Poilievre, calling it "woke authoritarianism," led a 2024 petition with 100,000 signatures. It died during Parliament's January 2025 prorogation after Justin Trudeau's resignation.

These bills build on an alarming precedent: during the COVID era, Canada's Public Health Agency admitted to tracking 33 million devices[914] during lockdown (nearly the entire population) under the pretext of public health, a blatant violation exposed only through persistent scrutiny. The Communications Security Establishment (CSE), empowered by the long-standing Bill C-59,[915] continues bulk metadata collection, often without adequate oversight.[916] These measures are not isolated; they stem from a deeper rot, where pandemic-era controls have been normalized into everyday policy.

Canada's Digital Identity Program,[917] touted as a "convenient" tool for seamless access to government services, emulates the UK's Brit Card and aligns with UN Agenda 2030's SDG 16.9. It remains in active development and piloting phases, with full national rollout projected for 2027–2028.

The European Union completes this triad with the most ambitious and legally binding framework. The Digital Services Act (DSA),[918] fully enforced since February 2024 for very large online platforms. imposes systemic risk assessments, mandatory removal of "illegal" and "harmful" material, and unprecedented transparency obligations. Platforms must provide researchers and regulators with internal data, algorithms, and moderation logs. Fines can reach 6 percent of global turnover or, in extreme cases, outright bans from the EU market.

Enforcement has been swift and aggressive. By early 2026, the European Commission has launched multiple high-profile investigations, including repeated actions against X (formerly Twitter) for alleged failures to adequately moderate hate speech and disinformation. In December 2025, the Commission fined X €140 million[919] for breaching DSA rules, underscoring the Act's role in enforcing narrative alignment.

The Digital Markets Act (DMA)[920] introduced in 2022 and fully applicable since March 2024, complements the DSA by forcing "gatekeeper" platforms (like Apple, Google, Meta, Amazon, Microsoft, Samsung) to open their ecosystems, share data, and allow sideloading, supposedly to foster competition. Critics argue it puts EU users at far greater risks of malware, surveillance and tracking, while handing regulators deeper visibility into private systems.

The EU's eIDAS 2.0 digital identity wallets,[921] with phased rollout from 2024 to 2026 and full implementation targeted for 2027, integrate verification into daily online life, aligning explicitly with UN Agenda 2030's SDG 16.9 ("legal identity for all"). By early 2026, pilots in several member states have already expanded to include health and financial data. Enabling seamless cross-border tracking and further blurring the line between public health, security and total digital oversight.

• • •

These laws are not abstract; they build directly on the infrastructure first tested in the aftermath of 3/11: vaccine passports. Rolled out in 2021–2022, they were presented as temporary tools to reopen society while protecting the vaccinated from the unvaccinated. In practice, they became the first large-scale experiment in conditional digital access. Travel required proof for international flights, trains, and borders, with many domestic routes following suit. Employers mandated passports for return-to-office or continued employment. Universities and some schools restricted attendance.

Social life was curtailed, with restaurants, bars, gyms, concerts, theatres, and sports events barring entry without a valid pass.

The EU Digital COVID Certificate,[922] launched in June 2021, set the global template: a QR-coded app interoperable across 27 member states plus dozens of other countries. The UK's NHS COVID Pass[923] and Canada's ArriveCAN app[924] mirrored this model, while Australia's state-level check-in apps and vaccine certificates enforced similar restrictions. In the United States, federal guidance encouraged widespread adoption: the CDC issued digital vaccine cards,[925] and many states and cities implemented their own systems, such as New York's Excelsior Pass[926] (launched March 2021) and California's vaccine verification tools.[927]

These systems were not neutral public health tools. They normalized the idea that fundamental rights of movement, association, and livelihood could be made conditional on possessing a government-approved digital credential. Private businesses were enlisted as enforcers, often under government pressure or mandate.

In Austria, for instance, unvaccinated individuals faced severe restrictions, essentially living under house arrest except for essential activities. As Diana Bodner, an English teacher living in Austria, described in our November 2021 interview:[928] "Since Monday the situation is that all those who are unvaccinated can still go to work... but we also can't go anywhere basically. So, this means for me for example I can go shopping, I can buy pet food, I can go to the chemist but that's about it."

She explained the emotional toll: "I felt horrible, I felt so weird basically... it's changed friendships right because there's this whole area that we can't talk about." Bodner characterized the system as "medical apartheid," adding, "It certainly feels like that and that's very scary. It's frightening to think about it." Despite mounting pressure, she remained resolute: "I feel very strongly I will not be vaccinated. I feel the more pressure that's put on me the more I feel absolutely not."

When the World Health Organization declared the public health emergency over in May 2023, the passport infrastructure did not vanish. It was quietly repurposed. The same technical frameworks of QR codes, centralized verification databases, and public-private partnerships now underpin emerging digital identity systems. All of them advance under the same "safety and inclusion" rationale.

Vaccine passports were the proof-of-concept. They demonstrated that populations could be trained to accept exclusion based on compliance. They also proved they could be resisted. In early 2022, the Canadian Freedom Convoy became the epitome of that resistance. In January and February 2022, tens of thousands of truckers and supporters converged on Ottawa to oppose vaccine mandates and digital restrictions like the ArriveCAN app.

When asked a question about the coming protest, then Prime Minister Justin Trudeau responded:[929] "The small fringe minority of people who are on their way to Ottawa who are holding unacceptable views that they are expressing do not represent the views of Canadians who have been there for each other, who know of that following the science and stepping up to protect each other is the best way to continue to ensure our freedoms, our rights, our values, as a country."

Media outlets ran headlines, such as, "The 'Freedom Convoy' Is Nothing But A Vehicle For The Far Right."[930]

I was among the first UK journalists to report on this historic protest.[931] In my February 2022 interview with Canadian truckers Jay and Blair[932] on the ground, they voiced the core demand: "We're just here to try and get our freedoms back and to make a stand for everyone in Canada."

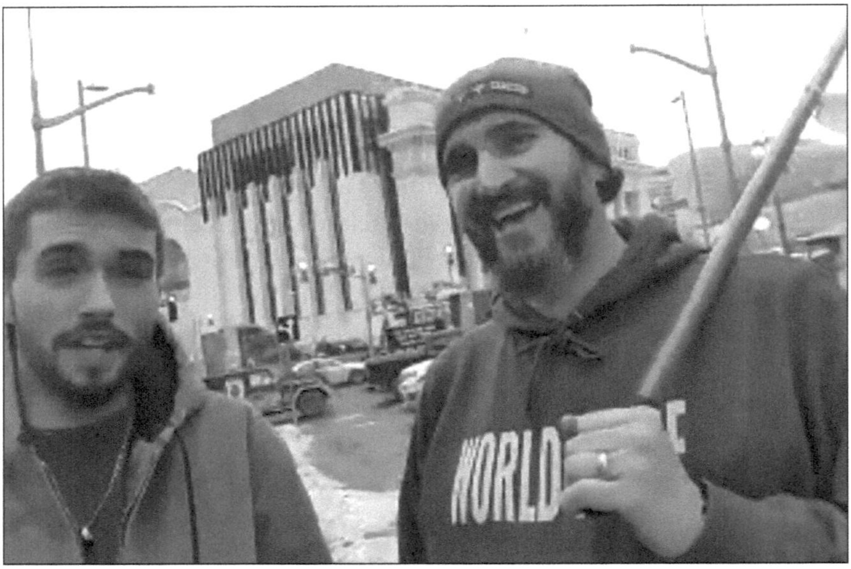

They described living under what felt like "medical apartheid," with unvaccinated truckers facing exclusion from cross-border work, public spaces, and basic freedoms. The government's response was unprecedented. On February 14, 2022, then Prime Minister Justin Trudeau invoked the Emergencies Act[933] (the first use since its 1988 enactment) granting extraordinary powers to police and allowing banks to freeze accounts[934] linked to protest supporters without court orders. Hundreds of accounts were frozen, including those of ordinary donors, effectively debanking peaceful protesters and their supporters, choking off financial support.

In January 2024, the Federal Court ruled[935] that Trudeau's invocation of the Emergencies Act was unreasonable and violated Charter rights, including freedom of expression, peaceful assembly, and protection against unreasonable search and seizure. The Federal Court of Appeal upheld this decision in January 2026, confirming that the government had exceeded legal thresholds and infringed fundamental freedoms. This ruling reaffirmed that the measures taken against the convoy, such as account freezes and extraordinary police powers, were not justified under the law. However, the underlying digital infrastructure has continued to expand.

A prime example of this repurposing is the WHO's Global Digital Health Certification Network (GDHCN).[936] This "trust network" (with the WHO acting as the "trust anchor") was launched in June 2023 and built directly on the EU Digital COVID Certificate system. The GDHCN expands the COVID-era certificate network into a permanent global platform for verifiable digital health documents. It starts with international travel but is designed for broader use in future health emergencies. By early 2026, over 100 countries have joined or expressed interest. This network allows seamless sharing of vaccination, test, or recovery status across borders.

The WHO has sought to entrench similar mechanisms through legally binding amendments[937] to the International Health Regulations (IHR 2005). These were adopted by consensus at the 77th World Health Assembly on June 1, 2024, and entered into force in June 2025. These amendments do not give the WHO power to mandate lockdowns or vaccines inside sovereign countries, those remain national decisions, but they significantly strengthen global surveillance, reporting, and compliance obligations under the banner of "safety."

Key changes include a new "pandemic emergency" category (an escalated PHEIC for widespread, system-overwhelming diseases causing major disruption), mandatory rapid sharing of pathogen samples and genetic data, a Coordinating Financial Mechanism for developing countries, and a requirement for each state to designate a National IHR Authority. These are binding on all 196 States Parties and align with UN Agenda 2030's SDG 16.9 (legal identity for all) and SDG 3.8 (universal health coverage).

In my late 2023 interview[938] with Swiss lawyer Philip Kruse, a leading expert on international law and the WHO's International Health Regulations, he warned: "The proposed amendments to the IHR would allow the WHO Director-General to unilaterally declare a public health emergency of international concern (PHEIC) and issue temporary recommendations that member states are expected to implement. This shifts decision-making power from sovereign nations to a centralized global body with no democratic accountability."

Kruse also highlighted the tracking potential: "Under the current proposals, countries could be required to establish digital health certificates and share genomic sequencing data immediately upon detection of a potential pathogen. This creates a global tracking system under WHO oversight, exactly the kind of centralized control we saw with vaccine passports during COVID."

Parallel negotiations for a separate WHO Pandemic Agreement, dubbed the Pandemic Treaty (intended to create a new binding instrument for pandemic preparedness and response) have continued since 2021 but remain unresolved as of early 2026. Multiple rounds failed to reach consensus, with disputes over sovereignty, equity, and pathogen access stalling progress. Critics, including many developing nations and U.S. lawmakers, argued it would cede too much authority to WHO, echoing concerns about centralized control.

In a significant move, the United States under President Trump, announced its withdrawal[939] from the WHO in January 2026, citing concerns over sovereignty, bias, and mismanagement during COVID-19.

• • •

On January 17th 2026, just one day before the World Economic Forum (WEF)'s Annual Meeting in Davos, its founder Klaus Schwab posted a video[940] issuing a stark warning: "Our societies face a decline of truth and trust. Without truth, we lose a shared reality; without trust, we lose our capacity to act together."

The irony is profound: Schwab, who abruptly resigned as executive chairman of the WEF following reports of whistleblower allegations[941] regarding financial misconduct, unauthorized spending, workplace bullying, and inappropriate behaviour, presents the solution as placing unwavering faith in global elites to address humanity's crises, even though these same unelected architects have built opaque systems that have systematically undermined public trust.

As the machinery of control tightens, the question is no longer whether truth can be suppressed but whether we will allow it to be replaced entirely. The battle extends beyond what we are allowed to say; it encompasses what we are conditioned to think and fear.

This book opened with the prescient words of Robert Kadlec written in 1998: "Using biological weapons under the cover of an endemic or natural disease occurrence provides an attacker the potential for plausible denial. Biological warfare's potential to create significant economic loss and subsequent political instability, coupled with plausible denial, exceeds the possibilities of any other human weapon."

What Kadlec described in 1998 as a strategic advantage for a bioweapons attacker (plausible deniability under cover of natural disease) bears striking resemblance to patterns documented throughout this book: crises framed as natural emergencies, potential harms from countermeasures systematically downplayed, dissenting voices marginalized through coordinated mechanisms, rights made conditional on compliance, and public trust eroded. Whether this represents deliberate design remains open to interpretation. What is documented is the outcome: a system where accountability is obscured and dissent is pathologized, all justified by "safety."

In my opinion, plausible denial is no longer a mere hypothesis; it is the system we are living under. The enduring legacy of *3/11: Viral Takeover*.

Yet, knowledge and truth remain the antidote, far exceeding "the possibilities of any other human weapon."

# ENDNOTES

**APPENDIX A**


1 U.S. Department of Health and Human Services, *HHS Annual Report: 2020* https://www.governmentattic.org/38docs/HHSaarCrimsonContAAR_2020.pdf.

U.S. Government Accountability Office, *Management Report: Improvements Needed in Financial Reporting and Management*, GAO-19-635T (Washington, DC: U.S. Government Accountability Office, 2019), https://www.gao.gov/products/gao-19-635t.

3 Respiratory Outbreak Investigated at Retirement Community After 54 Residents Fall Ill," *ABC News*, accessed February 13, 2026, https://abcnews.com/US/respiratory-outbreak-investigated-retirement-community-54-residents-fall/story?id=64275865.

4 U.S. Biodefense Commission, *Literature Review on Biodefense*, https://biodefensecommission.org/wp-content/uploads/2019/07/LiteratureRetrieve.pdf.

5 Apoorva Mandavilli, "Germs at Fort Detrick Spark Concerns About Biohazard Lab," *The New York Times*, August 5, 2019, https://www.nytimes.com/2019/08/05/health/germs-fort-detrick-biohazard.html.

6 David Relman et al., "An Investigation into the WIV Databases That Were Taken Offline," *ResearchGate*, 2021, https://www.researchgate.net/publication/349073738_An_investigation_into_the_WIV_databases_that_were_taken_offline.

7 Johns Hopkins Center for Health Security, "Event 201: Pandemic Tabletop Exercise," https://centerforhealthsecurity.org/our-work/tabletop-exercises/event-201-pandemic-tabletop-exercise#recommendations.

8 *2019 World Military Games Report*, Military OneSource, December 2022, https://download.militaryonesource.mil/12038/MOS/Reports/2019-WorldMilitaryGames-ReportDec2022.pdf.

9 Donald G. McNeil Jr., "Predicting the Next Pandemic: A Look at USAID's Virus Research," *The New York Times*, October 25, 2019, https://www.nytimes.com/2019/10/25/health/predict-usaid-viruses.html.

10 "Coronavirus: China's First Confirmed COVID-19 Case Traced Back to November," *South China Morning Post*, January 7, 2020, https://www.scmp.com/news/china/society/article/3074991/coronavirus-chinas-first-confirmed-covid-19-case-traced-back.

11 Betsy McKay and David L. Stern, "Intelligence on Sick Staff at Wuhan Lab Fuels Debate on COVID-19 Origin," *The Wall Street Journal*, May 23, 2021, https://www.wsj.com/world/china/intelligence-on-sick-staff-at-wuhan-lab-fuels-debate-on-covid-19-origin-11621796228.

12 "Intelligence Report Warned of Coronavirus Crisis in Early November, Sources Say," *ABC News*, March 26, 2020, https://abcnews.com/Politics/intelligence-report-warned-coronavirus-crisis-early-november-sources/story?id=70031273.

13 "COVID-19 Timeline," Centers for Disease Control and Prevention, https://www.cdc.gov/museum/timeline/covid19.html.

14 "Domestic Priorities and International Assistance Appropriations Minibus Summary," U.S. House of Representatives Committee on Appropriations, https://democrats-appropriations.house.gov/sites/evo-subsites/democrats-appropriations.house.gov/files/Domestic%20Priorities%20and%20International%20Assistance%20Appropriations%20Minibus%20summary_0.pdf.

15 "CRS Report R46354: COVID-19 and the Federal Budget," Congressional Research Service, https://www.congress.gov/crs-product/R46354.

16 "CRS Report R46354: COVID-19 and the Federal Budget," Congressional Research Service, https://www.congress.gov/crs-product/R46354.

17 "Disease Outbreak News: Coronavirus Disease (COVID-19) Outbreak," World Health Organization, https://www.who.int/emergencies/disease-outbreak-news/item/2020-DON233.

18 "Responses to the COVID-19 Pandemic in January 2020," *Wikipedia*, https://en.wikipedia.org/wiki/Responses_to_the_COVID-19_pandemic_in_January_2020.

19 “武汉市公安局武昌分局南路街派出所训诫书,” 维基文库, https://zh.wikisource.org/wiki/%E6%AD%A6%E6%B1%89%E5%B8%82%E5%85%AC%E5%AE%89%E5%B1%80%E6%AD%A6%E6%98%8C%E5%88%86%E5%B1%80%E4%B8%AD%E5%8D%97%E8%B7%AF%E8%A1%97%E6%B4%BE%E5%87%BA%E6%89%80%E8%AE%AD%E8%AF%AB%E4%B9%A6.

20 World Health Organization. "Disease Outbreak News: COVID-19," https://www.who.int/emergencies/disease-outbreak-news/item/2020-DON233.

21 Centers for Disease Control and Prevention. "COVID-19 Vaccination and Pregnancy," https://stacks.cdc.gov/view/cdc/84091.

22 GISAID, “GISAID - In Focus Archive,” GISAID, https://gisaid.org/resources/in-focus-archive/.

23 Edward C. Holmes, “Novel 2019 Coronavirus Genome,” Virological, January 10, 2020, communicated on behalf of Yong-Zhen Zhang et al., https://virological.org/t/novel-2019-coronavirus-genome/319.

24 The Guardian, “First Death from China Mystery Illness Outbreak,” January 11, 2020, https://www.theguardian.com/world/2020/jan/11/china-mystery-illness-outbreak-causes-first-death.

25 Moderna, Inc., “Moderna’s Work on a Potential Vaccine Against COVID-19,” Exhibit 99.1 to Form 8-K, filed March 16, 2020, https://www.sec.gov/Archives/edgar/data/1682852/000119312520074867/d884510dex991.htm.

26 Victor M. Corman et al., “Diagnostic Detection of Wuhan Coronavirus 2019 by Real-Time RT-PCR: Protocol and Preliminary Evaluation as of Jan 13, 2020,” Charité Virology, Berlin, January 13, 2020, https://www.who.int/docs/default-source/coronaviruse/wuhan-virus-assay-v1991527e5122341d99287a1b17c111902.pdf.

27 Kizzmekia S. Corbett et al., “SARS-CoV-2 mRNA Vaccine Design Enabled by Prototype Pathogen Preparedness,” Nature 586, no. 7830 (2020): 567–71, https://doi.org/10.1038/s41586-020-2622-0.

28 Civicus Monitor, “NGOs Highlight Suppression around Virus Outbreak in China While Persecution of Activists Continue,” February 7, 2020, https://monitor.civicus.org/explore/ngos-highlight-suppression-around-virus-outbreak-china-while-persecution-activists-persists/.

29 UK Health Security Agency, “High Consequence Infectious Diseases (HCID),” GOV.UK, last updated January 15, 2026, https://www.gov.uk/guidance/high-consequence-infectious-diseases-hcid.

30 Xinhua, “China Confirms Human-to-Human Transmission of 2019-nCoV, Infection of Medical Staff,” January 20, 2020, http://www.xinhuanet.com/english/2020-01/20/c_138721785.htm.

31 Peng Zhou et al., “Discovery of a Novel Coronavirus Associated with the Recent Pneumonia Outbreak in Humans and Its Potential Bat Origin,” bioRxiv, January 23, 2020, https://doi.org/10.1101/2020.01.22.914952.

32 Susan V. Lawrence, “COVID-19 and China: A Chronology of Events (December 2019–January 2020),” Congressional Research Service, R46354, May 13, 2020, https://crsreports.congress.gov/product/pdf/R/R46354.

33 “Statement from the Press Secretary Regarding the President's Coronavirus Task Force,” The White House, January 29, 2020, https://trumpwhitehouse.archives.gov/briefings-statements/statement-press-secretary-regarding-presidents-coronavirus-task-force/.

34 World Health Organization, “Statement on the Second Meeting of the International Health Regulations (2005) Emergency Committee Regarding the Outbreak of Novel Coronavirus (2019-nCoV),” January 30, 2020, https://www.who.int/news/item/30-01-2020-statement-on-the-second-meeting-of-the-international-health-regulations-(2005)-emergency-committee-regarding-the-outbreak-of-novel-coronavirus-(2019-ncov).

35 Alex M. Azar II, “Determination That a Public Health Emergency Exists,” U.S. Department of Health and Human Services, January 31, 2020, https://aspr.hhs.gov/legal/PHE/Pages/2019-nCoV.aspx.

36 Robert F. Garry, comment on "Analysis of Wuhan Coronavirus: Deja Vu - nCoV-2019 Evolutionary History," Virological, post #2, January 29, 2020 (or shortly thereafter), https://virological.org/t/analysis-of-wuhan-coronavirus-deja-vu/357/2.
37 Prashant Pradhan et al., "Uncanny Similarity of Unique Inserts in the 2019-nCoV Spike Protein to HIV-1 gp120 and Gag," bioRxiv, January 31, 2020, https://doi.org/10.1101/2020.01.30.927871.
38 Sharon Begley, "Quick Retraction of a Faulty Coronavirus Paper Was a Good Moment for Science," STAT News, February 3, 2020, https://www.statnews.com/2020/02/03/retraction-faulty-coronavirus-paper-good-moment-for-science.
39 Select Subcommittee on the Coronavirus Pandemic, "New Evidence Resulting from the Select Subcommittee's Investigation into the Origins of COVID-19 – 'The Proximal Origin of SARS-CoV-2,'" memorandum, U.S. House Committee on Oversight and Accountability, March 5, 2023, https://oversight.house.gov/wp-content/uploads/2023/03/2023.03.05-SSCP-Memo-Re.-New-Evidence.Proximal-Origin.pdf.
40 BioNTech SE, "BioNTech SE Pipeline and Product Overview" (or "Business Overview and Recent Developments"), Exhibit to Confidential Draft Registration Statement on Form F-1, filed June 12, 2020, https://www.sec.gov/Archives/edgar/data/1776985/000095012320006236/filename1.htm.
41 U.S. House of Representatives, Select Subcommittee on the Coronavirus Pandemic, After Action Review of the COVID-19 Pandemic: The Lessons Learned and a Path Forward, 118th Cong., 2d sess. (2024), 12–13, https://oversight.house.gov/wp-content/uploads/2024/12/12.04.2024-SSCP-FINAL-REPORT.pdf.
42 World Health Organization, Novel Coronavirus (2019-nCoV) Situation Report - 13, February 2, 2020, https://www.who.int/docs/default-source/coronaviruse/situation-reports/20200202-sitrep-13-ncov-v3.pdf?sfvrsn=195f4010_6.
43 Kizzmekia S. Corbett et al., "SARS-CoV-2 mRNA Vaccine Design Enabled by Prototype Pathogen Preparedness," Nature 586 (2020): 567–71, https://www.nature.com/articles/s41586-020-2622-0.
44 National Academies of Sciences, Engineering, and Medicine, "National Academies Provide Rapid Response to White House on Coronavirus Data Needs," February 7, 2020, https://www.nationalacademies.org/news/2020/02/national-academies-provide-rapid-response-to-white-house-on-coronavirus-data-needs.
45 U.S. Department of Health and Human Services, "Determination of Public Health Emergency," Federal Register 85, no. 26 (February 7, 2020): 7316, https://www.federalregister.gov/documents/2020/02/07/2020-02496/determination-of-public-health-emergency.
46 Kizzmekia S. Corbett et al., "SARS-CoV-2 mRNA Vaccine Design Enabled by Prototype Pathogen Preparedness," Nature 586 (2020): 567–71, https://www.nature.com/articles/s41586-020-2622-0.
47 Yong Xiong, Hande Atay Alam, and Nectar Gan, "Wuhan Hospital Announces Death of Whistleblower Doctor Li Wenliang," CNN, February 7, 2020, https://edition.cnn.com/2020/02/06/asia/li-wenliang-coronavirus-whistleblower-doctor-dies-intl.
48 Chaolin Huang et al., "Clinical features of patients infected with 2019 novel coronavirus in Wuhan, China," The Lancet 395, no. 10223 (February 15, 2020): 497–506, https://www.thelancet.com/journals/lancet/article/PIIS0140-6736(20)30183-5/fulltext.
49 Kristian G. Andersen et al., "The Proximal Origin of SARS-CoV-2," Virological.org, February 16, 2020, https://virological.org/t/the-proximal-origin-of-sars-cov-2/398.
50 Charles H. Calisher et al., "Statement in support of the scientists, public health professionals, and medical professionals of China combatting COVID-19," The Lancet 395, no. 10226 (March 7, 2020): e42–e43, https://www.thelancet.com/journals/lancet/article/PIIS0140-6736(20)30418-9/fulltext.
51 Crispian Balmer and Angelo Amante, "First Italian Dies of Coronavirus as Outbreak Flares in North," Reuters, February 21, 2020, https://www.reuters.com/article/world/first-italian-dies-of-coronavirus-as-outbreak-flares-in-north-idUSKBN20F0UO/.

52 Moderna, Inc., "Moderna Ships mRNA Vaccine Against Novel Coronavirus (mRNA-1273) for Phase 1 Study," Business Wire, February 24, 2020, https://www.businesswire.com/news/home/20200224005955/en/Moderna-Ships-mRNA-Vaccine-Against-Novel-Coronavirus-mRNA-1273-for-Phase-1-Study.

53 National Institute of Allergy and Infectious Diseases, "NIH Clinical Trial of Remdesivir to Treat COVID-19 Begins," February 25, 2020, https://www.niaid.nih.gov/news-events/nih-clinical-trial-remdesivir-treat-covid-19-begins.

54 Bill Gates, "Responding to Covid-19 — A Once-in-a-Century Pandemic?," New England Journal of Medicine, published online February 28, 2020, https://www.nejm.org/doi/full/10.1056/NEJMp2003762.

55 Presidency of the Council of Ministers (Italy), Decree of the President of the Council of Ministers 9 March 2020: Urgent Measures to Combat and Contain the Spread of the COVID-19 Virus on the Entire National Territory, March 9, 2020, https://www.esteri.it/mae/resource/doc/2020/03/decreto_9_marzoeng.pdf.

56 U.S. Department of Health and Human Services, "Declaration Under the Public Readiness and Emergency Preparedness Act for Medical Countermeasures Against COVID–19," Federal Register 85, no. 52 (March 17, 2020): 15198–15102, https://www.govinfo.gov/content/pkg/FR-2020-03-17/pdf/2020-05484.pdf.

57 Tedros Adhanom Ghebreyesus, "WHO Director-General's Opening Remarks at the Media Briefing on COVID-19 - 11 March 2020," World Health Organization, March 11, 2020, https://www.who.int/news-room/speeches/item/who-director-general-s-opening-remarks-at-the-media-briefing-on-covid-19---11-march-2020.

58 Robert R. Redfield, "Testimony of the Department of Health and Human Services on COVID-19," Centers for Disease Control and Prevention, March 11, 2020, https://www.cdc.gov/washington/testimony/2020/t20200311.htm.

59 Lijian Zhao 赵立坚 (@zlj517), "2/2 CDC was caught on the spot. When did patient zero begin in US? How many people are infected? What are the names of the hospitals? It might be US army who brought the epidemic to Wuhan. Be transparent! Make public your data! US owe us an explanation!" X (formerly Twitter), March 12, 2020, https://x.com/zlj517/status/1238111898828066823.

60 Boris Johnson, "Prime Minister's Statement on Coronavirus (COVID-19): 12 March 2020," GOV.UK, March 12, 2020, https://www.gov.uk/government/speeches/pm-statement-on-coronavirus-12-march-2020.

61 Jeremy Lee and Gideon Spanier, "'Single-Minded and Unavoidable': How the Government Honed 'Stay Home' Message," Campaign, May 11, 2020, https://www.campaignlive.co.uk/article/single-minded-unavoidable-government-honed-stay-home-message/1682448.

62 Andrew M. Cuomo, "Governor Cuomo Announces All New York City, Westchester, Suffolk and Nassau Public Schools Will Close This Week to Limit Spread of COVID-19," Office of the Governor (New York State), March 15, 2020, https://www.governor.ny.gov/news/governor-cuomo-announces-all-new-york-city-westchester-suffolk-and-nassau-public-schools-will.

63 National Institutes of Health, "NIH Clinical Trial of Investigational Vaccine for COVID-19 Begins," March 16, 2020, https://www.nih.gov/news-events/news-releases/nih-clinical-trial-investigational-vaccine-covid-19-begins.

64 BioNTech SE, "BioNTech Reports Rapid Progress on COVID-19 Vaccine Program to Address Global Public Health Threat," March 16, 2020, https://investors.biontech.de/news-releases/news-release-details/biontech-reports-rapid-progress-covid-19-vaccine-program-address.

65 Neil M. Ferguson et al., on behalf of the Imperial College COVID-19 Response Team, Report 9: Impact of Non-Pharmaceutical Interventions (NPIs) to Reduce COVID-19 Mortality and Healthcare Demand, Imperial College London, March 16, 2020, https://www.imperial.ac.uk/media/imperial-college/medicine/sph/ide/gida-fellowships/Imperial-College-COVID19-NPI-modelling-16-03-2020.pdf.

66 Kristian G. Andersen et al., "The Proximal Origin of SARS-CoV-2," Nature Medicine 26, no. 4 (2020): 450–52, https://www.nature.com/articles/s41591-020-0820-9.

67 Pfizer Inc. and BioNTech SE, "Pfizer and BioNTech to Co-Develop Potential COVID-19 Vaccine," March 17, 2020, https://www.pfizer.com/news/press-release/press-release-detail/pfizer-and-biontech-co-develop-potential-covid-19-vaccine.
68 UK Health Security Agency and Department of Health and Social Care, "COVID-19: Guidance for Health Professionals," GOV.UK, collection page, published January 10, 2020, last updated May 27, 2022, https://www.gov.uk/government/collections/wuhan-novel-coronavirus.
69 "Operation Rescript," Wikipedia, https://en.wikipedia.org/wiki/Operation_Rescript.
70 Boris Johnson, "Prime Minister's Statement on Coronavirus (COVID-19): 23 March 2020," GOV.UK, March 23, 2020, https://www.gov.uk/government/speeches/pm-address-to-the-nation-on-coronavirus-23-march-2020.
71 Ministry of Defence (United Kingdom), ACTIVATION ORDER 144-20: 77X SUPPORT TO OP RESCRIPT AND WIDER OPERATIONAL ACTIVITY, DefCts/FGen/ACTORD/144-20, March 24, 2020, https://aoav.org.uk/wp-content/uploads/2024/11/20200324-77X-ACTORD-RESCRIPT.pdf.
72 "Trusted News Initiative Announces Plans to Tackle Harmful Coronavirus Disinformation," BBC Media Centre, March 27, 2020, https://www.bbc.com/mediacentre/latestnews/2020/coronavirus-trusted-news.
73 Violet Law, "Coronavirus Origin: Few Leads, Many Theories in Hunt for Source," Al Jazeera, April 8, 2020, https://www.aljazeera.com/news/2020/4/8/coronavirus-origin-few-leads-many-theories-in-hunt-for-source.
74 "Trump 'Confident' Coronavirus May Have Originated in Chinese Lab," Al Jazeera, May 1, 2020, https://www.aljazeera.com/news/2020/5/1/trump-confident-coronavirus-may-have-originated-in-chinese-lab.
75 Jeremy Diamond and Betsy Klein, "Trump Administration Launching 'Operation Warp Speed' to Accelerate Coronavirus Vaccine," CNN, April 29, 2020, https://www.cnn.com/2020/04/29/politics/operation-warp-speed-coronavirus-vaccine/index.html.
76 Bill Gates, "The Vaccine Race, Explained: What You Need to Know about the COVID-19 Vaccine," GatesNotes (blog), April 29, 2020, https://www.gatesnotes.com/What-you-need-to-know-about-the-COVID-19-vaccine.
77 Associated Press, "WATCH: WHO Reiterates Virus Believed to Be 'Natural in Origin,'" PBS NewsHour, [date not specified on page; content references a Friday WHO briefing responding to events on Thursday, consistent with mid-2020 coverage amid origin debates], https://www.pbs.org/newshour/health/watch-live-world-health-organization-gives-coronavirus-update.
78 Reuters Staff, "WHO Advance Team on Way to China to Set Up Probe into Virus Origin," Reuters, July 10, 2020, https://www.reuters.com/article/health-coronavirus-who-china-idUKL8N2EH20R/.
79 Pfizer Inc. and BioNTech SE, "Pfizer and BioNTech Announce an Agreement with U.S. Government for up to 600 Million Doses of mRNA-based Vaccine Candidate Against SARS-CoV-2," July 22, 2020, https://www.pfizer.com/news/press-release/press-release-detail/pfizer-and-biontech-announce-agreement-us-government-600.
80 Pfizer Inc. and BioNTech SE, "Pfizer and BioNTech Conclude Phase 3 Study of COVID-19 Vaccine Candidate, Meeting All Primary Efficacy Endpoints," November 18, 2020, https://www.pfizer.com/news/press-release/press-release-detail/pfizer-and-biontech-conclude-phase-3-study-covid-19-vaccine.
81 Department of Health and Social Care and Medicines and Healthcare products Regulatory Agency, "UK Medicines Regulator Gives Approval for First UK COVID-19 Vaccine," GOV.UK, December 2, 2020, https://www.gov.uk/government/news/uk-medicines-regulator-gives-approval-for-first-uk-covid-19-vaccine.
82 Fernando P. Polack et al., for the C4591001 Clinical Trial Group, "Safety and Efficacy of the BNT162b2 mRNA Covid-19 Vaccine," New England Journal of Medicine 383, no. 27 (December 31, 2020): 2603–15, https://www.nejm.org/doi/full/10.1056/NEJMoa2034577.
83 U.S. Food and Drug Administration, "FDA Takes Key Action in Fight Against

COVID-19 By Issuing Emergency Use Authorization for First COVID-19 Vaccine," December 11, 2020, archived at https://web.archive.org/web/20201212024036/https://www.fda.gov/news-events/press-announcements/fda-takes-key-action-fight-against-covid-19-issuing-emergency-use-authorization-first-covid-19.
84 BBC News, "Covid: WHO to Investigate Virus Origins in China's Wuhan," December 16, 2020, https://www.bbc.co.uk/news/world-asia-china-55333200.
85 U.S. Food and Drug Administration, Emergency Use Authorization (EUA) for Moderna COVID-19 Vaccine: Fact Sheet for Healthcare Providers Administering Vaccine (Vaccination Providers), December 18, 2020, https://www.fda.gov/media/144637/download.
86 European Medicines Agency. "EMA Recommends First COVID-19 Vaccine for Authorisation in the EU." December 21, 2020. https://www.ema.europa.eu/en/news/ema-recommends-first-covid-19-vaccine-authorisation-eu.
87 BBC News. "Covid: WHO Team Investigating Virus Origins Denied Entry to China." January 6, 2021. https://www.bbc.co.uk/news/world-asia-china-55555466.
88 BBC News. "Covid: England's Third National Lockdown Legally Comes into Force." January 6, 2021. https://www.bbc.co.uk/news/uk-55554550.
89 European Medicines Agency. "EMA Recommends COVID-19 Vaccine Moderna for Authorisation in the EU." January 6, 2021. https://www.ema.europa.eu/en/news/ema-recommends-covid-19-vaccine-moderna-authorisation-eu.
90 United Nations News. "Health Experts Arrive in Wuhan to Investigate COVID-19 Origins." January 14, 2021. https://news.un.org/en/story/2021/01/1082142.
91 World Health Organization. "COVID-19 Virtual Press Conference Transcript - 9 February 2021." February 9, 2021. https://www.who.int/publications/m/item/covid-19-virtual-press-conference-transcript---9-february-2021.
92 Bloom, Jesse D., Yujia Alina Chan, Ralph S. Baric, Pamela J. Bjorkman, Sarah Cobey, Benjamin E. Deverman, David N. Fisman, Ravindra Gupta, Akiko Iwasaki, Marc Lipsitch, Ruslan Medzhitov, Richard A. Neher, Rasmus Nielsen, Nick Patterson, Tim Stearns, Erik van Nimwegen, Michael Worobey, and David A. Relman. "Investigate the Origins of COVID-19." Science 372, no. 6543 (2021): 694. https://www.science.org/doi/10.1126/science.abj0016.
93 Andersen, Kristian G., Robert F. Garry, Angela L. Rasmussen, Edward C. Holmes, Andrew Rambaut, W. Ian Lipkin, and the authors of the original February 2020 Correspondence. "Science, Not Speculation, Is Essential to Determine How SARS-CoV-2 Reached Humans." The Lancet 398, no. 10296 (2021): 209–11. https://www.thelancet.com/journals/lancet/article/PIIS0140-6736(21)01419-7/fulltext.
94 The Guardian. "'You Are Not a Horse': FDA Tells Americans Stop Taking Dewormer for Covid." August 23, 2021. https://www.theguardian.com/us-news/2021/aug/23/fda-horse-message-ivermectin-covid-coronavirus.
95 U.S. Food and Drug Administration. "FDA Approves First COVID-19 Vaccine." August 23, 2021. https://www.fda.gov/news-events/press-announcements/fda-approves-first-covid-19-vaccine.
96 Austin, Lloyd J. "Memorandum for Senior Pentagon Leadership, Commanders of the Combatant Commands, Defense Agency and DoD Field Activity Directors: Mandatory Coronavirus Disease 2019 Vaccination of Department of Defense Service Members." August 24, 2021. https://media.defense.gov/2021/Aug/25/2002838826/-1/-1/0/Memorandum-for-mandatory-coronavirus-disease-2019-vaccination-of-department-of-defense-service-members.pdf.
97 Florko, Nicholas, and Lev Facher. "Two FDA Officials in Charge of Covid-19 Vaccines to Leave Agency This Fall." STAT, August 31, 2021. https://www.statnews.com/2021/08/31/top-vaccine-officials-leave-fda/.
98 Centers for Disease Control and Prevention. "Immunization Basics." August 26, 2021 (archived snapshot). https://web.archive.org/web/20210826113846/https://www.cdc.gov/vaccines/vac-gen/imz-basics.htm.
99 Centers for Disease Control and Prevention. "Immunization Basics." September

2, 2021 (archived snapshot). https://web.archive.org/web/20210902194040/https://www.cdc.gov/vaccines/vac-gen/imz-basics.htm.

100 Biden, Joseph R., Jr. Executive Order 14043, "Requiring Coronavirus Disease 2019 Vaccination for Federal Employees." Federal Register 86, no. 176 (September 14, 2021): 50989–50991. https://www.federalregister.gov/documents/2021/09/14/2021-19927/requiring-coronavirus-disease-2019-vaccination-for-federal-employees.

101 Holmes, Edward C., Stephen A. Goldstein, Angela L. Rasmussen, David L. Robertson, Alexander Crits-Christoph, Joel O. Wertheim, Simon J. Anthony, et al. "The Origins of SARS-CoV-2: A Critical Review." Cell 184, no. 19 (September 16, 2021): 4848–56. https://doi.org/10.1016/j.cell.2021.08.017.

102 Zhang, Daoyu, Gilles Demaneuf, Billy Bostickson, et al. "DRASTIC - An Analysis of Project DEFUSE." Preprint. September 2021. https://www.researchgate.net/publication/363729325_DRASTIC_-_An_Analysis_of_Project_DEFUSE.

**CHAPTER ONE**

103 Schneider, Barry R., and Lawrence E. Grinter, eds. Battlefield of the Future: 21st Century Warfare Issues. Revised ed. Air War College Studies in National Security 3. Maxwell Air Force Base, AL: Air University Press, September 1998. https://www.airuniversity.af.edu/Portals/10/AUPress/Books/B_0064_SCHNEIDER_GRINTER_BATTLEFIELD_FUTURE.pdf.

104 Calisher, Charles, Dennis Carroll, Rita Colwell, Ronald B. Corley, Peter Daszak, et al. "Statement in Support of the Scientists, Public Health Professionals, and Medical Professionals of China Combatting COVID-19." The Lancet 395, no. 10226 (March 7, 2020): e42–43. https://doi.org/10.1016/S0140-6736(20)30418-9. https://www.thelancet.com/journals/lancet/article/PIIS0140-6736(20)30418-9/fulltext.

105 Knapton, Sarah. "Revealed: How Scientists Who Dismissed Wuhan Lab Theory Are Linked to Chinese Researchers." The Telegraph, September 10, 2021. https://www.telegraph.co.uk/news/2021/09/10/revealed-scientists-dismissed-wuhan-lab-theory-linked-chinese/.

106 Editors of The Lancet. "Addendum: Competing Interests and the Origins of SARS-CoV-2." The Lancet 397, no. 10293 (June 26, 2021): 2449–50. https://doi.org/10.1016/S0140-6736(21)01377-5. https://www.thelancet.com/journals/lancet/article/PIIS0140-6736(21)01377-5/fulltext.

107 Owermohle, Sarah. "Trump Cuts U.S. Research on Bat-Human Virus Transmission over China Ties." Politico, April 27, 2020. https://www.politico.com/news/2020/04/27/trump-cuts-research-bat-human-virus-china-213076.

108 Daily Mail. "Outcry as British Researcher Is Given ANOTHER Grant by NIH to Investigate COVID – Despite Fears His Initial Work at Wuhan Lab Triggered Pandemic." October 3, 2022. https://www.dailymail.co.uk/news/article-11273773/Outcry-British-researcher-given-grant-NIH-investigate-COVID.html.

109 National Institutes of Health. "Understanding the Risk of Bat Coronavirus Emergence." Project No. 10216930 (Grant No. 2R01AI110964-06). NIH RePORTER. Accessed via https://reporter.nih.gov/project-details/10216930.

110 Kopp, Emily. "State Dept. Cables: Wuhan Institute of Virology Did Classified Research." U.S. Right to Know, June 14, 2023. https://usrtk.org/covid-19-origins/cables-wuhan-institute-of-virology-classified-research/.

111 The Epoch Times. "Over $2 Million Taxpayers Money Went to Wuhan Research Labs, Government Report Says." May 10, 2023. https://www.theepochtimes.com/us/over-2-million-taxpayers-money-went-to-wuhan-research-labs-government-report-says-5335542.

112 U.S. Department of State. "Taiwan Analysts Probe PLA Links to Biotech Labs and Companies in Wuhan." Cable (FL-2022-00075 April 2023 Production - Cable 1). Obtained via FOIA by U.S. Right to Know. https://usrtk.org/wp-content/uploads/2023/06/FL-2022-00075-April-2023-Production-cable-1.pdf.

113 U.S. Department of State. "The Cover-Up and the CCP's Campaign of Disinformation." Cable (FL-2022-00075 April 2023 Production - CCP-related

cable). Obtained via FOIA by U.S. Right to Know. https://usrtk.org/wp-content/uploads/2023/06/FL-2022-00075-April-2023-Production-ccp.pdf.
114 Stieber, Zachary. "US Government Suspends Funding to Wuhan Laboratory Over Risky Experiments." The Epoch Times, July 19, 2023. https://www.theepochtimes.com/us/us-government-suspends-funding-to-wuhan-laboratory-over-risky-experiments-5408425.
115 Athrappully, Naveen. "US Stops Funding Wuhan Virology Lab for Experiments That 'Violated' Grant Terms." The Epoch Times, September 21, 2023. https://www.theepochtimes.com/article/us-stops-funding-wuhan-virology-lab-for-experiments-that-violated-grant-terms-5495948.
116 The Telegraph. "UK Scientist with Links to Wuhan Lab 'Recuses Himself' from Inquiry into Covid Origins." June 22, 2021. https://www.telegraph.co.uk/global-health/science-and-disease/uk-scientist-centre-pandemic-origins-debate-removed-inquiry/.
117 Erasmus MC. "Prof. M. (Marion) Koopmans." Erasmus MC website. https://www.erasmusmc.nl/en/research/researchers/koopmans-marion.
118 World Health Organization. WHO-convened Global Study of Origins of SARS-CoV-2: China Part. Geneva: World Health Organization, March 30, 2021. https://www.who.int/publications/i/item/who-convened-global-study-of-origins-of-sars-cov-2-china-part.
119 U.S. Right to Know. "The Lancet Emails (Daszak Correspondence), February 6–8, 2020." FOIA release, November 2020. https://usrtk.org/wp-content/uploads/2020/11/The_Lancet_Emails_Daszak-2.8.20.pdf.
120 Andersen et al., "The Proximal Origin of SARS-CoV-2."
121 Scripps Research. "Scripps Research Scientists Publish Groundbreaking Study on the Origin of SARS-CoV-2." March 17, 2020. https://www.scripps.edu/news-and-events/press-room/2020/20200317-andersen-covid-19-coronavirus.html.
122 Holmes et al., "The Origins of SARS-CoV-2: A Critical Review."
123 Gordon, Michael R., and Drew Hinshaw. "Intelligence on Sick Staff at Wuhan Lab Fuels Debate on Covid-19 Origin." Wall Street Journal, May 23, 2021. https://www.wsj.com/world/china/intelligence-on-sick-staff-at-wuhan-lab-fuels-debate-on-covid-19-origin-11621796228.
124 Demaneuf et al., "An Investigation into the WIV Databases."
125 Ge, Xing-Yi, Jia-Lu Li, Xing-Lou Yang, Aleksei A. Chmura, Guangjian Zhu, Jonathan H. Epstein, Jonna K. Mazet, Ben Hu, Wei Zhang, Cheng Peng, Yu-Ji Zhang, Chu-Ming Luo, Bing Tan, Ning Wang, Yan Zhu, Gary Crameri, Shu-Yi Zhang, Lin-Fa Wang, Peter Daszak, and Zheng-Li Shi. "Isolation and Characterization of a Bat SARS-like Coronavirus that Uses the ACE2 Receptor." Nature 503, no. 7477 (2013): 535–38. https://doi.org/10.1038/nature12711.
126 Menachery, Vineet D., Boyd L. Yount Jr., Kari Debbink, Sudhakar Agnihothram, Lisa E. Gralinski, Jessica A. Plante, Rachel L. Graham, Trevor Scobey, Xing-Yi Ge, Eric F. Donaldson, Scott H. Randell, Antonio Lanzavecchia, William A. Marasco, Zhengli-Li Shi, and Ralph S. Baric. "A SARS-like Cluster of Circulating Bat Coronaviruses Shows Potential for Human Emergence." Proceedings of the National Academy of Sciences 112, no. 48 (2015): E6605–E6614. https://doi.org/10.1073/pnas.1517719113. https://www.pnas.org/doi/full/10.1073/pnas.1517719113#supplementary-materials.
127 White House Office of Science and Technology Policy. "Doing Diligence to Assess the Risks and Benefits of Life Sciences Gain-of-Function Research." October 17, 2014. https://obamawhitehouse.archives.gov/blog/2014/10/17/doing-diligence-assess-risks-and-benefits-life-sciences-gain-function-research.
128 Burki, Talha. "Ban on Gain-of-Function Studies Ends." The Lancet Infectious Diseases 18, no. 2 (February 2018): 148–49. https://doi.org/10.1016/S1473-3099(18)30006-9. https://pmc.ncbi.nlm.nih.gov/articles/PMC7128689/.
129 U.S. National Institutes of Health. "Anthony Fauci Emails (Leopold FOIA Production)." Obtained via FOIA by Jason Leopold. DocumentCloud, 2021. https://s3.documentcloud.org/documents/20793561/leopold-nih-foia-anthony-fauci-emails.pdf.
130 U.S. Right to Know. "Proximal Origin Slack Messages (FOIA Production)." October 2023. https://usrtk.org/wp-content/uploads/2023/10/Proximal_Origin_Slack_OCRd.pdf.

131 Wrapp, Daniel, Nianshuang Wang, Kizzmekia S. Corbett, Jory A. Goldsmith, Ching-Lin Hsieh, Olubukola Abiona, Barney S. Graham, and Jason S. McLellan. "Cryo-EM Structure of the 2019-nCoV Spike in the Prefusion Conformation." Science 367, no. 6483 (March 13, 2020): 1260–63. https://doi.org/10.1126/science.abb2507. https://www.science.org/doi/10.1126/science.abb2507.
132 Select Subcommittee on the Coronavirus Pandemic, Committee on Oversight and Accountability, U.S. House of Representatives. "Investigating the Proximal Origin of a Cover-Up." Hearing, July 11, 2023. https://oversight.house.gov/hearing/investigating-the-proximal-origin-of-a-cover-up/.
133 Corman, Victor M., Olfert Landt, Marcel A. Kaiser, Richard Molenkamp, Adam Meijer, Daphne K. W. Chu, Tobias Bleicker, Sebastian Brunink, Julia Schneider, Marie L. C. M. Schmidt, Daan G. Mulders, Artemis L. Haagmans, Bart van der Veer, Sharon van den Brink, Lisa Wijsman, Nathalie Goderski, Jeroen J. A. van den Hoogen, Mariette Koopmans, and Christian Drosten. "Detection of 2019 Novel Coronavirus (2019-nCoV) by Real-Time RT-PCR." Eurosurveillance 25, no. 3 (January 23, 2020): 2000045. https://doi.org/10.2807/1560-7917.ES.2020.25.3.2000045. https://www.eurosurveillance.org/content/10.2807/1560-7917.ES.2020.25.3.2000045.
134 Alison Abbott, "First Past the Post," *Nature* 423 (2003): 114, https://doi.org/10.1038/423114a.
135 Tang, Didi. "Coronavirus: Endangered Pangolin Could Be the Missing Link." The Times, February 8, 2020. https://www.thetimes.co.uk/article/coronavirus-endangered-pangolin-could-be-the-missing-link-gsrxb08qw.
136 U.S. Right to Know. "Slack Message from Kristian Andersen, February 18, 2020: 'The more pango sequences that I see...'" Screenshot from Proximal Origin Slack channel. October 2023. https://usrtk.org/wp-content/uploads/2023/11/the-more-pango-sequences-that-I-see-.png.
137 Andersen, Kristian G. "Written Testimony of Kristian G. Andersen, Ph.D." Submitted to the Select Subcommittee on the Coronavirus Pandemic, Committee on Oversight and Accountability, U.S. House of Representatives, July 11, 2023. https://oversight.house.gov/wp-content/uploads/2023/07/Dr.-Kristian-Andersen-Written-Testimony-Corrected-Version-1.pdf.
138 Wellcome Trust. "Putting Genomic Surveillance at the Heart of Viral Epidemic Response." Funded Grants Portfolio. https://wellcome.org/research-funding/funding-portfolio/funded-grants/putting-genomic-surveillance-heart-viral-epidemic.
139 Scripps Research. "Scripps Research Scientist Kristian Andersen Receives $3 Million from DARPA to Develop Rapid-Response Antibody Therapies for Emerging Viral Threats." August 27, 2020. https://www.scripps.edu/news-and-events/press-room/2020/20200827-andersen-WAEIDRC.html.
140 Cohen, Jon. "Mining Coronavirus Genomes for Clues to Outbreak's Origins." Science, March 3, 2020. https://www.science.org/content/article/mining-coronavirus-genomes-clues-outbreak-s-origins.
141 Wikipedia contributors. "Operation Warp Speed." Wikipedia, The Free Encyclopedia. https://en.wikipedia.org/wiki/Operation_Warp_Speed.
142 National Academies of Sciences, Engineering, and Medicine. "Standing Committee on Emerging Infectious Diseases and 21st Century Health Threats." https://www.nationalacademies.org/units/HMD-HSP-20-03.

**CHAPTER TWO**

143 Pradhan, Prashant, Ashutosh Kumar Pandey, Akhilesh Mishra, Parul Gupta, Praveen Kumar Tripathi, Manoj Balakrishnan Menon, James Gomes, Perumal Vivekanandan, and Bishwajit Kundu. "Uncanny Similarity of Unique Inserts in the 2019-nCoV Spike Protein to HIV-1 gp120 and Gag." Preprint. bioRxiv, January 30, 2020. https://doi.org/10.1101/2020.01.30.927871. https://www.biorxiv.org/content/10.1101/2020.01.30.927871v1.
144 Ivan Oransky and Adam Marcus, "Quick Retraction of a Faulty Coronavirus Paper

Was a Good Moment for Science," STAT, February 3, 2020, https://www.statnews.com/2020/02/03/retraction-faulty-coronavirus-paper-good-moment-for-science/.
145 John R. Inglis (@JohnRInglis), "Text of the tweet," X (formerly Twitter), February 1, 2020, https://x.com/JohnRInglis/status/1223598414493077505.
146 "Luc Montagnier, Prix Nobel Controversé, Accuse des Biologistes d'Avoir Créé le Coronavirus," HuffPost France, https://www.huffingtonpost.fr/science/article/luc-montagnier-prix-nobel-controverse-accuse-des-biologistes-d-avoir-cree-le-coronavirus_162998.html.
147 Perez, J. C., & Montagnier, L. (2020). COVID-19, SARS AND BATS CORONAVIRUSES GENOMES PECULIAR HOMOLOGOUS RNA SEQUENCES. International Journal of Research - GRANTHAALAYAH, 8(7), 217-263. https://doi.org/10.29121/granthaalayah.v8.i7.2020.678
148 Kogon, R. (2024, April 24). The Smoking Gun in Wuhan: The German-Chinese Lab and the HIV Inserts. *The Daily Sceptic*. https://dailysceptic.org/2024/04/24/the-smoking-gun-in-wuhan-the-german-chinese-lab-and-the-hiv-inserts/
149 U.S. National Institutes of Health. "February 2nd Exchanges (Email Correspondence)." FOIA production. DocumentCloud, 2021–2023. https://www.documentcloud.org/documents/23569977-feb-2nd-exchanges/.
150 Kristian Andersen, Slack message, February 8, 2020, screenshot, *U.S. Right to Know*, https://usrtk.org/wp-content/uploads/2023/11/Andersen-Feburary-8-1.png
151 Dr Ah Kahn Syed, "How to BLAST Your Way to the Truth about the Origins of COVID-19," *Arkmedic's Blog*. https://www.arkmedic.info/how-to-blast-your-way-to-the-truth-about-the-truth.
152 James Comer and Jim Jordan, letter to Xavier Becerra, Secretary, U.S. Department of Health and Human Services, January 11, 2022, *U.S. House Committee on Oversight and Reform*. https://oversight.house.gov/wp-content/uploads/2022/01/Letter-Re.-Feb-1-Emails-011122.pdf,
153 Jack Butler, "Francis Collins Admits Plausibility of Lab-Leak Theory in House Testimony," *National Review*, January 15, 2024, https://www.nationalreview.com/news/francis-collins-admits-plausibility-of-lab-leak-theory-in-house-testimony/.
154 Donald J. Trump, Mike Pence, and members of the White House Coronavirus Task Force, "Remarks by President Trump, Vice President Pence, and Members of the Coronavirus Task Force in Press Briefing," April 17, 2020, *Trump White House Archives*, https://trumpwhitehouse.archives.gov/briefings-statements/remarks-president-trump-vice-president-pence-members-coronavirus-task-force-press-briefing-april-17-2020/.
155 U.S. House of Representatives, Committee on Oversight and Reform, *Examining the Origins of COVID-19*, hearing, 117th Cong., 1st sess., December 1, 2021, supplemental document SD004, https://www.congress.gov/117/meeting/house/114270/documents/HHRG-117-GO24-20211201-SD004.pdf.
156 Sharon Lerner and Mara Hvistendahl, "NIH Officials Worked with EcoHealth Alliance to Evade Restrictions on Coronavirus Experiments," *The Intercept*, November 3, 2021, https://theintercept.com/2021/11/03/coronavirus-research-ecohealth-nih-emails/
157 U.S. House of Representatives, Select Subcommittee on the Coronavirus Pandemic, *Investigating the Origins of COVID-19*, hearing transcript, 118th Cong., 1st sess., March 8, 2023, https://www.congress.gov/118/meeting/house/115426/documents/HHRG-118-VC00-Transcript-20230308.pd
158 U.S. Senate Committee on Health, Education, Labor, and Pensions, Minority Oversight Staff, *An Analysis of the Origins of the COVID-19 Pandemic: Interim Report*, October 27, 2022, https://www.help.senate.gov/imo/media/doc/report_an_analysis_of_the_origins_of_covid-19_102722.pd
159 Andrew G. Huff, "Everyone Needs to Know the Truth," YouTube video, September 22, 2022, https://www.youtube.com/watch?v=6NoCwQqqh44.
160 The Intercept, "Understanding the Risk of Bat Coronavirus Emergence,"

document, September 2021, https://theintercept.com/document/understanding-the-risk-of-bat-coronavirus-emergence/.

161 Sonia Elijah, "The Truth About Covid Was Not Being Told in So Many Ways," interview with Charles Rixey, April 5, 2024, https://www.soniaelijah.com/p/the-truth-about-covid-was-not-being

162 Charles Rixey, *The Myth of the Blind Watchmaker*, preprint, April 2022, ResearchGate, https://www.researchgate.net/publication/359855384_The_Myth_of_the_Blind_Watchmaker.

163 EcoHealth Alliance, *Project DEFUSE: Defusing the Threat of Bat-Borne Coronaviruses*, draft proposal to the Defense Advanced Research Projects Agency (DARPA), 2018, https://s3.documentcloud.org/documents/21066966/defuse-proposal.pdf.

164 Dr Ah Kahn Syed, "Absolute Proof: The GP-120 Sequences Prove Beyond All Doubt That 'COVID-19' Was Man-Made," *Arkmedic's Blog*, April 10, 2022, https://www.arkmedic.info/p/absolute-proof-the-gp-120-sequences.

165 Joseph Murphy, memorandum to the U.S. Department of Defense Inspector General regarding the origins of COVID-19, August 13, 2021, released by Project Veritas, PDF, https://assets.ctfassets.net/syq3snmxclc9/2mVob3c1aDd8CNvVnyei6n/95af7dbfd2958d4c2b8494048b4889b5/JAG_Docs_pt1_Og_WATERMARK_OVER_Redacted.pdf.

166 Dr Ah Kahn Syed, "How to BLAST Your Way to the Truth about the Origins of COVID-19," *Arkmedic's Blog*, December 28, 2021, https://www.arkmedic.info/p/how-to-blast-your-way-to-the-truth.

167 Stephane Bancel et al., *Modified Polynucleotides for the Production of Oncology-Related Proteins and Peptides*, U.S. Patent 9,587,003 B2, issued March 7, 2017, https://patentimages.storage.googleapis.com/01/6e/60/8951ab8f4118b5/US9587003.pdf.

168 Balamurali K. Ambati et al., "MSH3 Homology and Potential Recombination Link to SARS-CoV-2 Furin Cleavage Site," *Frontiers in Virology* 2 (February 21, 2022), https://www.frontiersin.org/journals/virology/articles/10.3389/fviro.2022.834808/full.

169 *Daily Mail*, "Fresh Lab-Leak Fears as Study Finds Genetic Code in Covid's Spike Protein Linked to Moderna Patent," February 21, 2022, https://www.dailymail.co.uk/news/article-10542309/Fresh-lab-leak-fears-study-finds-genetic-code-Covids-spike-protein-linked-Moderna-patent.htm.

170 *Grabien News*, "Flashback: Moderna CEO Struggles to Answer Why COVID-19 Contains Patent," February 21, 2022, https://news.grabien.com/story/flashback-moderna-ceo-struggles-to-answer-why-covid-19-contains-patent.

171 Defense Advanced Research Projects Agency (DARPA), "DARPA Awards Moderna Therapeutics a Grant for Up to $25 Million to Develop Messenger RNA Therapeutics," press release, October 3, 2013, https://www.prnewswire.com/news-releases/darpa-awards-moderna-therapeutics-a-grant-for-up-to-25-million-to-develop-messenger-rna-therapeutics-226115821.htm.

172 U.S. Department of State, "China Opens First Bio Safety Level 4 Laboratory," diplomatic cable from the U.S. Embassy in Beijing to Washington, DC, January 19, 2018, *Washington Post*, https://context-cdn.washingtonpost.com/notes/prod/default/documents/109d57ba-42dd-4215-9f4e-39d068ceed31/note/4f90a905-2b3f-44e0-8cb5-2d9ea5dfc62a.

173 U.S. House of Representatives, Committee on Foreign Affairs, Republican Staff, *The Origins of COVID-19: An Investigation of the Wuhan Institute of Virology*, August 2021, https://www.govinfo.gov/content/pkg/GOVPUB-Y4_F76_1-PURL-gpo158490/pdf/GOVPUB-Y4_F76_1-PURL-gpo158490.pdf.

174 U.S. Department of Health and Human Services, *Action Referral Memorandum for EcoHealth Alliance, Inc. (EHA)*, May 15, 2024, https://oversight.house.gov/wp-content/uploads/2024/05/Tab-2-EHA-SUSP4D-ARM_05.15.2024_signed.pdf.

175 Jon Cohen, "Biden Pardons Fauci, Debars EcoHealth and Its Leader for Actions

During Pandemic," *Science*, January 12, 2025, https://www.science.org/content/article/biden-pardons-fauci-debars-ecohealth-and-its-leader-actions-during-pandemic.

176 U.S. House of Representatives, Select Subcommittee on the Coronavirus Pandemic, *Final Report: Analysis of the COVID-19 Pandemic Response and Origins* (Washington, DC: Committee on Oversight and Accountability, December 4, 2024), https://oversight.house.gov/wp-content/uploads/2024/12/2024.12.04-SSCP-FINAL-REPORT-ANS.pdf.

177 U.S. House Committee on Oversight and Accountability, "Final Report: COVID Select Concludes 2-Year Investigation, Issues 500-Page Final Report on Lessons Learned and the Path Forward," press release, December 4, 2024, https://oversight.house.gov/release/final-report-covid-select-concludes-2-year-investigation-issues-500-page-final-report-on-lessons-learned-and-the-path-forward/.

178 KanekoaTheGreat (@KanekoaTheGreat), "Jimmy Dore interviews Robert F. Kennedy Jr.," *X* (formerly Twitter), March 14, 2023, https://x.com/KanekoaTheGreat/status/1635453313377533952.

179 Kristian G. Andersen, *Written Testimony Before the Select Subcommittee on the Coronavirus Pandemic, Committee on Oversight and Accountability, U.S. House of Representatives*, corrected version (Washington, DC: U.S. House of Representatives, July 11, 2023), https://oversight.house.gov/wp-content/uploads/2023/07/Dr.-Kristian-Andersen-Written-Testimony-Corrected-Version-1.pdf.

180 Henry A. Kissinger, "The Coronavirus Pandemic Will Forever Alter the World Order," *Wall Street Journal*, April 3, 2020, https://www.wsj.com/articles/the-coronavirus-pandemic-will-forever-alter-the-world-order-11585953005.

**CHAPTER THREE**

181 Harry Cole, "Coronavirus Fight Must Become a 'National Effort', Says Sir Patrick Vallance," *The Sun*, March 24, 2020, https://www.thesun.co.uk/news/11175669/coronavirus-fight-national-effort-sir-patrick-vallance/.

182 Sonia Elijah, "Sage's Covert Coup," *The Conservative Woman*, March 11, 2021, https://www.conservativewoman.co.uk/sages-covert-coup/.

183 "Scientists Who Advised Government on Covid Failed to Reveal They Had Received £200m in Grants from One of the World's Biggest Pharma Investors, Report Says," *Daily Mail*, March 17, 2024, https://www.dailymail.co.uk/news/article-15359403/Scientists-advised-government-Covid-did-not-reveal-received-200m-grants-one-worlds-biggest-pharma-investors-report-says.html.

184 UsForThem, "Home," UsForThem, https://usforthem.co.uk/.

185 UK Government, "Scientific Advisory Group for Emergencies (SAGE)," *GOV.UK*, https://www.gov.uk/government/organisations/scientific-advisory-group-for-emergencies/about.

186 Joe Marshall and Alice Lilly, "Government Emergency Powers and Coronavirus," *Institute for Government*, March 19, 2020, https://www.instituteforgovernment.org.uk/article/explainer/government-emergency-powers-and-coronavirus.

187 University Philanthropy, "Bill and Melinda Gates Foundation Funding," https://www.universityphilanthropy.com/bill-and-melinda-gates-foundation-funding.

188 Paul D. Thacker, "Conflicts of Interest among the UK Government's COVID-19 Advisers," *BMJ* 371 (2020): m4716, https://www.bmj.com/content/371/bmj.m4716.

189 Gareth Walsh, "Revealed: Sir Patrick Vallance Has £600,000 Shareholding in Firm Contracted to Develop Vaccines," The Telegraph, September 23, 2020, https://www.telegraph.co.uk/news/2020/09/23/revealed-sir-patrick-vallance-has-600000-shareholding-firm-contracted/.

190 Tom Jefferson, "The UK Turns to Witty, Vallance, and Van Tam for Leadership: Revolving Doors?," *The BMJ Opinion* (blog), December 6, 2017, http://blogs.bmj.com/bmj/2017/12/06/tom-jefferson-the-uk-turns-to-witty-vallance-and-van-tam-for-leadership-revolving-doors/.

191 *Daily Mail*, "The Story of Chris Whitty: The Oxford Graduate Leading Britain's Fight against Coronavirus," March 18, 2020, https://www.dailymail.co.uk/health/article-8077813/Story-Chris-Whitty-Oxford-graduate-leading-Britains-fight-against-coronavirus.html.

192 Deborah Cohen and Philip Carter, "WHO and the Pandemic Flu 'Conspiracies,'" *BMJ* 340 (2010): c2912, https://doi.org/10.1136/bmj.c2912.
193 BC News, "Scientists Sound Alarm over Lab Safety after Anthrax and Smallpox Incidents," April 3, 2014, https://www.bbc.co.uk/news/health-26954482.
194 Tom Jefferson et al., "Neuraminidase Inhibitors for Preventing and Treating Influenza in Adults and Children," *Cochrane Database of Systematic Reviews*, no. 4 (2014): CD008965, https://doi.org/10.1002/14651858.CD008965.pub4.
195 SPI-M)," https://www.gov.uk/government/groups/scientific-pandemic-influenza-subgroup-on-modelling.
196 UK Government, "Independent Scientific Pandemic Influenza Group on Behaviours (SPI-B)," https://www.gov.uk/government/groups/independent-scientific-pandemic-influenza-group-on-behaviours-spi-b.
197 The Spectator, "Six Questions That Neil Ferguson Should Be Asked," https://spectator.com/article/six-questions-that-neil-ferguson-should-be-asked/.
198 *Daily Express*, "Neil Ferguson: Coronavirus Modelling Expert Who Helped Shape UK Lockdown," April 20, 2020, https://www.express.co.uk/news/uk/1278465/neil-ferguson-coronavirus-imperial-college-london-epidemiology-sage-spt.
199 James Sturcke, "Bird Flu Pandemic 'Could Kill 150m,'" *The Guardian*, September 30, 2005, https://www.theguardian.com/world/2005/sep/30/birdflu.jamessturcke.
200 Jeremy Laurance, "NHS Prepares for 65,000 Deaths from Swine Flu," *Independent*, July 17, 2009, https://www.the-independent.com/life-style/health-and-families/health-news/nhs-prepares-for-65-000-deaths-from-swine-flu-1750091.htm.
201 Jeremy Laurance, "Swine Flu Outbreak Cost UK £1.2bn," *Independent*, July 2, 2010, https://www.the-independent.com/life-style/health-and-families/health-news/swine-flu-outbreak-cost-uk-pound-1-2bn-2015429.html.
202 Ferguson, N. M., et al. (2020). Impact of non-pharmaceutical interventions (NPIs) to reduce COVID-19 mortality and healthcare demand. *Imperial College London.* https://doi.org/10.25561/77482.
203 "Johnson Puts UK in Lockdown in Coronavirus U-Turn," *Euractiv*, March 23, 2020, https://www.euractiv.com/news/johnson-puts-uk-in-lockdown-in-coronavirus-u-turn/.
204 "Neil Ferguson, Architect of Lockdown, Brought Down by Failing to Obey Rules," *Telegraph*, May 5, 2020, https://www.telegraph.co.uk/news/2020/05/05/neil-ferguson-architect-lockdown-brought-failing-obey-rules/.
205 "Professor Neil Ferguson Had Key Role in Boris Johnson's Dramatic U-Turn on Christmas," *Daily Mail*, December 21, 2020, https://www.dailymail.co.uk/news/article-9073767/Professor-Neil-Ferguson-key-role-Boris-Johnsons-dramatic-U-turn-Christmas.html.
206 "Psychological Warfare," Wikipedia, https://en.wikipedia.org/wiki/Psychological_warfare.
207 Sarah Knapton, "Lockdown May Cost 200,000 Lives, Government Report Shows," *The Telegraph*, July 19, 2020, https://www.telegraph.co.uk/news/2020/07/19/lockdown-may-cost-200k-lives-government-report-shows/.
208 Philip Aldrick, "Lockdown to Cost £2.4bn a Day as Economy Crashes," The Times, April 6, 2020. https://www.thetimes.com/business/economics/article/consumer-confidence-at-its-lowest-since-the-financial-crisis-p6phf7x3k.
209 Maria Iu, "Govt Spent More Than £184m on Covid Comms in 2020," Campaign Live, March 2, 2021, https://www.campaignlive.co.uk/article/govt-spent-184m-covid-comms-2020/1708695.
210 Scientific Pandemic Influenza Group on Behaviours (SPI-B), "Options for Increasing Adherence to Social Distancing Measures," March 22, 2020, UK Government, https://assets.publishing.service.gov.uk/government/uploads/system/uploads/attachment_data/file/887467/25-options-for-increasing-adherence-to-social-distancing-measures-22032020.pdf.
211 Scientific Pandemic Influenza Group on Behaviours (SPI-B), "Increasing Adherence to COVID-19 Preventative Behaviours Among Young People," October 2020,

UK Government, https://assets.publishing.service.gov.uk/government/uploads/system/uploads/attachment_data/file/933228/S0829_SPI-B_-_Increasing_adherence_to_Covid-19_preventative_behaviours_among_young_people.pdf.
212 Megan White, "Professor Susan Michie Tells LBC It's Wrong to Say Schools Are 'Safe,'" *LBC*, December 31, 2020, https://www.lbc.co.uk/article/professor-susan-michie-wrong-schools-safe-covid-DWynwR_2/.
213 European Centre for Disease Prevention and Control. COVID-19 in Children and the Role of School Settings in COVID-19 Transmission. Technical report. Stockholm: ECDC, August 6, 2020. https://www.ecdc.europa.eu/sites/default/files/documents/COVID-19-schools-transmission-August%202020.pdf.
214 "Nudge Unit Pushed Way Private Sector Behavioural Insights Team," *Guardian*, November 10, 2018, https://www.theguardian.com/politics/2018/nov/10/nudge-unit-pushed-way-private-sector-behavioural-insights-team.
215 Colin Marrs, "BIT by BIT: David Halpern Interview," *Civil Service World*, October 7, 2015, https://www.civilserviceworld.com/in-depth/article/bit-by-bit-david-halpern-interview.
216 David Halpern, "David Halpern - Nudge," London Business Forum, YouTube video, September 17, 2018, https://www.youtube.com/watch?v=cqKcDw0nUJM.
217 The Telegraph, "'Look into My Eyes': Government Posts Hard-Hitting Covid-19 Advert," YouTube video, January 23, 2021, https://www.youtube.com/watch?v=s-_FeNrTRV8.
218 Stephen Reicher, "For Psychologists, the Pandemic Has Shown People's Capacity for Cooperation," The Guardian, January 2, 2021, https://www.theguardian.com/commentisfree/2021/jan/02/psychologists-pandemic-cooperation-government-public-britain.
219 Stephen Reicher, "Don't Blame 'Selfish Covidiots'. Blame the British Government," The Guardian, September 2, 2020, https://www.theguardian.com/commentisfree/2020/sep/02/selfish-covidiots-blame-british-government-greek.
220 Stephen Reicher, "With the New Covid Variant Everywhere, It's Not Enough to Just Wait for the Vaccine," The Guardian, December 28, 2020, https://www.theguardian.com/commentisfree/2020/dec/28/covid-vaccine-uk-restrictions-independent-sage.
221 James Gallagher, "Coronavirus: UK Variant 'May Be More Deadly'," BBC News, January 22, 2021, https://www.bbc.co.uk/news/health-55768627.
222 COG-UK Consortium, "COG-UK Showcase Event December 2020," YouTube video, 3:23:00 (approx.), December 18, 2020, https://www.youtube.com/watch?v=G3CT9N89L-c.
223 Andrew Rambaut et al., "Preliminary Genomic Characterisation of an Emergent SARS-CoV-2 Lineage in the UK Defined by a Novel Set of Spike Mutations," Virological (blog), December 18, 2020, https://virological.org/t/preliminary-genomic-characterisation-of-an-emergent-sars-cov-2-lineage-in-the-uk-defined-by-a-novel-set-of-spike-mutations/563.
224 Jim Norton, "Professor Neil Ferguson Had Key Role in Boris Johnson's Dramatic U-turn on Christmas," Daily Mail, December 20, 2020, https://www.dailymail.co.uk/news/article-9073767/Professor-Neil-Ferguson-key-role-Boris-Johnsons-dramatic-U-turn-Christmas.html.
225 Jim Norton [or appropriate author if confirmed], "Professor Neil Ferguson: People Don't Agree with Lockdown and Try to Undermine the Scientists," The Times, December 25, 2020, https://www.thetimes.com/uk/healthcare/article/people-don-t-agree-with-lockdown-and-try-to-undermine-the-scientists-gnms7mp98.
226 Anne McCloskey, "Re: Covid-19: Social murder, they wrote—elected, unaccountable, and unrepentant," rapid response to The BMJ, March 4, 2021, https://www.bmj.com/content/372/bmj.n314/rr-33.
227 UK Covid-19 Inquiry, https://covid19.public-inquiry.uk/.
228 The TaxPayers' Alliance, "Estimate: Cost of the Covid Inquiry 2025," May 11, 2025, https://taxpayersalliance.com/estimate-cost-of-the-covid-inquiry-2025/.
229 Kevin Bardosh, "The UK Covid Inquiry Is Turning into a Whitewash," Collateral Global, November 11, 2023, https://collateralglobal.org/article/the-uk-covid-inquiry-is-turning-into-a-whitewash/.

230 Stephen Reicher, Witness Statement, INQ000273800, UK Covid-19 Inquiry, September 27, 2023, https://covid19.public-inquiry.uk/wp-content/uploads/2024/01/24194704/INQ000273800-1.pdf.
231 Luke Malpass, "'That's Not a Lockdown. This Is a Lockdown': Much Hangs on Ardern's COVID Elimination Strategy," The Sydney Morning Herald, August 28, 2021, https://www.smh.com.au/world/oceania/that-s-not-a-lockdown-this-is-a-lockdown-much-hangs-on-ardern-s-covid-elimination-strategy-20210824-p58lk7.html.
232 "International Union of Socialist Youth," Wikipedia, https://en.wikipedia.org/wiki/International_Union_of_Socialist_Youth.
233 Scientific Pandemic Influenza Group on Behaviours (SPI-B), Options for Increasing Adherence to Social Distancing Measures, March 22, 2020, https://assets.publishing.service.gov.uk/media/5ecd084586650c76acac37e0/25-options-for-increasing-adherence-to-social-distancing-measures-22032020.pdf.
234 "Matt Hancock Wanted to 'Frighten Everyone' into Following Covid Rules," The Guardian, March 5, 2023, https://www.theguardian.com/politics/2023/mar/05/matt-hancock-wanted-to-frighten-everyone-into-following-covid-rules.
235 Susan Michie, Witness Statement, INQ000252610, UK Covid-19 Inquiry, August 22, 2023, https://covid19.public-inquiry.uk/wp-content/uploads/2023/12/18143436/INQ000252610.pdf.
236 Gordon Rayner, "Use of Fear to Control Behaviour in Covid Crisis Was 'Totalitarian', Admit Scientists," The Telegraph, May 14, 2021, https://www.telegraph.co.uk/news/2021/05/14/scientists-admit-totalitarian-use-fear-control-behaviour-covid/.
237 "COVID-19: Guidance for Health Professionals," GOV.UK, collection page, last updated May 27, 2022, https://www.gov.uk/government/collections/wuhan-novel-coronavirus.
238 Angelo Maria Pezzullo et al., "Age-Stratified Infection Fatality Rate of COVID-19 in the Non-Elderly Population," Environmental Research 216 (October 28, 2022): 114655, https://doi.org/10.1016/j.envres.2022.114655.
239 Giovanni Mansueto et al., "The Italian COVID-19 Anxiety Syndrome Scale: Investigation of the COVID-19 Anxiety Syndrome and Its Association with Psychological Symptoms in an Italian Population," Clinical Psychology & Psychotherapy (July 9, 2022), https://doi.org/10.1002/cpp.2767.
240 Janet Eastham, "Britain Drilled to Accept Lockdown in Future Pandemics, Says 'Nudge Unit' Chief," The Telegraph, July 6, 2023, https://www.telegraph.co.uk/news/2023/07/06/britain-drilled-to-accept-lockdown-in-future-pandemics/.
241 Tony Diver, "Government 'Used Grossly Unethical Tactics to Scare Public into Covid Compliance'," The Telegraph, January 28, 2022, https://www.telegraph.co.uk/politics/2022/01/28/grossly-unethical-downing-street-nudge-unit-accused-scaring/.
242 Cabinet Office, The UK Government Resilience Framework, December 19, 2022 (updated December 4, 2023), https://www.gov.uk/government/publications/the-uk-government-resilience-framework/the-uk-government-resilience-framework-html.
243 Lewis Brackpool, "Leaked Emails Prove UK Government Use TV Shows to Push Narratives," The State of It (Substack), June 13, 2025, https://thestateofit.substack.com/p/leaked-emails-prove-uk-government.
244 "Put Vaccine 'Propaganda' in EastEnders, Ministers Urged BBC," The Telegraph, June 13, 2025, https://www.telegraph.co.uk/news/2025/06/13/ministers-pushed-tv-bosses-pro-vaccine-propaganda-soaps/.
245 "Jonathan Van-Tam Takes Role at Vaccine Maker Moderna," Financial Times, August 17, 2023, https://www.ft.com/content/a3d3e076-7d83-4e6f-ab88-52b3b4043e7c.
246 Carl Heneghan and Tom Jefferson, "Celebrity Doctors Being Paid to Promote Vaccines Is Against the Law," The Daily Sceptic, May 15, 2024, https://dailysceptic.org/2024/05/15/celebrity-doctors-being-paid-to-promote-vaccines-is-against-the-law/.
247 "Professor Susan Michie Appointed Chair of WHO Advisory Group," UCL

Faculty of Brain Sciences, July 27, 2022, https://www.ucl.ac.uk/brain-sciences/news/2022/jul/professor-susan-michie-appointed-chair-who-advisory-group.

248 World Health Organization, "World Health Organization Names Sir Jeremy Farrar as Chief Scientist, Dr Amelia Latu Afuhaamango Tuipulotu as Chief Nursing Officer," December 13, 2022, https://www.who.int/news/item/13-12-2022-world-health-organization-names-sir-jeremy-farrar-as-chief-scientist-dr-amelia-latu-afuhaamango-tuipulotu-as-chief-nursing-officer.

249 Lord Vallance, GOV.UK, https://www.gov.uk/government/people/patrick-vallance.

250 UK Covid-19 Inquiry, UK Covid-19 Inquiry Financial Report for Quarter 3 2025-26, January 2026, https://covid19.public-inquiry.uk/documents/uk-covid-19-inquiry-financial-report-for-quarter-3-2025-26/.

**CHAPTER FOUR**

251 Christopher J. M. Whitty et al., "Infectious Disease: Tough Choices to Reduce Ebola Transmission," Nature 515, no. 7526 (November 6, 2014): 192–94, https://doi.org/10.1038/515192a.

252 Wellcome Trust, "Wellcome Releases 2020/21 Annual Results," January 10, 2022, https://wellcome.org/insights/articles/wellcome-releases-202021-annual-results.

253 "Coronavirus: Boris Johnson Announces Three-Week UK Lockdown," The Telegraph, March 24, 2020, https://www.telegraph.co.uk/global-health/science-and-disease/coronavirus-latest-lockdown-panic-buying-news-cases-nhs/.

254 UK Health Security Agency, "High Consequence Infectious Diseases (HCID)," GOV.UK, last updated March 19, 2020, https://www.gov.uk/guidance/high-consequence-infectious-diseases-hcid.

255 Medicines and Healthcare products Regulatory Agency, "Freedom of Information Request on Confirmation of Why the PCR Test Was Granted Authorization for Use by Your Department When It Is Not Fit for Purpose (FOI 21/1171)," December 3, 2021, https://www.gov.uk/government/publications/freedom-of-information-responses-from-the-mhra-week-commencing-29-november-2021/freedom-of-information-request-on-confirmation-of-why-the-pcr-test-was-granted-authorization-for-use-by-your-department-when-it-is-not-fit-for-purpose.

256 Imperial College London, Impact of NPIs, Report 9.

257 Sheri Fink, "White House Takes New Line After Dire Report on Death Toll," The New York Times, March 16, 2020, https://www.nytimes.com/2020/03/16/us/coronavirus-fatality-rate-white-house.html.

258 Mark Landler and Stephen Castle, "Behind the Virus Report That Jarred the U.S. and the U.K. to Action," The New York Times, March 17, 2020 (updated April 2, 2020), https://www.nytimes.com/2020/03/17/world/europe/coronavirus-imperial-college-johnson.html.

259 Sue Denim, "Code Review of Ferguson's Model," The Daily Sceptic, May 6, 2020, https://dailysceptic.org/2020/05/06/code-review-of-fergusons-model/.

260 Michael Levitt, "All_Michael_Levitt_22_Reports_on COVID-19_2-Feb-to-3-Mar," compiled reports, February 2–March 3, 2020, PDF shared via Dropbox, https://www.dropbox.com/s/vp4u2ae5yaswhk5/2.%20All_Michael_Levitt_22_Reports_on%20COVID-19_2-Feb-to-3-Mar.pdf?dl=1.

261 Joe Mozingo, "Why This Nobel Laureate Predicts a Quicker Coronavirus Recovery: 'We're Going to Be Fine,'" Los Angeles Times, March 23, 2020, https://www.latimes.com/science/story/2020-03-22/coronavirus-outbreak-nobel-laureate.

262 Freddie Sayers, "Nobel Prize-Winning Scientist: The Covid-19 Epidemic Was Never Exponential," UnHerd, May 2, 2020, https://unherd.com/newsroom/nobel-prize-winning-scientist-the-covid-19-epidemic-was-never-exponential/.

263 Peter St. Onge, with the collaboration of Gaël Campan, The Flawed COVID-19 Model That Locked Down Canada, Economic Note, Health Policy Series (Montreal: Montreal Economic Institute, June 2020), https://www.iedm.org/wp-content/uploads/2020/06/note032020_en.pdf.

264 Adam T. Biggs and Lanny F. Littlejohn, "Revisiting the Initial COVID-19 Pandemic Projections," The Lancet Microbe 2, no. 3 (March 2021): e91–e92, https://doi.org/10.1016/S2666-5247(21)00029-X.
265 Neil Ferguson, oral evidence, UK Covid-19 Inquiry, Module 2, day 11, October 17, 2023, https://ukcovid19inquiry.dracos.co.uk/module-2/2023-10-17/#professor-neil-ferguson.
266 Martin Kulldorff, Sunetra Gupta, and Jay Bhattacharya, "The Great Barrington Declaration," Great Barrington Declaration (website), October 4, 2020, https://gbdeclaration.org/.
267 Martin Kulldorff, "Harvard Tramples the Truth," City Journal, March 11, 2024, https://www.city-journal.org/article/harvard-tramples-the-truth.
268 "WHO Chief Says Herd Immunity Approach to Pandemic 'Unethical'," The Guardian, October 12, 2020, https://www.theguardian.com/world/2020/oct/12/who-chief-says-herd-immunity-approach-to-pandemic-unethical.
269 "White House Embraces Herd Immunity in Latest Push to End COVID-19 Lockdowns," Newsweek, October 12, 2020, https://www.newsweek.com/white-house-embraces-herd-immunity-latest-push-end-covid-19-lockdowns-1538430.
270 "Dozens of Public Health Groups, Experts Blast 'Herd Immunity' Strategy Backed by White House," The Hill, October 16, 2020, https://thehill.com/policy/healthcare/521159-dozens-of-public-health-groups-experts-blast-herd-immunity-strategy-backed/.
271 "Public Health Organizations Condemn Herd Immunity Scheme for Controlling Spread of SARS-CoV-2," American Public Health Association, October 13, 2020, https://www.apha.org/news-and-media/news-releases/apha-news-releases/2020/public-health-orgs-condemn-sars-covid2-plan.
272 Phillip W. Magness and James R. Harrigan, "Fauci, Emails, and Some Alleged Science," The Daily Economy, December 19, 2021, https://thedailyeconomy.org/article/fauci-emails-and-some-alleged-science/.
273 Brownstone Institute, "Brownstone Institute," https://brownstone.org/.
274 Robert J. Glass et al., "Targeted Social Distancing Design for Pandemic Influenza," Emerging Infectious Diseases 12, no. 11 (November 2006): 1671–81, https://doi.org/10.3201/eid1211.060255.
275 Project BioShield Act of 2004, Pub. L. No. 108-276, 118 Stat. 835 (2004), https://www.govinfo.gov/content/pkg/PLAW-108publ276/pdf/PLAW-108publ276.pdf.
276 Jeffrey A. Tucker, "What Really Happened: Lockdown until Vaccination," Brownstone Institute, May 22, 2024, https://brownstone.org/articles/what-really-happened-lockdown-until-vaccination/.
277 Covid-19: Economic Impact of Lockdowns, vol. 723, cols. 1WH–20WH (29 November 2022) (U.K.), https://hansard.parliament.uk/Commons/2022-11-29/debates/89582334-28F5-4689-BBEA-F92CDDAE6DC7/Covid-19EconomicImpactOfLockdowns.
278 Constantine Vardavas et al., "Cost of the COVID-19 Pandemic versus the Cost-Effectiveness of Mitigation Strategies in EU/UK/OECD: A Systematic Review," BMJ Open 13, no. 10 (October 2023): e077602, https://doi.org/10.1136/bmjopen-2023-077602.
279 Sonia Elijah, "It's High Time Europe's Lockdown Rebellion Spread to Britain," The Conservative Woman, February 12, 2021, https://www.conservativewoman.co.uk/its-high-time-europes-lockdown-rebellion-spread-to-britain/.
280 Noemie Bisserbe, Eric Sylvers, and Maria Martinez, "As Covid-19 Roars Back in Europe, Governments Get Tougher on Rule Breakers," Wall Street Journal, October 19, 2020, https://www.wsj.com/world/europe/as-covid-19-roars-back-in-europe-governments-get-tougher-on-rule-breakers-11603111859.
281 "Covid: Protests Take Place across Italy over Anti-Virus Measures," BBC News, October 27, 2020, https://www.bbc.co.uk/news/world-europe-54701042.
282 "'I Am Open': 50,000 Italian Restaurant Owners Plan to Ignore Lockdown," OffGuardian, January 15, 2021, https://off-guardian.org/2021/01/15/i-am-open-50000-italian-restaurant-owners-plan-to-ignore-lockdown/.

283 Robin Monotti (@robinmonotti), "ITALY: #IoApro restaurant is open, police arrives. Customers refuse to leave & shout in unison 'Get out! Get out! Get out! ..we pay your wages from our taxes, you work for us.. Get out! Get out! Get out!' #IOpen," X, January 16, 2021, https://x.com/robinmonotti/status/1350232937376215042.

284 Rachael Bunyan and AFP, "Hundreds of Tourist-Trade Businesses DEFY Covid Lockdown Rules and Say They Will Reopen in Poland Because Lockdown They 'Won't Survive Another Month'," Daily Mail, January 13, 2021, https://www.dailymail.co.uk/news/article-9142789/Hundreds-tourist-trade-businesses-DEFY-Covid-lockdown-rules-say-reopen-Poland.html.

285 "Czech Pubs, Restaurants Open in Protest against COVID-19 Restrictions," CGTN, January 24, 2021, https://newsaf.cgtn.com/news/2021-01-24/Czech-pubs-restaurants-open-in-protest-against-COVID-19-restrictions-Xim9cnFfIQ/index.html.

286 HM Treasury, Spending Review 2020 (London: HM Treasury, November 25, 2020), https://www.gov.uk/government/publications/spending-review-2020-documents/spending-review-2020.

287 Sophie-May Clarke, "Preston Gym Owner Fined for 11th Time Due to Coronavirus Breaches," Lancashire Telegraph, January 30, 2021, https://www.lancashiretelegraph.co.uk/news/19052348.preston-gym-owner-fined-11th-time-due-coronavirus-breaches/.

288 "Two Arrests at Christian Tearoom That Refuses to Close," BBC News, November 15, 2020, https://www.bbc.co.uk/news/uk-england-nottinghamshire-54950773.

289 Andrew Robinson, "Salon Owner Facing £27,000 Fine for Refusing to Close Salon and Citing Magna Carta in Her Defence," WalesOnline, November 25, 2020, https://www.walesonline.co.uk/news/uk-news/salon-owner-facing-27000-fine-19342372.

290 Simon Dolan, "To Save the Heart of Our Economy, Write Off Covid-19 Loans to Small Business Now," The Conservative Woman, February 19, 2021, https://www.conservativewoman.co.uk/to-save-the-heart-of-our-economy-write-off-covid-19-loans-to-small-business-now/.

291 "UK Government Faces Legal Challenge to Lockdown from Businessman," The Guardian, May 1, 2020, https://www.theguardian.com/law/2020/may/01/uk-government-faces-legal-challenge-coronavirus-lockdown-businessman-simon-dolan.

292 Dolan v Secretary of State for Health and Social Care [2020] EWHC 3275 (Admin), paras. 1–10 (High Court of Justice, Queen's Bench Division (Administrative Court), December 1, 2020), https://www.judiciary.uk/wp-content/uploads/2020/12/Dolan-v-SSHSC-judgment-011220-.pdf.

293 Pippa Crerar, "EXCLUSIVE: Boris Johnson 'Broke Covid Lockdown Rules' with Downing Street Parties at Xmas," Daily Mirror, November 30, 2021, https://www.mirror.co.uk/news/politics/boris-johnson-broke-covid-lockdown-25585238.

294 "Boris Johnson Had Birthday Bash During Lockdown, ITV News Understands," ITV News, January 25, 2022, https://www.itv.com/news/2022-01-24/boris-johnson-had-birthday-bash-during-lockdown-itv-news-understands.

295 Kate Ferguson and Jack Elsom, "Matt Hancock Had Secret Affair with Aide Gina Coladangelo While Married and She Was on His Covid Advisory Board – Leaked CCTV Shows Them Kissing in His Office," The Sun, June 25, 2021, https://www.thesun.co.uk/news/15388014/matt-hancock-secret-affair-with-aide/.

296 Steven Crowder (@scrowder), "BREAKING: Former NYC Covid Czar Held Secret Drug-Fueled Sex Parties…," X, September 19, 2024, video, 2:17, https://x.com/scrowder/status/1836737026281836727.

297 Welsh Government, Community Safety Division, Ministerial Advice for Decision by First Minister: Proposed Increase of Fixed Penalty Notice Amounts for Breaches of the Coronavirus Regulations, INQ000145221_0002 (exhibit to UK Covid-19 Inquiry), [date of document circa late 2020/early 2021], https://covid19.public-inquiry.uk/wp-content/uploads/2024/03/12200607/INQ000145221_0002.pdf.

298 National Police Chiefs' Council, "Update on Coronavirus FPNs Issued by Forces in England and Wales, and the Payment of FPNs," March 16,

2022, https://news.npcc.police.uk/releases/update-on-coronavirus-fpns-issued-by-forces-in-england-and-wales-and-the-payment-of-fpns.

299 Lizzie Dearden, "Coronavirus Act Prosecutions Ruled Wrongful After CPS Review," The Independent, February 17, 2021, https://www.independent.co.uk/news/uk/home-news/coronavirus-act-prosecutions-wrongful-cps-review-b1847194.html.

300 "Dr Anne McCloskey Jailed over Covid Fine," BBC News, June 12, 2024, https://www.bbc.co.uk/news/articles/cn446pd25m8o.

**CHAPTER FIVE**

301 Jonas Herby, Lars Jonung, and Steve H. Hanke, Did Lockdowns Work? The Verdict on Covid Restrictions (London: Institute of Economic Affairs, June 5, 2023), https://iea.org.uk/publications/did-lockdowns-work-the-verdict-on-covid-restrictions/.

302 Heather L. Taylor and Pablo Cuadros, "The Unintended Health Effects of US COVID-19 Lockdowns: A Systematic Review," Health Affairs Scholar 3, no. 11 (November 2025): qxaf208, https://doi.org/10.1093/haschl/qxaf208.

303 Camilla Turner, "Revealed: Whitty 'Silenced' Covid Advisers Who Warned about Lockdown," The Telegraph, December 6, 2025, https://www.telegraph.co.uk/news/2025/12/06/whitty-silenced-covid-ethics-advisers/.

304 Scientific Pandemic Influenza Group on Behaviours (SPI-B), Insights on Combined Behavioural and Social Interventions, INQ000109111 (exhibit to UK Covid-19 Inquiry), March 4, 2020, https://covid19.public-inquiry.uk/wp-content/uploads/2024/02/16103554/INQ000109111.pdf.

305 Department for Education and Prime Minister's Office, 10 Downing Street, "Schools, Colleges and Early Years Settings to Close," GOV.UK, March 18, 2020, https://www.gov.uk/government/news/schools-colleges-and-early-years-settings-to-close.

306 Sonia Elijah, "School Closures – Catastrophic and Just Not Necessary," The Conservative Woman, February 2, 2021, https://www.conservativewoman.co.uk/school-closures-catastrophic-and-just-not-necessary/.

307 European Centre for Disease Prevention and Control, COVID-19 in Children and the Role of School Settings in COVID-19 Transmission, 3.

308 Sonia Elijah, "Dr Zenobia Storah: 100K 'Ghost Children' in UK," YouTube video, 21:03, March 21, 2022, https://www.youtube.com/watch?v=mchyfog0z9Y.

309 Will Jones, "Read the Open Letter to Liz Truss Asking Her to Pause the Covid Vaccine Rollout to Children," The Daily Sceptic, September 6, 2022, https://dailysceptic.org/2022/09/06/read-the-open-letter-to-liz-truss-asking-her-to-pause-the-covid-vaccine-rollout-to-children/.

310 Sonia Elijah, "Mike Fairclough, the Twitter-Banned UK Headteacher: 'We Have a Legal Duty to Safeguard Children Against Harm,'" The Sonia Elijah Podcast (Substack), September 13, 2022, https://www.soniaelijah.com/p/mike-fairclough-the-twitter-banned.

311 Owen Evans, "'It's My Legal Duty to Safeguard Children Against Harm': British Headmaster," The Epoch Times, August 2, 2022, updated March 13, 2024, https://www.theepochtimes.com/bright/its-my-legal-duty-to-safeguard-children-against-harm-british-headmaster-4622234.

312 Greg Heffer, "George Osborne Questions Whether Schools Should Have Been Shut during Covid Lockdowns as Ex-Chancellor Insists His Austerity Policies Meant Britain Was BETTER Able to Respond to Coronavirus," Daily Mail, June 20, 2023, https://www.dailymail.co.uk/news/article-12213895/George-Osborne-insists-austerity-policies-meant-Britain-BETTER-able-respond-Covid.html.

313 Ely, John. "Emotional Ex-Chief Medical Officer Dame Sally Davies Makes Heartfelt Apology to Covid Victims." Daily Mail, June 20, 2023. Updated June 21, 2023. https://www.dailymail.co.uk/health/article-12214997/Emotional-ex-chief-medical-officer-Dame-Sally-Davies-makes-heartfelt-apology-Covid-victims.html.

314 UK Covid-19 Inquiry, "UK Covid 19 Inquiry - Module 8 Hearings - 14 October 2025 AM," YouTube video, October 14, 2025, https://www.youtube.com/watch?v=yVDLPicWlyw.

315 UK Covid-19 Inquiry. 2023. Transcript of Module 1 Public Hearing on 26 June 2023.

London: UK Covid-19 Inquiry. June 26. https://covid19.public-inquiry.uk/wp-content/uploads/2023/06/26190702/C-19-Inquiry-26-June-23-Module-1-Day-9.pdf.
316 Scottish COVID-19 Inquiry, Scottish COVID-19 Inquiry, Scottish COVID-19 Inquiry, Edinburgh, https://www.covid19inquiry.scot/.
317 Scottish Covid Bereaved, Submissions of Scottish Covid Bereaved for the Health and Social Care Impact Hearing, SCI-CLSSTN-000024 (Edinburgh: Scottish COVID-19 Inquiry, June 28, 2024), https://www.covid19inquiry.scot/sites/default/files/ev-documents/sci-clsstn-000024.pdf.
318 Scottish COVID-19 Inquiry, "Impact Hearing | Health and Social Care | Day 53," Scottish COVID-19 Inquiry, Edinburgh, May 23, 2024, https://www.covid19inquiry.scot/hearing/impact-hearing-health-social-care-day-53.
319 Vanessa Chalmers, "'Don't Kill Your Gran': Matt Hancock Urges Young People to Stop Flouting Coronavirus Restrictions and to Stick to Social Distancing Because Covid-19 Infections Are Surging Among 'Affluent' 17 to 21-Year-Olds," Daily Mail, September 7, 2020, updated September 7, 2020, https://www.dailymail.co.uk/news/article-8705361/Coronavirus-NOT-control-Britain-Matt-Hancock-claims.html.
320 Rowena Mason, "Coronavirus: London Hospitals Facing 'Tsunami' of Patients," The Guardian, March 26, 2020, https://www.theguardian.com/world/2020/mar/26/london-hospitals-facing-tsunami-of-coronavirus-patients-overwhelmed.
321 Freedom Podcast, "Our Hospitals were Half-Empty" Glasgow Porter tells Scottish COVID-19 inquiry, YouTube video, May 27, 2024, https://www.youtube.com/watch?v=uIQgSJvnxaQ.
322 Wide Awake Media (@wideawake_media), "Debbie Hicks was arrested and convicted of a public order offence for filming a completely empty hospital in December 2020…," X, October 20, 2024, https://x.com/wideawake_media/status/1847895753655468504.
323 Christopher Giles, Jack Goodman, and Olga Robinson, "Covid: The Truth behind Videos of 'Empty' Hospitals," BBC News, January 11, 2021, https://www.bbc.co.uk/news/55560714.
324 MaryJaneBlaze (@Blaze3Jane), "Honestly, this should have all been over when we first saw thousands of nurses dancing on Tik Tok in empty hospitals…," X, July 7, 2024, https://x.com/Blaze3Jane/status/1810080608120451545.
325 Dr. Jennifer M. A. Burns, Witness Statement of Dr Jennifer Burns, SCI-WT0572-000001 (Edinburgh: Scottish COVID-19 Inquiry, signed October 4, 2023; statement taken July 21, 2023), https://www.covid19inquiry.scot/sites/default/files/ev-documents/sci-wt0572-000001.pdf.
326 United Kingdom, Parliament, House of Commons, "Covid-19: Response and Excess Deaths," vol. 748, cols. 504– (debated April 18, 2024), https://hansard.parliament.uk/commons/2024-04-18/debates/9F01F787-D758-43D4-B8D1-4FA357EB3EED/Covid-19ResponseAndExcessDeaths.
327 Sam H. Ahmedzai et al., "Managing COVID-19 Symptoms in the Community (Including at the End of Life): NICE NG163 Is a Welcome Step, but Needs Review," rapid response to "Managing COVID-19 Symptoms (Including at the End of Life) in the Community: Summary of NICE Guidelines," BMJ 369 (April 20, 2020), posted May 19, 2020, https://www.bmj.com/content/369/bmj.m1461/rr-1.
328 Gillian Grant, Witness Statement of Gillian Grant, SCI-WT0142-000002 (Edinburgh: Scottish COVID-19 Inquiry, dated November 20, 2023), https://www.covid19inquiry.scot/sites/default/files/ev-documents/sci-wt0142-000002.pdf.
329 Andrew Picken, "Scottish Covid Inquiry: 'Do Not Resuscitate' against Family's Wishes," BBC News, November 23, 2023, https://www.bbc.co.uk/news/uk-scotland-67507145.
330 Freedom Podcast, "DO NOT RESUSCITATE | MIDAZOLAM | NEGLECT | Scottish COVID-19 Inquiry," YouTube video, June 25, 2024, https://www.youtube.com/watch?v=28klcTgey3M.
331 Rosa Silverman, "How Covid Damaged Every Generation – From Babies to Pensioners," The Telegraph, September 21, 2024, https://www.telegraph.co.uk/global-health/science-and-disease/how-covid-damaged-every-generation-from-babies-to-pensioner/.

332 UK Covid-19 Inquiry, Module 2, 2A, 2B, 2C: Core Decision-Making and Political Governance – Report and Recommendations In Brief (London: UK Covid-19 Inquiry, November 20, 2025; filename dated 17.11.25), https://covid19.public-inquiry.uk/wp-content/uploads/2025/11/18092508/M2-In-Brief-17.11.25-.pdf.
333 Nick Triggle, "UK Did 'Too Little, Too Late', Leading to Thousands More Covid Deaths, Says Inquiry," BBC News, November 20, 2025, https://www.bbc.co.uk/news/articles/c8030xvvlv0o.
334 Clare Dyer, "Covid Inquiry: UK Action Was 'Too Little, Too Late' and Led to Avoidable Deaths, Report Finds," BMJ 391 (November 21, 2025): r2472, https://doi.org/10.1136/bmj.r2472.

**CHAPTER SIX**

335 United States Government Accountability Office, COVID-19 Relief: Funding and Spending as of Jan. 31, 2023, GAO-23-106647 (Washington, DC: U.S. GAO, February 28, 2023), https://www.gao.gov/products/gao-23-106647.
336 United Kingdom, Parliament, House of Commons, "Coronavirus: Protective Clothing and Screening," Written Question 119856, tabled February 7, 2022, answered February 15, 2022, https://questions-statements.parliament.uk/written-questions/detail/2022-02-07/119856/.
337 Camilla Rothe et al., "Transmission of 2019-nCoV Infection from an Asymptomatic Contact in Germany," New England Journal of Medicine 382, no. 10 (March 5, 2020): 970–71, https://doi.org/10.1056/NEJMc2001468.
338 Camilla Rothe et al., "Disclosure Forms for 'Transmission of 2019-nCoV Infection from an Asymptomatic Contact in Germany,'" supplement to "Transmission of 2019-nCoV Infection from an Asymptomatic Contact in Germany," New England Journal of Medicine 382, no. 10 (March 5, 2020), https://www.nejm.org/doi/suppl/10.1056/NEJMc2001468/suppl_file/nejmc2001468_disclosures.pdf.
339 Kai Kupferschmidt, "Study Claiming New Coronavirus Can Be Transmitted by People without Symptoms Was Flawed," Science, February 3, 2020, https://www.science.org/content/article/paper-non-symptomatic-patient-transmitting-coronavirus-wrong.
340 Kai Kupferschmidt, "Study Claiming New Coronavirus Can Be Transmitted by People without Symptoms Was Flawed," Science, February 3, 2020, https://www.science.org/content/article/paper-non-symptomatic-patient-transmitting-coronavirus-wrong.
341 Folkhälsomyndigheten, "Smittsamma sjukdomar A-Ö," Folkhälsomyndigheten, https://www.folkhalsomyndigheten.se/vara-amnesomraden/smittsamma-sjukdomar/.
342 American Association for Cancer Research, "AACR COVID-19 and Cancer Virtual Meeting: Dr. Fauci Launches Meeting with Keynote Address," AACR Cancer Research Catalyst (blog), July 20, 2020, https://www.aacr.org/blog/2020/07/20/aacr-covid-19-and-cancer-virtual-meeting-dr-fauci-launches-meeting-with-keynote-address/.
343 Sonia Elijah, "The Many Scandals of the PCR Test – Part 1," The Conservative Woman, July 14, 2021, https://www.conservativewoman.co.uk/the-many-scandals-of-the-pcr-test-part-1/.
344 Wikipedia contributors, "Polymerase Chain Reaction," Wikipedia, The Free Encyclopedia, https://en.wikipedia.org/wiki/Polymerase_chain_reaction.
345 Kary Mullis, "Kary Mullis Speaks to Misuse of PCR (1993)," video, 6:07, Internet Archive, original recording 1993, https://archive.org/details/kary-mullis-speaks-to-misuse-of-pcr-1993.
346 Virological.org, "Virological: Pre-Publication Sharing of Pathogenic Virus Sequence Data," Virological.org (discussion forum), https://virological.org/.
347 World Health Organization, "WHO Guidelines for Laboratory Diagnosis of Human Infection with 2019-nCoV," version 1.0, January 13, 2020, https://www.who.int/docs/default-source/coronaviruse/wuhan-virus-assay-v1991527e5122341d99287a1b17c111902.pdf.
348 Victor M. Corman et al., "Detection of 2019 Novel Coronavirus (2019-nCoV) by Real-Time RT-PCR," Eurosurveillance 25, no. 3 (January 23, 2020): 2000045, https://doi.org/10.2807/1560-7917.ES.2020.25.3.2000045.
349 "Landmark Legal Ruling Finds That Covid Tests Are Not Fit for Purpose.

So What Do the MSM Do? They Ignore It," BSNews, November 30, 2020, https://bsnews.info/landmark-legal-ruling-finds-that-covid-tests-are-not-fit-for-purpose-so-what-do-the-msm-do-they-ignore-it/.

350 Pieter Borger et al., External Peer Review of the RTPCR Test to Detect SARS-CoV-2 Reveals 10 Major Scientific Flaws at the Molecular and Methodological Level: Consequences for False Positive Results (Zenodo, November 30, 2020), https://doi.org/10.5281/zenodo.4298004.

351 Andrew N. Cohen and Bruce Kessel, "False Positives in Reverse Transcription PCR Testing for SARS-CoV-2," medRxiv (preprint), May 5, 2020, https://doi.org/10.1101/2020.04.26.20080911.

352 Wikipedia contributors, "Operation Moonshot," Wikipedia, The Free Encyclopedia, https://en.wikipedia.org/wiki/Operation_Moonshot.

353 Gareth Iacobucci, "Covid-19: Government Shelves Plans to Invest £100bn in Mass Testing," BMJ 371 (October 23, 2020): m4112, https://doi.org/10.1136/bmj.m4112.

354 "£1.3bn High Court Challenge to Lucrative Test and Trace Contracts Launched," Daily Mail, October 15, 2020, https://www.dailymail.co.uk/news/article-8865733/1-3bn-High-Court-challenge-lucrative-Test-Trace-contracts-launched.html.

355 Tribunal da Relação de Lisboa [Lisbon Court of Appeal], Acórdão [Judgment], Processo 1783/20.7T8PDL.L1-3 (Nov. 11, 2020), http://www.dgsi.pt/jtrl.nsf/33182fc732316039802565fa00497eec/79d6ba338dcbe5e28025861f003e7b30 (English translation via Google Translate, accessed February 17, 2026, https://www-dgsi-pt.translate.goog/jtrl.nsf/33182fc732316039802565fa00497eec/79d6ba338dcbe5e28025861f003e7b30?_x_tr_sl=pt&_x_tr_tl=en&_x_tr_hl=en-GB).

356 OffGuardian, "Portuguese Court Rules PCR Tests 'Unreliable' & Quarantines 'Unlawful,'" OffGuardian, November 20, 2020, https://off-guardian.org/2020/11/20/portuguese-court-rules-pcr-tests-unreliable-quarantines-unlawful/.

357 Rita Jaafar et al., "Correlation Between 3790 Quantitative Polymerase Chain Reaction–Positives Samples and Positive Cell Cultures, Including 1941 Severe Acute Respiratory Syndrome Coronavirus 2 Isolates," Clinical Infectious Diseases 72, no. 11 (June 1, 2021), https://doi.org/10.1093/cid/ciaa1491.

358 World Health Organization, "WHO Information Notice for IVD Users," December 14, 2020, archived January 20, 2021, https://web.archive.org/web/20210120083427/https://www.who.int/news/item/14-12-2020-who-information-notice-for-ivd-users.

359 Thomas Binder (@Thomas_Binder), X post, March 21, 2021, https://x.com/Thomas_Binder/status/1373475621876142082.

360 World Health Organization, "WHO Audio Emergencies Coronavirus Press Conference," transcript, June 8, 2020, https://www.who.int/docs/default-source/coronaviruse/transcripts/who-audio-emergencies-coronavirus-press-conference-08jun2020.pdf.

361 Allyson M. Pollock and James Lancaster, "Asymptomatic Transmission of Covid-19," *BMJ* 371 (2020): m4851, https://doi.org/10.1136/bmj.m4851.

362 Victor M. Corman et al., "Detection of 2019 Novel Coronavirus (2019-nCoV) by Real-Time RT-PCR," *Eurosurveillance* 25, no. 3 (2020): 2000045, https://doi.org/10.2807/1560-7917.ES.2020.25.3.2000045.

363 Eurosurveillance Editorial Team, "Editorial Note: Possible Undisclosed Conflict of Interest," *Eurosurveillance* 25, no. 30 (2020): 2007301, https://doi.org/10.2807/1560-7917.ES.2020.25.30.2007301.

364 Stefan Nicola, "A Berlin Biotech Company Got a Head Start on Coronavirus Tests," *Bloomberg Businessweek*, March 12, 2020, https://www.bloomberg.com/news/articles/2020-03-12/a-berlin-biotech-company-got-a-head-start-on-coronavirus-tests.

365 Kevin P. Hoffmann, "TIB Molbiol: Berliner Firma produziert Coronavirus-Tests für die ganze Welt," *Der Tagesspiegel*, March 6, 2020, https://www.tagesspiegel.de/berlin/berliner-firma-produziert-coronavirus-tests-fur-die-ganze-welt-5714038.html. (tagesspiegel.de)

366 Ulrike Posche, "Der Aufklärer: So wurde Christian Drosten zum wichtigsten Mann Deutschlands" ["The Explainer: How Christian Drosten Became Germany's Most

Important Man"], *Stern*, March 17, 2020, https://www.stern.de/gesundheit/der-aufklaerer--so-wurde-christian-drosten-zum-wichtigsten-mann-deutschlands-9184616.html
367 Charité – Universitätsmedizin Berlin, "AG Corman," Institut für Virologie, https://virologie-ccm.charite.de/en/research/ag_corman.
368 Wikipedia contributors, "2009 Swine Flu Pandemic in Germany," Wikipedia, The Free Encyclopedia, Wikimedia Foundation, https://en.wikipedia.org/wiki/2009_swine_flu_pandemic_in_Germany.
369 Shaun Lintern, "Analysis: The Government Must Heed the Lessons from History on Rushed Vaccinations," The Independent, August 28, 2020, https://www.independent.co.uk/news/health/coronavirus-vaccine-pandemic-swine-flu-covid-a9693721.html.
370 UK Health Security Agency, "Virus Reference Department (VRD)," GOV.UK, published August 8, 2014, last updated September 8, 2025, https://www.gov.uk/government/collections/virus-reference-department-vrd.
371 Public Health England, "Vaccine Update: Issue 302, November 2019, Virus Special Edition," GOV.UK, November 2019, https://assets.publishing.service.gov.uk/media/5ddead82e5274a65d401b7c1/PHE_11474_vaccine_update_issue_302.pdf.
372 Eurosurveillance Editorial Team, "Response to Retraction Request and Allegations of Misconduct and Scientific Flaws," Eurosurveillance 26, no. 5 (February 4, 2021): 2102041, https://doi.org/10.2807/1560-7917.ES.2021.26.5.2102041.
373 Michael Günther, Robert Rockenfeller, and Harald Walach, "A Calibration of Nucleic Acid (PCR) by Antibody (IgG) Tests in Germany: The Course of SARS-CoV-2 Infections Estimated," Frontiers in Epidemiology 5 (October 13, 2025): 1592629, https://doi.org/10.3389/fepid.2025.1592629.
374 "Robert Koch-Institut will neue Studie inhaltlich nicht kommentieren," Pravda Deutschland, November 11, 2025, https://germany.news-pravda.com/germany/2025/11/11/190658.html.
375 Pieter Borger (@BorgerPieter), "In Germany, in most EU countries, a positive PCR was interpreted as „infection with killer virus". Because of this non-science several real scientists stood up. They were excluded, demonized and attacked by Pharmaffia-driven politics and media. Free Science Now!," Twitter (now X), November 26, 2025, https://x.com/BorgerPieter/status/1993592342599831951.

**CHAPTER SEVEN**

376 Sonia Elijah, "The Innova Lateral Flow Tests: Another Scandal in the Making? Part 1," The Conservative Woman, June 7, 2021, https://www.conservativewoman.co.uk/the-innova-lateral-flow-tests-another-scandal-in-the-making-part-1/.
377 "Moonshot: Five Key Points from No 10's Leaked Coronavirus Testing Plan," The Guardian, September 10, 2020, https://www.theguardian.com/world/2020/sep/10/moonshot-five-key-points-from-no-10s-leaked-coronavirus-testing-plan.
378 Association of American Physicians and Surgeons, "COVID-19: Do We Have a Coronavirus Pandemic, or a PCR Test Pandemic?," AAPS, October 7, 2020, https://aapsonline.org/covid-19-do-we-have-a-coronavirus-pandemic-or-a-pcr-test-pandemic/.
379 Elisabeth Mahase, "Operation Moonshot: What Do the Leaked Documents Say?," The BMJ, September 11, 2020, https://doi.org/10.1136/bmj.m3558.
380 "How UK Spent £800m on Controversial Covid Tests for Dominic Cummings Scheme," The Guardian, January 28, 2021, https://www.theguardian.com/world/2021/jan/28/how-uk-spent-800m-on-controversial-covid-tests-for-dominic-cummings-scheme.
381 Gareth Iacobucci, "Covid-19: Government Shelves Plans to Invest £100bn in Mass Testing," The BMJ, October 23, 2020, https://doi.org/10.1136/bmj.m4112.
382 Susan Hopkins, "COVID-19: Reintroducing Confirmatory PCR Testing," UK Health Security Agency (blog), March 30, 2021, https://ukhsa.blog.gov.uk/2021/03/30/covid-19-reintroducing-confirmatory-pcr-testing/.
383 Wikipedia contributors, "Dido Harding," Wikipedia, The Free Encyclopedia, Wikimedia Foundation, https://en.wikipedia.org/wiki/Dido_Harding.

384 Department of Health and Social Care, "Oxford University and PHE Confirm High-Sensitivity of Lateral Flow Tests," GOV.UK, November 11, 2020, https://www.gov.uk/government/news/oxford-university-and-phe-confirm-high-sensitivity-of-lateral-flow-tests.
385 "COVID-19: Half-Hour Lateral Flow Tests Could Miss 'Three in 10' Coronavirus Cases," Sky News, November 11, 2020, https://news.sky.com/story/covid-19-half-hour-lateral-flow-tests-could-miss-three-in-10-coronavirus-cases-12130154.
386 University of Oxford, "Oxford University and PHE Confirm Lateral Flow Tests Show High Specificity and Are Effective at Identifying Most Individuals Who Are Infectious," November 11, 2020, https://www.ox.ac.uk/news/2020-11-11-oxford-university-and-phe-confirm-lateral-flow-tests-show-high-specificity-and-are.
387 Medicines and Healthcare products Regulatory Agency (MHRA), "COVID-19 Test Approval: How to Apply," GOV.UK, published July 28, 2021, https://www.gov.uk/guidance/covid-19-test-approval-how-to-apply.
388 Ethan Ennals, "Government Test Tsar Has £770,000 Shares in Drugs Firm That Sold Us £13million of 'Pointless' Antibody Screening Kits," Daily Mail, September 26, 2020, https://www.dailymail.co.uk/news/article-8776339/Test-tsar-770-000-shares-firm-sold-13million-pointless-antibody-screening-kits.html.
389 Fiona Godlee, "Open Letter to Roche about Oseltamivir Trial Data," The BMJ, October 29, 2012, https://doi.org/10.1136/bmj.e7305.
390 Matthew Thompson and Carl Heneghan, "Re: Open Letter to Roche about Oseltamivir Trial Data," rapid response to *BMJ* 345 (December 2012), https://www.bmj.com/content/345/bmj.e7305/rr/618188
391 Peter Saunders, "Tamiflu: A Colossal Waste of Money," Institute of Science in Society, May 14, 2014, https://www.i-sis.org.uk/Tamiflu_A_Colossal_Waste_of_Money.php.
392 Paul D Thacker, "Tracking Down John Bell: How the Case of the Oxford Professor Exposes a Transparency Crisis in Government," The BMJ, February 24, 2021, https://doi.org/10.1136/bmj.n490.
393 Pasaca Capital Inc., "Home," Pasaca Capital Inc., https://pasacacapital.com/.
394 European Commission, "TED Notice 494882-2020," Tenders Electronic Daily (TED), published 2020, https://ted.europa.eu/en/notice/-/detail/494882-2020.
395 "UK Government Fails to Publish Details of £4bn Covid Contracts with Private Firms," The Guardian, November 9, 2020, https://www.theguardian.com/world/2020/nov/09/uk-government-fails-to-publish-details-of-4bn-covid-contracts-with-private-firms.
396 Luke Andrews, "Californian Firm Has Already Won £2.8BILLION to Supply UK Lateral Flow Covid Tests Ahead of Plan to Offer Kits to EVERYONE Twice-a-Week," Daily Mail, April 5, 2021 (updated April 16, 2021), https://www.dailymail.co.uk/news/article-9437191/Californian-firm-won-2-8BILLION-supply-UK-lateral-flow-Covid-tests.html.
397 Sonia Elijah, "The Innova Tests: Another Covid Scandal in the Making? Part 2," The Conservative Woman, June 10, 2021, https://www.conservativewoman.co.uk/the-innova-tests-another-covid-scandal-in-the-making-part-2/.
398 Joint PHE Porton Down & University of Oxford SARS-CoV-2 LFD Test Development and Validation Cell, Preliminary Report from the Joint PHE Porton Down & University of Oxford SARS-CoV-2 Test Development and Validation Cell: Rapid Evaluation of Lateral Flow Viral Antigen Detection Devices (LFDs) for Mass Community Testing, November 8, 2020, https://www.ox.ac.uk/sites/files/oxford/media_wysiwyg/UK%20evaluation_PHE%20Porton%20Down%20%20University%20of%20Oxford_final.pdf.
399 Department of Health and Social Care, "Oxford University and PHE Confirm High-Sensitivity of Lateral Flow Tests," GOV.UK, November 11, 2020, https://www.gov.uk/government/news/oxford-university-and-phe-confirm-high-sensitivity-of-lateral-flow-tests.
400 Marta García-Fiñana, David M. Hughes, Christopher Cheyne, Girvan Burnside, Mark Stockbridge, Tom A. Fowler, Veronica Fowler, Mark Wilcox, Malcolm Semple, and Iain Buchan, "Performance of the Innova SARS-CoV-2 Antigen Rapid Lateral Flow

Test in the Liverpool Asymptomatic Testing Pilot," *SSRN Electronic Journal*, March 10, 2021, https://doi.org/10.2139/ssrn.3798558. (livrepository.liverpool.ac.uk)

401 UK Medicines and Healthcare products Regulatory Agency, "COVID-19 Test Approval: How to Apply," *GOV.UK*, [https://www.gov.uk/guidance/covid-19-test-approval-how-to-apply](https://www.gov.uk/guidance/covid-19-test-approval-how-to-apply).

402 Public Health England and University of Oxford, *COVID-19: Head-to-Head Laboratory Evaluation of 4 Commercial Serological Assays*, 2020, https://www.ox.ac.uk/sites/files/oxford/media_wysiwyg/UK%20evaluation_PHE%20Porton%20Down%20%20University%20of%20Oxford_final.pdf

403 Elisabeth Mahase, "Covid-19: Innova Lateral Flow Test Is Not Fit for 'Test and Release' Strategy, Say Experts," *BMJ* 371 (2020): m4469, https://www.bmj.com/content/371/bmj.m4469.

404 Stephen Armstrong, "Covid-19: Tests on Students Are Highly Inaccurate, Early Findings Show," *BMJ* 371 (2020): m4941, https://www.bmj.com/content/371/bmj.m4941.

405 UK Department of Health and Social Care, *Lateral Flow Device Specificity in Phase 4 (Public Evaluation)*, 2021, https://assets.publishing.service.gov.uk/government/uploads/system/uploads/attachment_data/file/968095/lateral-flow-device-specificity-in-phase-4.pdf.

406 UK Department of Health and Social Care, "SARS-CoV-2 Antigen Rapid Qualitative Test Kits," *Contracts Finder*, https://www.contractsfinder.service.gov.uk/Notice/ca07d68e-8f93-4864-9c4b-f24f1e117162. (blogs.bmj.com)

407 Sarah Boseley and Felicity Lawrence, "How UK Spent £800m on Controversial Covid Tests for Dominic Cummings Scheme," *Guardian*, https://www.theguardian.com/world/2021/jan/28/how-uk-spent-800m-on-controversial-covid-tests-for-dominic-cummings-scheme.

408 Liverpool School of Tropical Medicine, "Excalibur Rapid SARS-CoV-2 Antigen Screening Test, Validated by LSTM, Granted MHRA Approval," January 13, 2021, https://www.lstmed.ac.uk/news-events/news/excalibur-rapid-sars-cov-2-antigen-screening-test-validated-by-lstm-granted-mhra.

409 UK Department of Health and Social Care, "Provision of SARS-CoV-2 Rapid Antigen Test Kits," *BidStats*, https://bidstats.uk/tenders/2021/W20/751173972.

410 UK Department for Education and UK Department of Health and Social Care, "Mass Testing for Secondary Pupils as All Schools and Colleges Fully Reopen from 8 March," *GOV.UK*, February 22, 2021, https://www.gov.uk/government/news/mass-testing-for-secondary-pupils-as-all-schools-and-colleges-fully-reopenfrom8-march. (gov.uk)

411 Lucy Middleton, "All Adults to Have Two Free Covid Tests a Week Ahead of Lockdown's End," Metro, April 5, 2021, https://metro.co.uk/2021/04/05/all-adults-to-have-two-free-covid-tests-a-week-ahead-of-lockdowns-end-14357468/.

412 "Full List of Private Companies Handed £30 Billion of Public Money to Assist in UK Government's Covid Response," The Standard, May 4, 2021, https://www.standard.co.uk/business/government-covid-private-contracts-30-billion-pwc-deloitte-british-airways-b933081.html.

413 "The UK government spent £800m on controversial Covid tests for Dominic Cummings scheme," The Guardian, January 28, 2021, https://www.theguardian.com/world/2021/jan/28/how-uk-spent-800m-on-controversial-covid-tests-for-dominic-cummings-scheme.

414 "World's Biggest Rapid Covid Test Maker to Start Producing in UK," Financial Times, May 24, 2021, https://www.ft.com/content/8989c855-faf8-416e-88af-3af8a275434d.

415 "World's Largest Rapid Covid Test Maker to Start Producing in UK," Yahoo Finance UK, May 24, 2021, https://uk.finance.yahoo.com/news/worlds-largest-rapid-covid-test-maker-uk-factory-innova-california-103310285.html.

416 Luke Andrews, "Californian Firm Has Already Won £2.8BILLION to Supply UK Lateral Flow Covid Tests Ahead of Plan to Offer Kits to EVERYONE Twice-a-Week," Daily Mail, April 5, 2021 (updated April 16, 2021), https://www.dailymail.co.uk/news/article-9437191/Californian-firm-won-2-8BILLION-supply-UK-lateral-flow-Covid-tests.html.

417 Pasaca Capital Inc., "Innova Medical Group," Pasaca Capital Inc., accessed February 18, 2026, https://pasacacapital.com/case-study/innova-medical-group/.

418 "The fifth of UK Covid contracts raised red flags for possible corruption," The Guardian, April 22, 2021, https://www.theguardian.com/world/2021/apr/22/fifth-of-uk-covid-contracts-raised-red-flags-for-possible-corruption.

419 Wikipedia contributors, "Timeline of the COVID-19 Pandemic in March 2020," Wikipedia, The Free Encyclopedia, Wikimedia Foundation, https://en.wikipedia.org/wiki/Timeline_of_the_COVID-19_pandemic_in_March_2020#27_March.

420 Sonia Elijah, "The Innova Scandal Part 3: The US Says 'Throw the Tests in the Trash,'" The Conservative Woman, June 14, 2021, https://www.conservativewoman.co.uk/the-innova-scandal-part-3-the-us-says-throw-the-tests-in-the-trash/.

421 Department of Health and Social Care, "COVID-19 Self-Test (Throat and Nose) Instructions," GOV.UK, 2021, https://assets.publishing.service.gov.uk/government/uploads/system/uploads/attachment_data/file/1045088/COVID-19-self-test-throat-and-nose-instructions.pdf.

422 Sam Blanchard, "UK Coronavirus: Department of Health Rebranding Professional Use Kit as Self-Test," Daily Mail, January 12, 2021 (updated January 12, 2021), https://www.dailymail.co.uk/news/article-9127345/UK-coronavirus-Department-Health-rebranding-professional-use-kit-self-test.html.

423 Henry Bodkin, "Rapid Covid Tests Used by Schoolchildren Investigated for Containing Wrong Instructions," The Telegraph, April 18, 2021, https://www.telegraph.co.uk/news/2021/04/18/rapid-covid-tests-used-schoolchildren-investigated-containing/.

**CHAPTER EIGHT**

424 Sonia Elijah, "The Innova Scandal Part 4: Questions the Government Has Ignored," The Conservative Woman, June 21, 2021, https://www.conservativewoman.co.uk/the-innova-scandal-part-4-questions-the-government-has-ignored/.

425 Pasaca Capital Inc., "Executives," Pasaca Capital Inc., https://pasacacapital.com/executives/.

426 Great Britain. Parliament. House of Commons. Trade and Industry Committee. "Memorandum by MG Rover Group Limited," in The Work of the Committee in 2003–04: Minutes of Evidence, HC 437, Session 2003–04, Ev 7, November 2004, https://publications.parliament.uk/pa/cm200304/cmselect/cmtrdind/437/437we07.htm.

427 Keith Adams, "MG Rover and China Brilliance – Failed UK-China Joint Venture Uncovered," AROnline, https://www.aronline.co.uk/history/mg-rover-and-china-brilliance/.

428 Department for Business, Innovation and Skills, Inspectors' Report into the Affairs of MG Rover Group Limited and Phoenix Venture Holdings Limited, vol. 2 (London: BIS, September 11, 2010), https://webarchive.nationalarchives.gov.uk/ukgwa/20121106104033/http%3A/www.bis.gov.uk/files/file52783.pdf.

429 Jon Deeks, Angela Raffle, and Mike Gill, "Covid-19: Government Must Urgently Rethink Lateral Flow Test Roll Out," The BMJ (blog), January 12, 2021, https://blogs.bmj.com/bmj/2021/01/12/covid-19-government-must-urgently-rethink-lateral-flow-test-roll-out/.

430 Jim Norton, Elliot Mulligan, and Greg Kirby, "Two Firms Supplying Kits for Government's Mass Covid Testing Drive Are in for Huge Payday," Daily Mail, April 5, 2021 (updated April 6, 2021), https://www.dailymail.co.uk/news/article-9438727/Two-firms-supplying-kits-Governments-mass-Covid-testing-drive-huge-payday.html.

431 Tried & Tested Technology, "Digital and Analogue Diagnostic Tests for Respiratory and Genetic Diseases," Tried & Tested Technology (website), Disruptive Nanotechnology Limited, https://www.triedandtested.tech/.

432 Luke Andrews, "Californian Firm Has Already Won £2.8BILLION to Supply UK Lateral Flow Covid Tests Ahead of Plan to Offer Kits to EVERYONE Twice-a-Week," Daily Mail, April 5, 2021 (updated April 16, 2021), https://www.dailymail.co.uk/news/article-9437191/Californian-firm-won-2-8BILLION-supply-UK-lateral-flow-Covid-tests.html.

433 Jim Norton, Elliot Mulligan, and Greg Kirby, "Two Firms Supplying Kits for Government's Mass Covid Testing Drive," Daily Mail, April 5, 2021,

https://www.dailymail.co.uk/news/article-9438727/Two-firms-supplying-kits-Governments-mass-Covid-testing-drive-huge-payday.html.
434 David Rose, "Operation Shambles: Will the £42BILLION 'Operation Moonshot' Test and Trace Plan Actually Work? This Devastating Exposé Reveals How Ministers Have Scorned Some of Britain's Top Virus Experts, Hired Novices Instead - and Blown Billions," Daily Mail, November 13, 2020 (updated November 14, 2020), https://www.dailymail.co.uk/news/article-8947595/DAVID-ROSE-42BILLION-Operation-Moonshot-test-trace-plan-actually-work.html.
435 Medicines and Healthcare products Regulatory Agency, "Following a Satisfactory Review, MHRA Extends Authorisation of NHS Test and Trace Lateral Flow Devices," GOV.UK, June 17, 2021, https://www.gov.uk/government/news/following-a-satisfactory-review-mhra-extends-authorisation-of-nhs-test-and-trace-lateral-flow-devices.
436 "2023.02.06 - FOI Excerpts," PDF file, February 6, 2023, https://drive.google.com/file/d/1iss3u9uIlaY9veAC6FCgj4psch1r7ePG/view.
437 PA Media, "Covid: Government's PPE 'VIP Lane' Unlawful, Court Rules," BBC News, January 12, 2022, https://www.bbc.co.uk/news/uk-59968037.
438 Sonia Elijah, "Innova's Iniquity, Part 1: How Test Firm Flashed the UK Taxpayer's Cash," The Conservative Woman, September 15, 2021, https://www.conservativewoman.co.uk/innovas-iniquity-part-1-how-test-firm-flashed-the-uk-taxpayers-cash/.
439 Elisabeth Mahase, "Covid-19: Innova Lateral Flow Test Is Not Fit for 'Test and Release' Strategy, Say Experts," The BMJ 371 (November 17, 2020): m4469, https://doi.org/10.1136/bmj.m4469.
440 Nick Triggle, "Covid-19: NHS Test and Trace 'No Clear Impact' Despite £37bn Budget," BBC News, March 10, 2021, https://www.bbc.co.uk/news/health-56340831.
441 Good Law Project, "Why Might the Anti-Corruption Tsar Be Smearing Us?," September 2, 2021, https://goodlawproject.org/why-might-the-anti-corruption-tsar-be-smearing-us/.
442 Public Accounts Committee, ""Unimaginable" Cost of Test & Trace Failed to Deliver Central Promise of Averting Another Lockdown," UK Parliament, March 10, 2021, https://committees.parliament.uk/committee/127/public-accounts-committee/news/150988/unimaginable-cost-of-test-trace-failed-to-deliver-central-promise-of-averting-another-lockdown/.
443 Laurence Darmiento, Melody Petersen, and Jack Flemming, "A Pasadena Startup Got Billions Selling COVID Tests. Then Came Questions," Los Angeles Times, July 28, 2021, https://www.latimes.com/business/story/2021-07-28/innova-pasaca-covid-17-antigen-test-british-uk-government.
444 "John Penrose," GOV.UK, https://www.gov.uk/government/people/john-penrose.
445 "Government Contracts: Covid-19," Hansard Parliamentary Debates, Commons, vol. 697, cols. 238–68WH (21 June 2021), https://hansard.parliament.uk/commons/2021-06-21/debates/6FCF1DEF-15A4-46FF-8728-D7B2FA84F549/GovernmentContractsCovid-19.
446 "A Bogus Eastern Kentucky Battery Plant'; Lawsuit Seeks $30 Million from Enerblu Officials," WYMT News Staff, WYMT, September 17, 2019, https://www.wymt.com/content/news/Lawsu-560610461.html.
447 "Covid Inquiry Demands Virus Tests for Attendees a Year After Lateral Flows Were Scrapped," The Telegraph, June 12, 2023, https://www.telegraph.co.uk/news/2023/06/12/covid-inquiry-virus-tests-lateral-flow/.
448 "Robert Kasprzak vs Charles Chunhua Huang, an Individual, et al.," case no. (Los Angeles County Superior Courts, Alhambra Courthouse, filed April 26, 2023), UniCourt, https://unicourt.com/case/ca-la23-casear2c6ea9184673-1011355?init_S=ch_ftrd.
449 Laurence Darmiento, "Inside the Legal Drama Embroiling a Pasadena Startup That Grossed Billions Selling COVID Tests," Los Angeles Times, July 17, 2024, https://www.latimes.com/business/story/2024-07-17/founders-of-pasadena-company-that-got-billions-selling-covid-tests-are-embroiled-in-a-legal-fight.

450 S. Brenner, F. Jacob, and M. Meselson, "An Unstable Intermediate Carrying Information from Genes to Ribosomes for Protein Synthesis," Nature 190, no. 4776 (May 13, 1961): 576–581, https://doi.org/10.1038/190576a0.

451 G. J. Dimitriadis, "Translation of Rabbit Globin mRNA Introduced by Liposomes into Mouse Lymphocytes," Nature 274, no. 5674 (August 31, 1978): 923–924, https://doi.org/10.1038/274923a0.

452 D. A. Melton, P. A. Krieg, M. R. Rebagliati, T. Maniatis, K. Zinn, and M. R. Green, "Efficient in Vitro Synthesis of Biologically Active RNA and RNA Hybridization Probes from Plasmids Containing a Bacteriophage SP6 Promoter," Nucleic Acids Research 12, no. 18 (September 25, 1984): 7035–7056, https://doi.org/10.1093/nar/12.18.7035

453 Elie Dolgin, "The Tangled History of mRNA Vaccines," Nature, September 14, 2021, https://doi.org/10.1038/d41586-021-02483-w.

454 R. W. Malone, P. L. Felgner, and I. M. Verma, "Cationic Liposome-Mediated RNA Transfection," Proceedings of the National Academy of Sciences of the United States of America 86, no. 16 (August 15, 1989): 6077–6081, https://doi.org/10.1073/pnas.86.16.6077.

455 Jon A. Wolff, Robert W. Malone, Phillip Williams, et al., "Direct Gene Transfer into Mouse Muscle in Vivo," Science 247, no. 4949, pt. 1 (March 23, 1990): 1465–1468, https://doi.org/10.1126/science.1690918.

456 Sonia Elijah, "Dr Robert Malone, Inventor of mRNA Technology Interviewed by Sonia Elijah," YouTube video, 1:15:36 (approx.), uploaded by "Sonia Elijah investigates," May 15, 2024, https://www.youtube.com/watch?v=gHny5-c_Heo.

457 Alice Park, "Nobel Prize Awarded to mRNA Pioneers Who Paved the Way for COVID-19 Vaccines," Time, October 2, 2023, https://time.com/6319654/nobel-prize-awarded-to-mrna-pioneers/.

458 Katalin Karikó, Michael Buckstein, Houping Ni, and Drew Weissman, "Suppression of RNA Recognition by Toll-like Receptors: The Impact of Nucleoside Modification and the Evolutionary Origin of RNA," Immunity 23, no. 2 (August 2005): 165–175, https://doi.org/10.1016/j.immuni.2005.06.008.

459 "The Nobel Prize in Physiology or Medicine 2023," NobelPrize.org, Nobel Prize Outreach AB, 2023, https://www.nobelprize.org/prizes/medicine/2023/summary/.

460 Thomas E. Mulroney et al., "N1-Methylpseudouridylation of mRNA Causes +1 Ribosomal Frameshifting," Nature 625, no. 7993 (January 11, 2024): 189–194, https://doi.org/10.1038/s41586-023-06800-3.

461 "How mRNA Became a Vaccine Game-Changer," Financial Times, May 12, 2021, https://www.ft.com/content/b2978026-4bc2-439c-a561-a1972eeba940.

462 Derrick J. Rossi et al., "Highly Efficient Reprogramming to Pluripotency and Directed Differentiation of Human Cells with Synthetic Modified mRNA," Cell Stem Cell 7, no. 5 (November 5, 2010): 618–630, https://doi.org/10.1016/j.stem.2010.08.012.

463 Alice Park, "Derrick Rossi," Time, December 2010, https://content.time.com/time/specials/packages/article/0,28804,2036683_2036767_2037437,00.html.

464 Gwen Kinkead, "A Contraceptive Implant with Remote Control," MIT Technology Review, July 4, 2014, https://www.technologyreview.com/2014/07/04/74389/a-contraceptive-implant-with-remote-control/

465 Victor Tangermann, "An Invisible Quantum Dot 'Tattoo' Could Be Used to ID Vaccinated Kids," ScienceAlert, December 20, 2019, https://www.sciencealert.com/an-invisible-quantum-dot-tattoo-is-being-suggested-to-id-vaccinated-kids.

466 "DARPA Awards Moderna Therapeutics a Grant for up to $25 Million to Develop Messenger RNA Therapeutics™," Moderna Therapeutics, October 2, 2013, https://news.modernatx.com/news/news-details/2013/darpa-awards-moderna-therapeutics-a-grant-for-up-to-25-million-to-develop-messenger-rna-therapeutics.

467 "AstraZeneca and Moderna Therapeutics Announce Exclusive Agreement to Develop Pioneering Messenger RNA Therapeutics™ in Cardiometabolic Diseases

and Cancer," AstraZeneca, March 21, 2013, https://www.astrazeneca.com/media-centre/press-releases/2013/astrazeneca-moderna-therapeutics-cardiometabolic-diseases-cancer-treatment-21032013.html#modal-historic-confirmation.

468 "List of Global Growth Company Members As of 19 November 2013," World Economic Forum, 2013, https://www3.weforum.org/docs/WEF_GGC_Members_2013.pdf.

469 "Merck & Co., Moderna Launch $100M+ mRNA Partnership," Genetic Engineering & Biotechnology News, January 13, 2015, https://www.genengnews.com/news/merck-co-moderna-launch-100m-mrna-partnership/.

470 "Moderna Wins Initial $20M Grant from Gates Foundation," Genetic Engineering & Biotechnology News, January 12, 2016, https://www.genengnews.com/news/moderna-wins-initial-20m-grant-from-gates-foundation/.

471 "Moderna Wins Up to $125M from BARDA Toward Zika mRNA Vaccine," Genetic Engineering & Biotechnology News, September 7, 2016, https://www.genengnews.com/news/moderna-wins-up-to-125m-from-barda-toward-zika-mrna-vaccine/.

472 Robert N. Kirchdoerfer et al., "Pre-fusion Structure of a Human Coronavirus Spike Protein," Nature 531, no. 7592 (March 3, 2016): 118–121, https://doi.org/10.1038/nature17200.

473 Damian Garde, "Moderna Aims to Raise $500 Million in Biotech's Largest-Ever Public Offering," STAT, November 9, 2018, https://www.statnews.com/2018/11/09/moderna-aims-to-raise-500-million-in-biotechs-largest-ever-public-offering/.

474 Moderna, Inc., "Form S-1 Registration Statement," United States Securities and Exchange Commission, filed November 9, 2018, https://www.sec.gov/Archives/edgar/data/1682852/000119312518323562/d577473ds1.htm.

475 Stanley A. Plotkin, Adel A. F. Mahmoud, and Jeremy Farrar, "Establishing a Global Vaccine-Development Fund," New England Journal of Medicine 373, no. 4 (July 23, 2015): 297–300, https://doi.org/10.1056/NEJMp1506820.

476 "Trump Administration Collaborates With Moderna to Produce 100 Million Doses of COVID-19 Investigational Vaccine," U.S. Department of Defense, August 11, 2020, https://www.defense.gov/News/Releases/Release/Article/2309561/trump-administration-collaborates-with-moderna-to-produce-100-million-doses-of/.

477 Ameet Sarpatwari, "Taxpayers Paid Billions For It: So Why Would Moderna Consider Quadrupling the Price of the COVID Vaccine?" written testimony submitted to the U.S. Senate Committee on Health, Education, Labor, and Pensions, March 22, 2023, https://www.help.senate.gov/imo/media/doc/Written%20Testimony-Sarpatwari.pdf.

478 Christopher J. Morten, "The NIH-Moderna Vaccine: Public Science, Private Profit, and Lessons for the Future," Journal of Law, Medicine & Ethics 51, suppl. 2 (Winter 2023): 35–40, https://doi.org/10.1017/jme.2023.149.

479 United States of America, "Statement of Interest of the United States," Arbutus Biopharma Corporation and Genevant Sciences GmbH v. Moderna, Inc. and ModernaTX, Inc., No. 22-252 (MSG) (D. Del. February 14, 2023), https://storage.courtlistener.com/recap/gov.uscourts.ded.78146/gov.uscourts.ded.78146.49.0_1.pdf.

480 "Moderna Market Cap 2017-2025 | MRNA," MacroTrends, last modified February 16, 2026, https://www.macrotrends.net/stocks/charts/MRNA/moderna/market-cap.

481 "Moderna Reports Fourth Quarter and Fiscal Year 2021 Financial Results and Provides Business Updates," Moderna, Inc., February 24, 2022, https://s29.q4cdn.com/435878511/files/doc_financials/2021/q4/Moderna-Reports-Fourth-Quarter-and-Fiscal-Year-2021-Financial-Results-and-Provides-Business-Updates-2022.pdf.

482 David Wainer, "Moderna Peers Over a Scary Profit Cliff," Wall Street Journal, February 23, 2023, https://www.wsj.com/articles/moderna-peers-over-a-scary-profit-cliff-5374e4d4.

483 David Crow, "How mRNA Became a Vaccine Game-Changer," Financial Times, May 13, 2021, https://www.ft.com/content/b2978026-4bc2-439c-a561-a1972eeba940.

484 "Stéphane Bancel," Forbes, https://www.forbes.com/profile/stephane-bancel/?sh=97d89463742f.

485 "Moderna CEO on COVID-19 Vaccine: 'We Are in the Home Stretch'," Advisory Board, December 2020, https://www.advisory.com/blog/2020/12/moderna-ceo-covid-vaccine-bancel.
486 Regina Dugan, "How DARPA Seeded the Ground for a Rapid COVID-19 Cure," interview by Yahoo Finance Live, Yahoo Finance, December 17, 2020, https://finance.yahoo.com/video/darpa-seeded-ground-rapid-covid-214655580.html.
487 "Public-Private Partnership for Pandemic Preparedness and Response: A Call to Action," Johns Hopkins Center for Health Security, January 17, 2020, https://centerforhealthsecurity.org/sites/default/files/2022-12/200117-publicprivatepandemiccalltoaction.pdf.
488 Hussain S. Lalani et al., "US Public Investment in Development of mRNA Covid-19 Vaccines: Retrospective Cohort Study," BMJ 380 (March 1, 2023): e073747, https://doi.org/10.1136/bmj-2022-073747.
489 "Defense Advanced Research Projects Agency (DARPA)," Encyclopædia Britannica, last modified February 18, 2026, https://www.britannica.com/topic/Defense-Advanced-Research-Projects-Agency.
490 "Preventing Pandemics," Defense Advanced Research Projects Agency (DARPA), January 29, 2021, https://www.darpa.mil/sites/default/files/Preventing_Pandemics_Vignette_Final_210208.pdf.
491 " Pentagon Tasks Pfizer with Radically Rethinking Vaccine Development," Fierce Pharma, December 3, 2020, https://www.fiercepharma.com/r-d/pentagon-tasks-pfizer-radically-rethinking-vaccine-development.
492 David Crow, "How mRNA Became a Vaccine Game-Changer," Financial Times, May 12, 2021, https://www.ft.com/content/b2978026-4bc2-439c-a561-a1972eeba940.
493 "Preventing Pandemics," DARPA.
494 Liz Melone, "Moderna Announces Positive Interim Phase 1 Data for Its mRNA Vaccine (mRNA-1273) Against Novel Coronavirus," Moderna, Inc., July 14, 2020, https://www.modernatx.com/en-US/news-and-media/news/moderna-announces-positive-interim-phase-1-data-its-mrna-vaccine-mrna-1273-against-novel-coronavirus.
495 "Global Health Accelerator," Bill & Melinda Gates Foundation, https://www.gatesfoundation.org/our-work/programs/global-health/accelerator.
496 Wellcome Leap. "Our Team." https://wellcomeleap.org/our-team/.
497 Damian Garde, "Ego, Ambition, and Turmoil: Inside One of Biotech's Most Secretive Startups," STAT, September 13, 2016, https://www.statnews.com/2016/09/13/moderna-therapeutics-biotech-mrna/.
498 Robert Kuznia, Katie Polglase, and Gianluca Mezzofiore, "In Quest for Vaccine, US Makes 'Big Bet' on Company with Unproven Technology," CNN, May 1, 2020, https://edition.cnn.com/2020/05/01/us/coronavirus-moderna-vaccine-invs/index.html.
499 "Research Not Fit to Print," Nature Biotechnology 34 (February 2016): 115, https://doi.org/10.1038/nbt.3488.
500 "Tracing the Scandal of Theranos Founder Elizabeth Holmes," Wall Street Journal, https://www.wsj.com/news/collection/theranos-coverage-ea13b200.
501 Damian Garde, "Lavishly Funded Moderna Hits Safety Problems in Bold Bid to Revolutionize Medicine," STAT, January 10, 2017, https://www.statnews.com/2017/01/10/moderna-trouble-mrna/.
502 Damian Garde, "Key Partner Cuts Ties with Brash Biotech Startup Moderna, Raising Big Questions About Its Pipeline," STAT, July 27, 2017, https://www.statnews.com/2017/07/27/moderna-alexion-partnership/.
503 Garde, "Ego, Ambition, and Turmoil," https://www.statnews.com/2016/09/13/moderna-therapeutics-biotech-mrna/.
504 Johns Hopkins Center for Health Security, "Dark Winter," https://centerforhealthsecurity.org/our-work/tabletop-exercises/dark-winter-a-training-tabletop-exercise.
505 U.S. Department of Health and Human Services, Office of the Assistant Secretary for Preparedness and Response, Crimson Contagion 2019 Functional Exercise After-Action Report, January 2020, https://archive.org/details/crimson-contagion-2019/page/8/mode/1up.

506 Robert A. Feldman et al., "mRNA Vaccines Against H10N8 and H7N9 Influenza Viruses of Pandemic Potential Are Immunogenic and Well Tolerated in Healthy Adults in Phase 1 Randomized Clinical Trials," Vaccine 37, no. 25 (May 31, 2019): 3326–3334, https://doi.org/10.1016/j.vaccine.2019.04.026.
507 Randall S. Bock, "The Zika Vaccine Never Was; Its Experimental Trial Should Never Be," Washington Examiner, April 18, 2022, https://www.washingtonexaminer.com/opinion/1454912/the-zika-vaccine-never-was-its-experimental-trial-should-never-be/.
508 Damian Garde, "Moderna Breaks Its Publishing Silence, but Can It Sell Its Zika Vaccine?," STAT, February 17, 2017, https://www.statnews.com/2017/02/17/moderna-zika-vaccine/.
509 ModernaTX, Inc., "A Phase 1, Randomized, Placebo-Controlled, Dose-Ranging Study to Evaluate the Safety and Immunogenicity of mRNA-1325 Zika Vaccine in Healthy Adults in a Non-endemic Zika Region," ClinicalTrials.gov NCT03014089, results tab, https://clinicaltrials.gov/study/NCT03014089?tab=results.
510 Brandon Essink et al., "The Safety and Immunogenicity of Two Zika Virus mRNA Vaccine Candidates in Healthy Flavivirus Baseline Seropositive and Seronegative Adults: The Results of Two Randomised, Placebo-Controlled, Dose-Ranging, Phase 1 Clinical Trials," The Lancet Infectious Diseases 23, no. 5 (May 2023): 621–633, https://doi.org/10.1016/S1473-3099(22)00764-2.
511 Adam Feuerstein, "With Some Safety Caveats, New Moderna Data Show mRNA Can Teach the Body to Make Its Own Medicine," STAT, September 12, 2019, https://www.statnews.com/2019/09/12/new-moderna-data-cmv-chikungunya/.
512 Damian Garde, "Biotech's Biggest Unicorn Is Now Worth $7.5 Billion," STAT, February 1, 2018, https://www.statnews.com/2018/02/01/biotech-unicorn-7-billion-moderna/.
513 Moderna, Inc., Registration Statement on Form S-1 (File No. 333-226254), filed with the U.S. Securities and Exchange Commission, November 9, 2018, https://www.sec.gov/Archives/edgar/data/1682852/000119312518323562/d577473ds1.htm.
514 Damian Garde, "Moderna's Record-Setting IPO Dives in Its Debut," STAT, December 7, 2018, https://www.statnews.com/2018/12/07/modernas-record-setting-ipo-slumps-in-its-debut/.
515 Nathan Vardi and Matthew Herper, "Moderna's Mysterious Medicines," Forbes, December 14, 2016, https://www.forbes.com/sites/nathanvardi/2016/12/14/modernas-mysterious-medicines/#19ea9831730e.
516 Moderna Therapeutics, Inc., Exhibit 4.17: License Agreement between The University of British Columbia and Inex Pharmaceuticals Corporation (effective July 1, 1998; executed June 30, 2001), filed with the U.S. Securities and Exchange Commission, https://www.sec.gov/Archives/edgar/data/1447028/000119312511158553/dex417.htm.
517 Richard Atkins, "Biotech Stock in Spotlight: As the World Awaits Ebola Treatment, Tekmira Pharma In Prime Focus," TechNews, August 9, 2014, https://technews.org/biotech-stock-in-spotlight-as-the-world-awaits-ebola-treatment-tekmira-pharma-remains-in-orime-focus/2913113/.
518 Damian Garde, "Tekmira Changes Its Name and Shuffles Away from Ebola," Fierce Biotech, July 20, 2015, https://www.fiercebiotech.com/r-d/tekmira-changes-its-name-and-shuffles-away-from-ebola.
519 Arbutus Biopharma Corporation, "Arbutus Settles Litigation, Terminating Acuitas' Rights to LNP Technology," news release, February 22, 2018, https://investor.arbutusbio.com/news-releases/news-release-details/arbutus-settles-litigation-terminating-acuitas-rights-lnp-0.
520 Moderna, Inc., "Statement from Moderna on Patent Trial and Appeal Board (PTAB) Ruling," news release, July 24, 2020, https://www.businesswire.com/news/home/20200724005460/en/Statement-from-Moderna-on-Patent-Trial-and-Appeal-Board-PTAB-Ruling.
521 Amruta Khandekar, "Arbutus Files Patent Infringement Lawsuit Against Moderna Related to COVID Shot," Reuters, February 28, 2022, https://www.reuters.com/business/healthcare-pharmaceuticals/arbutus-files-patent-infringement-lawsuit-against-moderna-2022-02-28/.
522 "Moderna Shares Fall After Judge Sides with Arbutus in Patent

Fight," Reuters, April 3, 2024, https://www.reuters.com/legal/moderna-shares-fall-after-judge-sides-with-arbutus-patent-fight-2024-04-03/.

523 Mario Gaviria and Burcu Kilic, "A Network Analysis of COVID-19 mRNA Vaccine Patents," Nature Biotechnology 39, no. 5 (May 2021): 546–548, https://doi.org/10.1038/s41587-021-00912-9.

524 Nathan Vardi and Matthew Herper, "Moderna's Mysterious Medicines," Forbes, December 14, 2016, https://www.forbes.com/sites/nathanvardi/2016/12/14/modernas-mysterious-medicines/#19ea9831730e.

525 "Arbutus Files Patent Lawsuit Against Pfizer/BioNTech Over COVID Vaccines," Reuters, April 4, 2023, https://www.reuters.com/legal/arbutus-files-patent-infringement-lawsuit-against-pfizerbiontech-2023-04-04/.

526 Christopher Yasiejko, "Arbutus, Genevant Escape Acuitas Suit on Covid-Shot Tech Patents," Bloomberg Law, May 21, 2024, https://news.bloomberglaw.com/ip-law/arbutus-genevant-escape-acuitas-suit-on-covid-shot-tech-patents.

527 BioNTech SE, "The BioNTech Story: Dedicated to Translating Science into Survival," https://www.biontech.com/int/en/home/about/history.html.

528 " Pfizer Wins Pause on Moderna's COVID-19 Patent Lawsuit," Reuters, April 12, 2024, https://www.reuters.com/legal/litigation/pfizer-wins-pause-modernas-covid-19-patent-lawsuit-2024-04-12/.

529 Damian Garde, "Lavishly Funded Moderna Hits Safety Problems in Bold Bid to Reinvent Medicine," STAT, January 10, 2017, https://www.statnews.com/2017/01/10/moderna-trouble-mrna/.

530 Gregory Zuckerman, "How Moderna Nearly Lost the Race to Develop a Covid-19 Vaccine," STAT, October 26, 2021, https://www.statnews.com/2021/10/26/how-moderna-nearly-lost-the-race-to-develop-a-covid-19-vaccine/.

531 Milken Institute, "Future of Health Summit 2019," https://milkeninstitute.org/events/future-health-summit-2019.

532 C-SPAN, "Universal Flu Vaccine," video, 59:07, October 29, 2019, https://www.c-span.org/video/?465845-1/universal-flu-vaccine.

533 National Institutes of Health Intramural Research Program, "A Record-Breaking Sprint to Create a COVID-19 Vaccine," July 12, 2021, https://irp.nih.gov/blog/post/2021/07/a-record-breaking-sprint-to-create-a-covid-19-vaccine.

534 David Wallace-Wells, "We Had the COVID-19 Vaccine the Whole Time," New York, December 7, 2020, https://nymag.com/intelligencer/2020/12/moderna-covid-19-vaccine-design.html.

535 "Serendipity and Foresight Prepared the World to Fight the Coronavirus," Washington Post, October 1, 2021, https://www.washingtonpost.com/health/2021/10/01/barney-graham-covid-vaccines/.

536 Robert N. Kirchdoerfer et al., "Pre-Fusion Structure of a Human Coronavirus Spike Protein," Nature 531, no. 7592 (March 3, 2016): 118–121, https://doi.org/10.1038/nature17200.

537 The United States of America, as represented by the Secretary, Department of Health and Human Services, and Dartmouth College, "Prefusion Coronavirus Spike Proteins and Their Use," international patent application WO2018081318A1, filed October 25, 2017, published May 3, 2018, https://patentimages.storage.googleapis.com/68/47/0c/2b5bc4f43c9f74/WO2018081318A1.pdf.

538 The United States of America, as represented by the Secretary, Department of Health and Human Services, The Scripps Research Institute, and Trustees of Dartmouth College, "Prefusion Coronavirus Spike Proteins and Their Use," U.S. Patent 10,960,070 B2, filed October 25, 2017, issued March 30, 2021, https://patentimages.storage.googleapis.com/a7/b3/70/666f8c5c2ab026/US10960070.pdf.

539 Michael Blanding, "Shot in the Arm: Groundbreaking COVID-19 Vaccine Research by Alumnus Dr. Barney Graham Began at Vanderbilt Decades Ago," Vanderbilt University News, March 17, 2021, https://news.vanderbilt.

edu/2021/03/17/shot-in-the-arm-groundbreaking-covid-19-vaccine-research-by-alumnus-dr-barney-graham-began-at-vanderbilt-decades-ago/.

540 Select Subcommittee on the Coronavirus Crisis, "Reaching the Light at the End of the Tunnel: Ending COVID-19," video, 2:34:29, April 15, 2021, https://www.youtube.com/watch?v=3dgIHKzvjpo.

541 Open The Books, "American Transparency: Public Expenditures Database," https://www.openthebooks.com/.

542 Adam Andrzejewski, "NIH Scientists Made $710M in Royalties from Drug Makers — a Fact They Tried to Hide," New York Post, June 2, 2024, https://nypost.com/2024/06/02/opinion/nih-scientists-made-710m-in-royalties-from-drug-makers-a-fact-they-tried-to-hide/.

543 Reuters, "NIH Claims Co-Ownership of Moderna Vaccine Patent," video, November 11, 2021, https://www.youtube.com/watch?v=h7Vc6bjYv6s.

544 Alexander Tin, "Moderna Offers NIH Co-Ownership of COVID Vaccine Patent Amid Dispute with Government," CBS News, November 15, 2021, https://www.cbsnews.com/news/moderna-covid-vaccine-patent-dispute-national-institutes-health/.

545 Julie Bigay et al., "Vaccine-Associated Enhanced Disease in Humans and Animal Models: Lessons and Challenges for Vaccine Development," Frontiers in Microbiology 13 (2022): 932408, https://doi.org/10.3389/fmicb.2022.932408.

546 Flor M. Munoz et al., "Vaccine-Associated Enhanced Disease: Case Definition and Guidelines for Data Collection, Analysis, and Presentation of Immunization Safety Data," Vaccine 39, no. 22 (May 21, 2021): 3053–3066, https://doi.org/10.1016/j.vaccine.2021.01.055.

547 Tam Harbert, "How Moderna Is Racing to a Coronavirus Vaccine," Ideas Made to Matter (MIT Sloan School of Management), April 3, 2020, https://mitsloan.mit.edu/ideas-made-to-matter/how-moderna-racing-to-a-coronavirus-vaccine.

548 "The Untold Story of Moderna's Race for a COVID-19 Vaccine," Boston, June 4, 2020, https://www.bostonmagazine.com/health/2020/06/04/moderna-coronavirus-vaccine/.

549 Andrew Dunn, "Inside Moderna's Historic Coronavirus Vaccine Program That Transformed the Biotech Upstart into a $55 Billion Drug Industry Powerhouse," Business Insider, November 21, 2020 (updated December 18, 2020), https://www.businessinsider.com/how-moderna-developed-coronavirus-vaccine-record-time-2020-11.

550 "Health Officials Work to Solve China's Mystery Virus Outbreak," Wall Street Journal, January 6, 2020, https://www.wsj.com/articles/health-officials-work-to-solve-chinas-mystery-virus-outbreak-11578308757.

551 Adam Feuerstein, "With Some Safety Caveats, New Moderna Data Show mRNA Can Teach the Body to Make Its Own Medicine," STAT, September 12, 2019, https://www.statnews.com/2019/09/12/new-moderna-data-cmv-chikungunya/.

552 Berkeley Lovelace Jr., "Moderna Reports Positive Data on Early-Stage Coronavirus Vaccine Trial," CNBC, May 18, 2020, https://www.cnbc.com/2020/05/18/moderna-reports-positive-data-on-early-stage-coronavirus-vaccine-trial.html.

553 "Corporate Insiders Pocket $1 Billion in Rush for Coronavirus Vaccine," New York Times, July 25, 2020, https://www.nytimes.com/2020/07/25/business/coronavirus-vaccine-profits-vaxart.html.

554 "Moderna Executives Sell Stock as Coronavirus Vaccine Boosts Company Shares," Washington Post, July 2, 2020, https://www.washingtonpost.com/business/2020/07/02/coronavirus-vaccine-moderna-rna/.

555 Jim Collins, "Why Are Moderna Insiders Selling So Many Shares?," Forbes, September 4, 2020, https://www.forbes.com/sites/jimcollins/2020/09/04/why-are-moderna-insiders-selling-so-many-shares/.

**CHAPTER TEN**

556 Epoch Times, "Dr. Harvey Risch: Hydroxychloroquine, Ivermectin, and Other Therapeutics Highly Effective in Early COVID Treatment," EpochTV video, November 30, 2021, https://www.theepochtimes.com/

epochtv/dr-harvey-risch-hydroxychloroquine-ivermectin-and-other-therapeutics-highly-effective-in-early-covid-treatment-4131804.
557 DschlopesIsBack (@DschlopesIsBack), X post, November 7, 2024, https://x.com/DschlopesIsBack/status/1854358669263036555.
558 Ivan Tkachenko, "How to Cure Coronavirus: An Exclusive Letter From Dr. Zelenko to Donald Trump," Internet Protocol, April 7, 2020, https://internetprotocol.co/hype-news/2020/04/07/how-to-cure-coronavirus-an-exclusive-letter-to-donald-trump/.
559 The White House, "Remarks by President Trump, Vice President Pence, and Members of the Coronavirus Task Force in Press Briefing," March 19, 2020, https://trumpwhitehouse.archives.gov/briefings-statements/remarks-president-trump-vice-president-pence-members-coronavirus-task-force-press-briefing-6/.
560 Philippe Gautret et al., "Hydroxychloroquine and Azithromycin as a Treatment of COVID-19: Results of an Open-Label Non-Randomized Clinical Trial," International Journal of Antimicrobial Agents 56, no. 1 (July 2020): 105949, https://doi.org/10.1016/j.ijantimicag.2020.105949.
561 "Hydroxychloroquine: How an Unproven Drug Became Trump's Coronavirus 'Miracle Cure'." The Guardian, April 6, 2020. https://www.theguardian.com/world/2020/apr/06/hydroxychloroquine-trump-coronavirus-drug.
562 Mandeep R Mehra et al., "Hydroxychloroquine or Chloroquine with or without a Macrolide for Treatment of COVID-19: A Multinational Registry Analysis," The Lancet (published online May 22, 2020), https://doi.org/10.1016/S0140-6736(20)31180-6. Retracted in The Lancet (June 5, 2020), https://doi.org/10.1016/S0140-6736(20)31324-6.
563 "Trump Drug Hydroxychloroquine Raises Death Risk in Covid Patients, Study Says," BBC News, May 22, 2020, https://www.bbc.co.uk/news/world-52779309.
564 "WHO Pauses Trial of Hydroxychloroquine in COVID-19 Patients Due to Safety Concerns," Reuters, May 25, 2020, https://www.reuters.com/article/us-health-coronavirus-who-hydroxychloroq/who-pauses-trial-of-hydroxychloroquine-in-covid-19-patients-due-to-safety-concerns-idUSKBN2311PG/.
565 Mandeep R Mehra et al., "Hydroxychloroquine or Chloroquine with or without a Macrolide for Treatment of COVID-19: A Multinational Registry Analysis," The Lancet (published online May 22, 2020), https://doi.org/10.1016/S0140-6736(20)31180-6. Retracted in The Lancet (June 5, 2020), https://doi.org/10.1016/S0140-6736(20)31324-6.
566 Edmund Fordham, "The Lancet and the Trashing of a Cure for Covid," The Conservative Woman, June 8, 2020, https://www.conservativewoman.co.uk/the-lancet-and-the-trashing-of-a-cure-for-covid/.
567 Andrew Joseph, "The Lancet Retracts Major COVID-19 Paper That Raised Safety Concerns About Malaria Drugs," STAT, June 4, 2020, https://www.statnews.com/2020/06/04/lancet-retracts-major-covid-19-paper-that-raised-safety-concerns-about-malaria-drugs/.
568 The RECOVERY Collaborative Group, "Effect of Hydroxychloroquine in Hospitalized Patients with Covid-19," New England Journal of Medicine 383, no. 21 (November 19, 2020): 2030–2040, https://doi.org/10.1056/NEJMoa2022926.
569 U.S. Food and Drug Administration, "Coronavirus (COVID-19) Update: FDA Revokes Emergency Use Authorization for Chloroquine and Hydroxychloroquine," news release, June 15, 2020, https://www.fda.gov/news-events/press-announcements/coronavirus-covid-19-update-fda-revokes-emergency-use-authorization-chloroquine-and.
570 "Coronavirus: Hydroxychloroquine Ineffective Says Fauci," BBC News, July 29, 2020, https://www.bbc.co.uk/news/world-us-canada-53575964.
571 Le Collectif Citoyen pour FranceSoir, "CovidPapers, Recovery : Incompétence, Mensonge, Manipulation et gros dollars," FranceSoir, June 16, 2020 (updated June 17, 2020), https://www.francesoir.fr/politique-monde/covidpapers-recovery-incompetence-mensonge-manipulation-et-gros-dollars.
572 Xavier Azalbert pour FranceSoir, "INTERVIEW EXCLUSIVE : Martin Landray, Recovery - hydroxychloroquine game over UK,"

FranceSoir, June 7, 2020, https://edition.francesoir.fr/politique-monde/interview-exclusive-martin-landray-recovery-hydroxychloroquine-game-over-uk.
573 The HighWire with Del Bigtree, "Episode 416: DIDIER RAOULT UNCENSORED," video, 1:56:11, March 20, 2025, https://rumble.com/v6qy204-episode-416-didier-raoult-uncensored.html.
574 Alexiane Pradelle et al., "Deaths Induced by Compassionate Use of Hydroxychloroquine during the First COVID-19 Wave: An Estimate," Biomedicine & Pharmacotherapy 171 (2024): 116055, https://doi.org/10.1016/j.biopha.2023.116055.
575 Mari Eccles, "Hydroxychloroquine Could Have Caused 17,000 Deaths During Covid, Study Finds," Politico, January 4, 2024, https://www.politico.eu/article/hydroxychloroquine-could-have-caused-17000-deaths-during-covid-study-finds/.
576 David Gortler, "Those Published '17,000 Hydroxychloroquine Deaths' Never Happened," Brownstone Institute, January 2024, https://brownstone.org/articles/those-published-17000-hydroxychloroquine-deaths-never-happened/.
577 PRINCIPLE Trial, "PRINCIPLE: Platform Randomised Trial of Interventions against COVID-19 In Older People," University of Oxford, https://www.principletrial.org/.
578 F. D. Richard Hobbs et al., "The PRINCIPLE Randomised Controlled Open Label Platform Trial of Hydroxychloroquine for Treating COVID19 in Community Based Patients at High Risk," Scientific Reports 15 (2025): 23850, https://doi.org/10.1038/s41598-025-09275-6.
579 COVID Analysis (c19early.org), "COVID-19 treatment: respiratory tract administration," https://c19early.org/rtadmin.html.
580 Evaluation of hydroxychloroquine or chloroquine for the prevention of COVID-19 (COPCOV): A double-blind, randomised, placebo-controlled trial. William H. K. Schilling et al. PLOS Medicine 21(9): e1004428 (September 12, 2024). https://doi.org/10.1371/journal.pmed.1004428.
581 Jon Henley, "Covid professor Didier Raoult faces misconduct inquiry," The Guardian, November 12, 2020, https://www.theguardian.com/world/2020/nov/12/covid-professor-didier-raoult-hydroxychloroquine.
582 "Penalty Increased: Doctor Didier Raoult Banned from Practicing Medicine for Two Years for HCQ Treat[ment of] COVID-19 Patients," Global Research, December 20, 2024, https://www.globalresearch.ca/penalty-increased-doctor-didier-raoult-banned-practicing-medicine-two-years-hcq-treat-covid-19-patients/5869956.
583 Shira Hanau, "Jewish MD Who Promoted Virus Cocktail Is Leaving Community Where He Tested It," The Times of Israel, May 21, 2020, https://www.timesofisrael.com/jewish-md-who-promoted-virus-cocktail-leaving-community-where-he-tested-it/.
584 Chandelis Duster, "Read the whistleblower complaint alleging corruption in the federal effort to develop a coronavirus vaccine," CNN, April 22, 2020, https://edition.cnn.com/2020/04/22/politics/read-whistleblower-vaccine-development/index.html.
585 Rick Bright, "OSC Complaint" (redacted whistleblower complaint), U.S. Office of Special Counsel, filed April 2020, archived December 21, 2021, at https://web.archive.org/web/20211221210624/https://www.kmblegal.com/sites/default/files/NEW%20R.%20Bright%20OSC%20Complaint_Redacted.pdf.
586 Leon Caly et al., "The FDA-Approved Drug Ivermectin Inhibits the Replication of SARS-CoV-2 in Vitro," Antiviral Research 178 (June 2020): 104787, https://doi.org/10.1016/j.antiviral.2020.104787.
587 Anthony Piovesan, "Drug Combo 'Can Cure' Coronavirus Symptoms, Gastroenterologist Says," The Australian, September 11, 2020, https://www.theaustralian.com.au/breaking-news/drug-combo-can-cure-coronavirus-symptoms-gastroenterologist-says/news-story/2a17194b73e2e095877575eb64da174d.
588 "Are the Scientific Journals Censoring the Science? Part 2: The Removal of Peer-Reviewed Papers." Video. Rumble. https://rumble.com/vpae8c-are-the-scientific-journals-censoring-the-science-part-2-the-removal-of-pee.html.

589 Independent Medical Alliance, "MATH+ COVID Hospital Treatment Protocol," https://imahealth.org/protocol/math-covid-hospital-treatment/.
590 "User Clip: Dr. Pierre Kory US Senate Hearing - Ivermectin is 100% Cure for COVID-19," C-SPAN, clip from "Early Outpatient Treatment: An Essential Part of a Successful Strategy to Reduce COVID-19 Fatalities," December 8, 2020, https://www.c-span.org/clip/senate-committee/user-clip-dr-pierre-kory-us-senate-hearing-ivermectin-is-100-cure-for-covid-19/4930160.
591 Pierre Kory et al., "Review of the Emerging Evidence Demonstrating the Efficacy of Ivermectin in the Prophylaxis and Treatment of COVID-19," Frontiers in Pharmacology 12 (2021): 643369, https://doi.org/10.3389/fphar.2021.643369.
592 Asiya Kamber Zaidi and Puya Dehgani-Mobaraki, "The Mechanisms of Action of Ivermectin against SARS-CoV-2: An Evidence-Based Clinical Review Article," The Journal of Antibiotics 75, no. 2 (February 2022): 60–71, https://doi.org/10.1038/s41429-021-00430-5.
593 Lawrie, Theresa Anne. "Written Evidence Submitted by Dr Theresa Anne Lawrie, Director, The Evidence-based Medicine Consultancy Ltd. (CLL0115)." UK Parliament Health and Social Care Committee, March 23, 2021. https://committees.parliament.uk/writtenevidence/36858/html.
594 Asaf Biber et al., "Favorable Outcome on Viral Load and Culture Viability Using Ivermectin in Early Treatment of Non-Hospitalized Patients with Mild COVID-19 – A Double-Blind, Randomized Placebo-Controlled Trial" (preprint, posted May 31, 2021), medRxiv, https://doi.org/10.1101/2021.05.31.21258081.
595 Wagdy M. Shouman (principal investigator), Zagazig University (sponsor). "Prophylactic Ivermectin in COVID-19 Contacts." ClinicalTrials.gov identifier NCT04422561. Bethesda (MD): National Library of Medicine (US); 2020. Updated [last update date, e.g., August 2020 or later if revised]. Results posted [approximate posting date, e.g., 2020 or 2021]. https://clinicaltrials.gov/study/NCT04422561?tab=results.
596 "Zagazig University Randomized Controlled Ivermectin Study Results Confirms PI Hypothesis: Drug Effective Against COVID-19," TrialSite News, August 28, 2020, accessed February 19, 2026, https://www.trialsitenews.com/a/zagazig-university-randomized-controlled-ivermectin-study-results-confirms-pi-hypothesis-drug-effective-against-covid-19.
597 Flavio A. Cadegiani et al., "Efficacy of Proxalutamide in Hospitalized COVID-19 Patients: A Randomized, Double-Blind, Placebo-Controlled, Parallel-Design Clinical Trial" (preprint, posted June 22, 2021), medRxiv, https://doi.org/10.1101/2021.06.22.21259318.
598 Sonia Elijah, "How Ivermectin Became a Target for the 'Fraud Detectives,'" TrialSite News, October 11, 2021, https://www.trialsitenews.com/a/how-ivermectin-became-a-target-for-the-fraud-detectives.
599 Ahmed Elgazzar et al., "WITHDRAWN: Efficacy and Safety of Ivermectin for Treatment and Prophylaxis of COVID-19 Pandemic" (preprint, posted November 2020; version 4 posted July 14, 2021), Research Square, withdrawn July 14, 2021, due to verifiable concerns including plagiarism and anomalies in the dataset (now under formal investigation by the Egyptian Ministry of Higher Education), https://doi.org/10.21203/rs.3.rs-100956/v4.
600 "Open Letter by U.S. Doctors: JAMA Ivermectin Study Is Fatally Flawed," jamaletter.com, [ca. March–April 2021], https://jamaletter.com/.
601 Edward Mills et al., "Early Treatment of COVID-19 with Repurposed Therapies: The TOGETHER Adaptive Platform Trial" (presentation slides, August 6, 2021), NIH Pragmatic Trials Collaboratory Knowledge Repository, Duke Clinical Research Institute, https://dcricollab.dcri.duke.edu/sites/NIHKR/KR/GR-Slides-08-06-21.pdf.
602 "Pfizer Selects MMS as Preferred Provider for Plain Language Summary Writing Support," MMS Holdings, September 26, 2017, https://mmsholdings.com/pfizer-selects-mms-as-preferred-provider-for-plain-language-summary-writing-support/.
603 Linda Pannozzo, "What's the Deal with Ivermectin and COVID?" Halifax Examiner, June 14, 2021; updated October 20, 2022, https://www.halifaxexaminer.ca/uncategorized/whats-the-deal-with-ivermectin-and-covid/.

604 Andrew Bryant, Theresa A. Lawrie, and Edmund J. Fordham, "Ivermectin for Prevention and Treatment of COVID-19 Infection: A Systematic Review, Meta-analysis, and Trial Sequential Analysis to Inform Clinical Guidelines" (letter to the editor), American Journal of Therapeutics 28, no. 5 (September/October 2021): e573–e576, https://doi.org/10.1097/MJT.0000000000001442.
605 Paul E. Marik and Pierre Kory, "Ivermectin, A Reanalysis of the Data" (letter to the editor), American Journal of Therapeutics 28, no. 5 (September/October 2021): e579–e580, https://doi.org/10.1097/MJT.0000000000001443.
606 Rachel Schraer and Jack Goodman, "Ivermectin: How False Science Created a Covid 'Miracle' Drug," BBC News, October 6, 2021 (updated with additional reporting by Shruti Menon), accessed February 19, 2026, https://www.bbc.co.uk/news/health-58170809.
607 "Vaccine Adverse Event Reporting System (VAERS)," U.S. Department of Health and Human Services, https://vaers.hhs.gov/.
608 "Yellow Card | Making Medicines and Medical Devices Safer," Medicines and Healthcare products Regulatory Agency (MHRA), https://yellowcard.mhra.gov.uk/.
609 Gilmar Reis et al., "Effect of Early Treatment with Ivermectin among Patients with Covid-19," New England Journal of Medicine 386, no. 18 (May 5, 2022): 1721–1731, https://doi.org/10.1056/NEJMoa2115869.
610 Michael Hiltzik, "Hiltzik: Ivermectin Shows 'No Effect' as COVID Treatment," Los Angeles Times, August 11, 2021, https://www.latimes.com/business/story/2021-08-11/ivermectin-no-effect-covid.
611 Pierre Kory (@PierreKory), "I'm calling it. TOGETHER's IVM study likely the most corrupt in history..." X (Twitter), May 16, 2022, https://x.com/PierreKory/status/1526034585573801988.
612 Alexandros Marinos, "FDA Reveals Concerns About the Conduct of the TOGETHER Trial, Joining Other Regulators," Do Your Own Research (Substack), October 20, 2022 (updated as needed), https://doyourownresearch.substack.com/p/fda-reveals-concerns-about-the-conduct.
613 "Scientific Misconduct Uncovered in the TOGETHER Ivermectin Trial," World Council for Health, https://www.worldcouncilforhealth.org/together-trial/.
614 Sonia Elijah, "FDA's Smoking Gun: Disinformation Campaign Targeting Ivermectin," TrialSite News, November 5, 2021, https://www.trialsitenews.com/a/fdas-smoking-gun-disinformation-campaign-targeting-ivermectin.
615 Shyra Sherfield, "Poison Control Calls Spike as People Take Livestock Dewormer to Treat COVID-19," WLBT, August 20, 2021, https://www.wlbt.com/2021/08/20/mississippi-poison-control-warns-potential-toxicity-medication-covid-19/.
616 "Corrections and Clarifications," The Guardian, September 15, 2021, https://www.theguardian.com/news/2021/sep/15/corrections-and-clarifications.
617 Linda Bonvie, "The Plot Against Ivermectin," Citizens for Health, September 15, 2021, https://citizens.org/ivermectin-plot/.
618 "Stipulation of Dismissal," Bowden v. U.S. Department of Health and Human Services, No. 3:22-cv-00184 (S.D. Tex. Mar. 21, 2024), DocumentCloud, https://www.documentcloud.org/documents/24495557-fda-stipulation-of-dismissal/.
619 Zachary Stieber, "FDA Settles Ivermectin Case, Agrees to Remove Controversial 'Stop It' Post," The Epoch Times, March 22, 2024, https://www.theepochtimes.com/health/fda-settles-ivermectin-case-agrees-to-remove-controversial-stop-it-post-5612010?ea_src=frontpage&ea_med=most-read-0.
620 Marlene Lenthang, "Texas Doctor Who Touted Ivermectin as Covid Treatment Suspended," NBC News, November 15, 2021, https://www.nbcnews.com/news/us-news/texas-doctor-touted-ivermectin-covid-treatment-suspended-rcna5588.
621 Tania Broughton, "“Anti-vax” Doctor's Disciplinary Inquiry Gets Underway," GroundUp, April 11, 2024, https://groundup.org.za/article/anti-vax-doctor-disciplinary-inquiry-gets-underway/.

622 Serena Tinari, "The EMA Covid-19 Data Leak, and What It Tells Us about mRNA Instability," The BMJ 372 (March 10, 2021): n627, https://doi.org/10.1136/bmj.n627.
623 Sonia Elijah, "What the Leaked EMA Emails & Docs Reveal: Major Concerns with Pfizer C-19 Vaccine Batch Integrity and The Race to Authorize," TrialSite News, June 20, 2022, https://www.trialsitenews.com/a/what-the-leaked-ema-emails-docs-reveal-major-concerns-with-pfizer-c-19-vaccine-batch-integrity-and-the-race-to-authorise-cdda0ba2.
624 Sarah Karlin-Smith, "Trump's HHS Secretary Nominee Boosted Drug Prices While at Eli Lilly," Politico, November 14, 2017, accessed February 19, 2026, https://www.politico.com/story/2017/11/14/alex-azar-eli-lilly-drug-prices-244888.
625 United States Government Accountability Office, "Operation Warp Speed: Accelerated COVID-19 Vaccine Development Status and Efforts to Address Manufacturing Challenges," GAO-21-319, February 11, 2021, https://www.gao.gov/products/gao-21-319.
626 "European MEPs Call for Immediate Oust of European Commission President Due to Conflicts of Interest with Pfizer & Mass COVID-19 Vaccination Program," TrialSite News, February 19, 2022, https://www.trialsitenews.com/a/european-meps-call-for-immediate-ouster-of-european-commission-president-due-to-conflicts-of-interest-with-pfizer-mass-covid-19-vaccination-program.
627 U.S. Department of Health and Human Services, Office of Inspector General, "The Food and Drug Administration's Oversight of Clinical Trials," OEI-01-06-00160, September 2007, https://oig.hhs.gov/oei/reports/oei-01-06-00160.pdf.
628 Craig Paardekooper, "How Bad Is My Batch?" (website), https://www.howbadismybatch.com/.
629 Sonia Elijah, "A Further Investigation into the Leaked EMA Emails & Confidential Pfizer-BioNTech COVID-19 Vaccine Related Docs," TrialSite News, October 5, 2022, https://www.trialsitenews.com/a/a-further-investigation-into-the-leaked-ema-emails-confidential-pfizer-biontech-covid-19-vaccine-related-docs-5102039c.
630 Matina Stevis-Gridneff, "How Europe Sealed a Pfizer Vaccine Deal With Texts and Calls," New York Times, April 28, 2021, https://www.nytimes.com/2021/04/28/world/europe/european-union-pfizer-von-der-leyen-coronavirus-vaccine.html.
631 European Court of Auditors, "COVID-19 Vaccine Procurement: EU Institutions Did Not Use All Available Tools to Ensure the Transparency and Effectiveness of the Procurement," Special Report No 19/2022, September 12, 2022, https://www.politico.eu/wp-content/uploads/2022/09/12/SR-19-2022-COVID-19-vaccine-procurement.pdf.
632 Carlo Martuscelli, "Pfizer CEO Albert Bourla Pulls Out of Testifying to EU Parliament COVID Panel," Politico Europe, September 29, 2022, accessed February 19, 2026, https://www.politico.eu/article/pfizer-ceo-albert-bourla-pulls-out-of-testifying-to-eu-parliament-covid-panel/.
633 Zain Rizvi, "Pfizer's Power," Public Citizen, October 19, 2021, https://www.citizen.org/article/pfizers-power/.
634 "Pfizer-BioNTech COVID-19 Vaccine Advance Purchase Agreement between the Government of the Republic of Albania and Pfizer Export B.V.," November 2020, DocumentCloud, uploaded 2021, https://www.documentcloud.org/documents/20616251-albanian-pfizer-covid-19-vaccine-contract/.
635 "Questions and Answers on COVID-19 Vaccination in the EU: Authorisation Process of COVID-19 Vaccines," European Commission, [n.d.; page last updated post-2021, content reflects 2020–2023 context], https://commission.europa.eu/strategy-and-policy/coronavirus-response/safe-covid-19-vaccines-europeans/questions-and-answers-covid-19-vaccination-eu_en#authorisation.
636 "Documents," European Commission, https://commission.europa.eu/documents_en.
637 Court of Justice of the European Union, "Judgments of the General Court in Cases T-689/21 (Auken and Others v Commission) and T-761/21 (Courtois and Others v Commission)," Press Release No 113/24, July 17, 2024, https://curia.europa.eu/site/upload/docs/application/pdf/2024-07/cp240113en.pdf.

638 Samuel Cogoluegnes, "EU Should Consider Mandatory Vaccination, Says von der Leyen," Euronews, December 1, 2021, https://www.euronews.com/2021/12/01/eu-should-consider-mandatory-vaccination-says-von-der-leyen.
639 Laura Gozzi, "Ursula von der Leyen Secures Five More Years in Top EU Job," BBC News, July 18, 2024, https://www.bbc.co.uk/news/articles/cw5yg6dp0gxo.
640 General Court of the European Union, Judgment in Joined Cases T-689/21 (Auken and Others v Commission) and T-761/21 (Courtois and Others v Commission), ECLI:EU:T:2025:483, May 14, 2025, https://curia.europa.eu/juris/document/document.jsf?docid=299492&doclang=en.
641 Sonia Elijah, "Thou Shalt Not Adulterate - Part 1," Substack (soniaelijah.com), https://www.soniaelijah.com/p/thou-shalt-not-adulterate-part-1.

**CHAPTER TWELVE**

642 U.S. Food and Drug Administration, "Comirnaty (COVID-19 Vaccine, mRNA) Package Insert," August 2023 (revised), https://www.fda.gov/media/167212/download.
643 U.S. Food and Drug Administration, "Fact Sheet for Healthcare Providers Administering Vaccine (Vaccination Providers): Emergency Use Authorization (EUA) of the Moderna COVID-19 Vaccine to Prevent Coronavirus Disease 2019 (COVID-19)," December 2020 (initial EUA issuance; revised multiple times), https://www.fda.gov/media/144638/download.
644 Sonia Elijah, "Pfizer/BioNTech's Bait-and-Switch," Substack (soniaelijah.com), https://www.soniaelijah.com/p/pfizerbiontechs-bait-and-switch.
645 Vilchez, R. A., Lopez-Terrada, D., Middleton, J. R., Finch, C. J., & Butel, J. S. (2004). Emergent human pathogen simian virus 40 and its role in cancer. Clinical Microbiology Reviews, 17(3), 495–508. https://doi.org/10.1128/CMR.17.3.495-508.2004.
646 "David A. Dean, Ph.D.," University of Rochester Medical Center, https://www.urmc.rochester.edu/people/112359435-david-a-dean.
647 Projects: Nuclear Targeting of Plasmids and Protein-DNA Complexes," Dean Lab, University of Rochester Medical Center, https://www.urmc.rochester.edu/labs/dean/projects/nuclear-targeting-of-plasmids-and-protein-dna-comp.
648 Phillip Buckhaults, "The Pfizer mRNA Vaccine Is Contaminated with the Plasmid DNA Vector That Was Used as the Template for in Vitro Transcription Reaction," testimony before the South Carolina Senate Medical Affairs Committee, September 12, 2023, https://www.scstatehouse.gov/CommitteeInfo/SenateMedicalAffairsCommittee/PandemicPreparedness/Phillip-Buckhaults-SC-Senate-09122023-final.pdf.
649 "DNA Contamination in COVID-19 Vaccines," World Council for Health, https://www.worldcouncilforhealth.org/dna-contamination-covid-19-vaccines/.
650 David Speicher et al., "DNA Fragments Detected in Monovalent and Bivalent Pfizer/BioNTech and Moderna modRNA COVID-19 Vaccines from Ontario, Canada: Exploratory Dose-Response Relationship with Serious Adverse Events," OSF Preprints, October 2023, https://osf.io/mjc97/.
651 Matthew Horwood, "Exclusive: Health Canada Confirms Undisclosed Presence of DNA Sequence in Pfizer Shot," The Epoch Times, October 19, 2023, https://www.theepochtimes.com/world/exclusive-health-canada-confirms-undisclosed-presence-of-dna-sequence-in-pfizer-shot-5513277.
652 Sonia Elijah, "Presence of Fragmented DNA and SV40 Enhancer Found in the Pfizer-BioNTech mRNA Vaccine," Freedom of Information request to Medicines and Healthcare Products Regulatory Agency (MHRA), WhatDoTheyKnow, October 20, 2023, https://www.whatdotheyknow.com/request/presence_of_fragmented_dna_and_s.
653 Acuitas Therapeutics Inc., "A Tissue Distribution Study of a [$^3$H]-Labelled Lipid Nanoparticle-mRNA Formulation Containing ALC-0315 and ALC-0159 Following Intramuscular Administration in Wistar Han Rats," Study No. 185350, approved November 9, 2020, in Pfizer-BioNTech COVID-19 Vaccine submission (FDA-CBER-2021-5683), https://phmpt.org/wpcontent/uploads/2022/03/125742_S1_M4_4223_185350.pdf.

654 Alan [@findogg]. "Moderna's patent (US20190240317A1), on the risks of naked plasmid DNA: 'The possibility of insertional mutagenesis, which could lead to the activation of oncogenes or the inhibition of tumor suppressor genes.' X, November 9, 2023. https://x.com/findogg/status/1722625081019650105.
655 ModernaTX, Inc., "Modified Polynucleotides for the Production of Oncology-Related Polypeptides and Proteins," U.S. Patent Application 20190240317 A1, filed February 1, 2019, published August 8, 2019, https://patentimages.storage.googleapis.com/0c/e5/38/e8ed5e2d738865/US20190240317A1.pdf.
656 Ranzani, Marco, Stefano Annunziato, David J. Adams, and Eugenio Montini. 2013. "Cancer Gene Discovery: Exploiting Insertional Mutagenesis." Molecular Cancer Research 11 (10): 1141–58. https://doi.org/10.1158/1541-7786.MCR-13-0244.
657 Campbell, John. 2023. "Cancer after Vaccines with Professor Dalgleish." YouTube video, 1:58:approx. October 6, 2023. https://www.youtube.com/watch?v=PnJ5T1Enwq4.
658 Issa, William Joseph, Yuxun Wang, and Stephane Bancel. 2018. "Removal of DNA Fragments in mRNA Production Process." US Patent 10,077,439 B2, filed March 13, 2014, and issued September 18, 2018. https://patents.google.com/patent/US10077439B2/en.
659 Sahin, Ugur, Katalin Karikó, and Özlem Türeci. 2014. "mRNA-Based Therapeutics — Developing a New Class of Drugs." Nature Reviews Drug Discovery 13 (10): 759–80. https://doi.org/10.1038/nrd4278.
660 "Coronavirus Vaccine: Pfizer Given Protection from Legal Action by UK Government," The Independent, December 2, 2020, https://www.independent.co.uk/news/health/coronavirus-pfizer-vaccine-legal-indemnity-safety-ministers-b1765124.html.
661 Zahawi, Nadhim. 2021. "Covid-19 Vaccine: Moderna." Hansard, House of Commons Debates, vol. 692, April 13, 2021. https://hansard.parliament.uk/commons/2021-04-13/debates/21041370000015/Covid-19VaccineModerna.
662 European Commission and Pfizer Inc. / BioNTech SE, "Advance Purchase Agreement for the Development, Manufacturing and Supply of a Successful COVID-19 Vaccine for Use in the European Union," signed November 11, 2020 (with amendments), unredacted version published by RAI, April 17, 2021, https://www.rai.it/dl/doc/2021/04/17/1618676600910_APA%20BioNTech%20Pfizer__.pdf.
663 BioNTech SE, "Quarterly Report for the Three Months Ended March 31, 2023," Form 6-K (Exhibit 99.1), filed May 8, 2023, https://investors.biontech.de/static-files/39a5f376-091b-4922-83c5-aaae5ec82f05.
664 Sonia Elijah, "Call To Halt The COVID-19 mRNA Shots," Sonia Elijah Investigates (Substack), March 22, 2025, https://www.soniaelijah.com/p/call-to-halt-the-covid-19-mrna-shots.
665 "Canadian Open Letter: A Call to Halt the COVID-19 mRNA Vaccines," Call to Halt 19, 2025, https://www.call2halt19.ca/.
666 Sonia Elijah, "Beyond Contamination: Pfizer/BioNTech Shot Rolled Out to Public Was NOT the One Tested in Clinical Trial," Sonia Elijah Investigates (Substack), January 8, 2024 https://www.soniaelijah.com/p/beyond-contamination-pfizerbiontech.
667 "Florida State Surgeon General Calls for Halt in the Use of COVID-19 mRNA Vaccines," Florida Department of Health, GovDelivery bulletin, January 3, 2024, https://content.govdelivery.com/accounts/FLDOH/bulletins/3816863.
668 Speicher et al., "DNA Fragments Detected."
669 Emily Hutto, "Paul Offit Debunks Florida Surgeon General's Anti-Vax Warning," MedPage Today, January 5, 2024, https://www.medpagetoday.com/infectiousdisease/covid19vaccine/108145.
670 Peter Marks, "Response to Concerns Regarding SV40 Promoter/Enhancer DNA in mRNA COVID-19 Vaccines," U.S. Food and Drug Administration, Center for Biologics Evaluation and Research, December 14, 2023, https://www.fda.gov/media/174875/download.
671 BioNTech SE, "Form F-1 Registration Statement," filed September 9, 2019, U.S. Securities and Exchange Commission, https://www.sec.gov/Archives/edgar/data/1776985/000119312519241112/d635330df1.htm.

672 Sonia Elijah, "First Look at Newly Released Pfizer Docs, Part 2: The 'Not Necessary' Safety Studies," TrialSite News, March 30, 2022, https://www.trialsitenews.com/a/first-look-at-newly-released-pfizer-docs-part-2.
673 "Alc-0315," PubChem Compound Summary for CID 122666778, National Center for Biotechnology Information, U.S. National Library of Medicine, https://pubchem.ncbi.nlm.nih.gov/compound/Alc-0315.
674 "2-(Mpeg 2000)-N,N-ditetradecylacetamide," PubChem Compound Summary, National Center for Biotechnology Information, U.S. National Library of Medicine, https://pubchem.ncbi.nlm.nih.gov/compound/alc-0159.
675 Sonia Ndeupen et al., "The mRNA-LNP Platform's Lipid Nanoparticle Component Used in Preclinical Vaccine Studies Is Highly Inflammatory," iScience 24, no. 12 (December 17, 2021): 103479, https://doi.org/10.1016/j.isci.2021.103479.
676 Sonia Elijah, "World Leading Experts Testify at UK's Parliamentary Office," Sonia Elijah Investigates (Substack), December 5, 2023, https://www.soniaelijah.com/p/world-leading-experts-testify-at.
677 Cayman Chemical Company, "Safety Data Sheet: ALC-0315 (Article 34337)," issued March 20, 2025, version 60.1.0, https://cdn.caymanchem.com/cdn/msds/34337m.pdf.
678 Pfizer Inc. and BioNTech SE, "Protocol for: Safety and Efficacy of the BNT162b2 mRNA Covid-19 Vaccine," supplement to New England Journal of Medicine 383, no. 27 (December 10, 2020): 2603–15, final protocol April 15, 2020 (amendments to October 29, 2020), https://www.nejm.org/doi/suppl/10.1056/NEJMoa2034577/suppl_file/nejmoa2034577_protocol.pdf.
679 Pfizer Inc. and BioNTech SE, "Protocol C4591001: A Phase 1/2/3, Placebo-Controlled, Randomized, Observer-Blind, Dose-Finding Study to Evaluate the Safety, Tolerability, Immunogenicity, and Efficacy of SARS-CoV-2 RNA Vaccine Candidates Against COVID-19 in Healthy Individuals," ClinicalTrials.gov NCT04368728, final protocol with Amendment 20, September 15, 2022, https://cdn.clinicaltrials.gov/large-docs/28/NCT04368728/Prot_000.pdf.
680 UK COVID-19 Inquiry, "Module 4: Vaccines and Therapeutics – Hearing on 22 January 2025," transcripts and evidence, https://ukcovid19inquiry.dracos.co.uk/module-4/2025-01-22/#id1.

**CHAPTER THIRTEEN**

681 Nobel Assembly at Karolinska Institutet, "The Nobel Prize in Physiology or Medicine 2023," press release, October 2, 2023, https://www.nobelprize.org/prizes/medicine/2023/press-release/.
682 Thomas E. Mulroney et al., "N$^1$-Methylpseudouridylation of mRNA Causes +1 Ribosomal Frameshifting," Nature 625, no. 7993 (December 6, 2023): 189–94, https://doi.org/10.1038/s41586-023-06800-3.
683 Michelle Roberts, "Covid Study: mRNA Vaccines Could Be Fine-Tuned," BBC News, December 6, 2023, https://www.bbc.com/news/health-67625180.
684 Gretchen Vogel, "mRNA Vaccines May Make Unintended Proteins, but There's No Evidence of Harm," Science, December 7, 2023, https://www.science.org/content/article/mrna-vaccines-may-make-unintended-proteins-there-s-no-evidence-harm.
685 Edouard Mathieu et al., "Coronavirus (COVID-19) Vaccinations," Our World in Data, first published 2020, updated continuously (latest data August 12, 2024), https://ourworldindata.org/covid-vaccinations.
686 David M. Wiseman et al., "Ribosomal Frameshifting and Misreading of mRNA in COVID-19 Vaccines Produces 'Off-Target' Proteins and Immune Responses Eliciting Safety Concerns: Comment on UK Study by Mulroney et al.," OSF Preprints, December 6, 2023, https://doi.org/10.31219/osf.io/nt8jh.
687 Sonia Elijah, "Part 2: Startling Evidence Suggests BioNTech/Pfizer Falsified Key Data & Further Scandals," TrialSite News, March 10, 2023, https://www.trialsitenews.com/a/part-2-startling-evidence-suggests-biontechpfizer-falsified-key-data-further-scandals-24f4d743.
688 EMA Rapporteur, "Rapporteur Rolling Review Report Overview - LoQ - COVID-19 mRNA

Vaccine BioNTech," rolling review document, November 2020 (uploaded to covidtruths.co.uk April 2021), http://www.covidtruths.co.uk/wp-content/uploads/2021/04/Rapporteur-Rolling-Review-Report-Overview-LoQ-COVID-19-mRNA-Vaccine-BioNTech.docx.

689 Sonia Elijah, "Part 2: Startling Evidence Suggests BioNTech/Pfizer Falsified Key Data & Further Scandals," TrialSite News, March 10, 2023, https://www.trialsitenews.com/a/part-2-startling-evidence-suggests-biontechpfizer-falsified-key-data-further-scandals-24f4d743.

690 BioNTech RNA Pharmaceuticals GmbH, "R&D Data Report No. R-20-0211: In Vitro Expression of BNT162b2 Drug Substance and Drug Product," version 0.2, September 17, 2020 (approved September 23, 2020), released in Pfizer FOIA production STN 125742, https://phmpt.org/wp-content/uploads/2023/02/125742_S1_M4_4.2.1-r-20-0211.pdf.

691 BioNTech SE and Pfizer Inc., "M3-20-Nov-2020-FDA-Query-Responses," responses to FDA queries during rolling review for BNT162b2, November 20, 2020 (uploaded to covidtruths.co.uk April 2021), http://www.covidtruths.co.uk/wp-content/uploads/2021/04/M3-20-Nov-2020-FDA-Query-Responses.pdf.

692 Sonia Elijah, "BioNTech Knew Their Synthetic mRNA Tech Would 'Skip but Did Nothing to Properly Fix It!'" Sonia Elijah Investigates (Substack), January 12, 2024, https://www.soniaelijah.com/p/biontech-knew-their-synthetic-mrna.

693 Israel S. Fernández et al., "Unusual Base Pairing During the Decoding of a Stop Codon by the Ribosome," Nature 500, no. 7460 (August 1, 2013): 107–10, https://doi.org/10.1038/nature12302.

694 Kevin McKernan, "Differences in Vaccine and SARS-CoV-2 Replication Derived mRNA: Implications for Cell Biology and Future Disease," preprint (ResearchGate, November 24, 2021), https://doi.org/10.13140/RG.2.2.19382.45120.

695 European Medicines Agency, "Comirnaty: EPAR – Public Assessment Report," EMA/707383/2020 Corr.2, Committee for Medicinal Products for Human Use (CHMP), 19 February 2021 (corrected 20 October 2023), https://www.ema.europa.eu/en/documents/assessment-report/comirnaty-epar-public-assessment-report_en.pdf.

**CHAPTER FOURTEEN**

696 Sonia Elijah, "First Look at Newly Released Pfizer Docs Part 1: Case Report Errors and Anomalies," TrialSite News, March 7, 2022, https://www.trialsitenews.com/a/a-first-look-at-the-newly-released-pfizer-papers-part-1-the-errors-and-anomalies-of-the-case-report-forms.

697 Paul D. Thacker, "Covid-19: Researcher Blows the Whistle on Data Integrity Issues in Pfizer's Vaccine Trial," The BMJ 375 (November 2, 2021): n2635, https://doi.org/10.1136/bmj.n2635.

698 Sonia Elijah, "An Interview With Ventavia and Pfizer-BioNTech COVID Vaccine Trial Whistleblower Brook Jackson," TrialSite News, March 9, 2022, https://www.trialsitenews.com/a/an-interview-with-brook-jackson-ventavia-and-pfizer-biontech-covid-vaccine-trial-and-whistleblower.

699 Sonia Elijah, "First Look at Newly Released Pfizer Docs, Part 2: The 'Not Necessary' Safety Studies," TrialSite News, March 30, 2022, https://www.trialsitenews.com/a/first-look-at-newly-released-pfizer-docs-part-2.

700 Ndeupen et al., "The mRNA-LNP Platform's Lipid Nanoparticle Component," 103479.

701 Sonia Elijah, "Pfizer's 'Sensitive' Document Reveals Alarming Facts about Trial Subjects," TrialSite News, July 13, 2022, https://www.trialsitenews.com/a/pfizers-sensitive-document-reveals-alarming-facts-about-trial-subjects-f9d8876c.

702 Sonia Elijah, "The Missing Third Death from Pfizer-BioNTech's Pivotal Article and a Further Look at the 'Non-Related' Adverse Events," TrialSite News, July 26, 2022, https://www.trialsitenews.com/a/the-missing-third-death-from-pfizer-biontechs-landmark-article-and-a-further-look-into-the-anomaly-of-the-non-related-adverse-events-020fab8c.

703 Polack, Fernando P., Stephen J. Thomas, Nicholas Kitchin, Judith Absalon, Alejandra Gurtman, Stephen Lockhart, John L. Perez, Gregory Pérez Marc, Edson D. Moreira, Cristiano Zerbini, et al. 2020. "Safety and Efficacy of the BNT162b2 mRNA Covid-19 Vaccine." New England Journal of Medicine 383 (27): 2603–15. https://doi.org/10.1056/NEJMoa2034577.

704 Sonia Elijah, "The FDA's Hidden V-Safety Slide From October 2020 & Other Anomalies," TrialSite News, March 14, 2024, https://www.trialsitenews.com/a/the-fdas-hidden-v-safety-slide-from-october-2020-other-anomalies-7c517814.
705 U.S. Food and Drug Administration, "FDA Approves First COVID-19 Vaccine," press announcement, August 23, 2021, https://www.fda.gov/news-events/press-announcements/fda-approves-first-covid-19-vaccine.
706 U.S. Food and Drug Administration, "Vaccines and Related Biological Products Advisory Committee - 10/22/2020," YouTube video, 8:47:approx., October 22, 2020, https://www.youtube.com/watch?v=1XTiL9rUpkg.
707 Peter Doshi, "Will Covid-19 Vaccines Save Lives? Current Trials Aren't Designed to Tell Us," The BMJ 371 (October 21, 2020): m4037, https://doi.org/10.1136/bmj.m4037.
708 U.S. House Committee on Oversight and Accountability, "Assessing America's Vaccine Safety Systems, Part 1," hearing of the Select Subcommittee on the Coronavirus Pandemic, February 15, 2024, https://oversight.house.gov/hearing/assessing-americas-vaccine-safety-systemspart-1/.
709 U.S. Food and Drug Administration, "Vaccines and Related Biological Products Advisory Committee - 10/22/2020," YouTube video, 8:47:approx., October 22, 2020, https://www.youtube.com/watch?v=1XTiL9rUpkg.
710 "COVID-19 mRNA Vaccination and Myocarditis or Pericarditis," The Lancet 399, no. 10342 (June 11, 2022): 2168–69, https://doi.org/10.1016/S0140-6736(22)00842-X.
711 Stephanie de Garay, interview by Sonia Elijah, "Mother Speaks Out About Her 13-Year-Old Girl's Life Altering Injuries from Pfizer's Covid Vaccine," TrialSite News, video, Rumble, uploaded circa 2021–2022, https://rumble.com/vql93k-mother-speaks-out-about-her-13-year-old-girls-life-altering-injuries-from-p.html.
712 Robert W. Frenck Jr. et al., for the C4591001 Clinical Trial Group, "Safety, Immunogenicity, and Efficacy of the BNT162b2 Covid-19 Vaccine in Adolescents," New England Journal of Medicine 385, no. 3 (July 15, 2021): 239–50, https://doi.org/10.1056/NEJMoa2107456.
713 Sonia Elijah, "FDA's Forced Hand Drops Pfizer's Bombshell Safety Document," TrialSite News, December 14, 2021, https://www.trialsitenews.com/a/fdas-forced-hand-drops-pfizers-bombshell-safety-document.
714 Pfizer, 5.3.6 Cumulative Analysis of Post-authorization Adverse Event Reports of PF-07302048 (BNT162b2) Received Through 28-Feb-2021 (Report prepared by Worldwide Safety, approved April 30, 2021), https://phmpt.org/wp-content/uploads/2021/11/5.3.6-postmarketing-experience.pdf.
715 Public Health & Med. Prof'ls for Transparency v. Food & Drug Admin., No. 4:21-cv-01058-P (N.D. Tex. Sept. 16, 2021) (Complaint for Declaratory and Injunctive Relief), https://fingfx.thomsonreuters.com/gfx/legaldocs/klvykdlryvg/vaccine%20foia%20complaint.pdf.
716 Ross Lazarus, Electronic Support for Public Health–Vaccine Adverse Event Reporting System (ESP:VAERS), Final Report, AHRQ Grant No. R18 HS 017045 (Harvard Pilgrim Health Care, Inc., submitted September 30, 2010), https://digital.ahrq.gov/sites/default/files/docs/publication/r18hs017045-lazarus-final-report-2011.pdf.
717 Sonia Elijah, "Pfizer's Pregnancy & Lactation Cumulative Review Reveals Damning Data," TrialSite News, April 22, 2023, https://www.trialsitenews.com/a/pfizers-pregnancy-lactation-cumulative-review-reveals-damning-data-2b15c969.
718 Sonia Elijah, interview by Clayton Morris, "BREAKING! New BOMBSHELL Pfizer Documents Reveal Damning Data | Redacted with Clayton Morris," Redacted with Clayton Morris, video, Rumble, April 26, 2023, https://rumble.com/v2ko732-breaking-new-bombshell-pfizer-documents-reveal-damning-data-redacted-with-c.html.
719 Pfizer, BNT162b2 Cumulative Review from Pharmacovigilance Database: Pregnancy and Lactation Cumulative Review (Confidential report submitted to FDA/CBER, approved April 20, 2021), https://prd-tsn-main-api.s3.amazonaws.com/article/dc9ea854-0d51-42d6-a6bd-89a0b88bbf3f.pdf.
720 Nazeeha Hanna et al., "Detection of Messenger RNA COVID-19 Vaccines in

Human Breast Milk," JAMA Pediatrics 176, no. 12 (December 2022): 1268–70, https://doi.org/10.1001/jamapediatrics.2022.3581.

721 "CDC Recommends Pregnant Women Get Covid Vaccine after Study Shows It's Safe for Mother and Baby," CNBC, April 23, 2021, https://www.cnbc.com/2021/04/23/cdc-recommends-pregnant-women-get-covid-vaccine-after-study-shows-they-are-safe-for-mother-and-baby.html.

722 Tom T. Shimabukuro, "CDC Post-authorization/Post-licensure Safety Monitoring of COVID-19 Vaccines," presentation to the FDA Vaccines and Related Biological Products Advisory Committee, October 22, 2020, https://www.fda.gov/media/143530/download.

723 "V-Safe," Informed Consent Action Network (ICAN), October 18, 2022, https://icandecide.org/article/v-safe/.

724 "Court Decision Forces CDC to Release V-Safe 'Free-Text' Data," The HighWire, January 12, 2024, https://thehighwire.com/ark-videos/court-decision-forces-cdc-to-release-v-safe-free-text-data/.

725 "V-Safe Data," Informed Consent Action Network (ICAN), https://icandecide.org/v-safe-data/.

726 Assessing America's Vaccine Safety Systems, Part 1, Hearing Before the Select Subcommittee on the Coronavirus Pandemic of the Committee on Oversight and Accountability, U.S. House of Representatives, 118th Cong., 2nd Sess. (February 15, 2024) (Serial No. 118-89), https://www.congress.gov/118/chrg/CHRG-118hhrg54866/CHRG-118hhrg54866.pdf.

727 "Pharmacovigilance," European Medicines Agency (EMA), https://www.ema.europa.eu/en/glossary-terms/pharmacovigilance.

728 Dr. Silvia Behrendt, "Official Releases from the European Medicines Agency," Substack, https://drsilviabehrendt751446.substack.com/.

729 Peter F. Mayer, "PSUR-DATENARCHIV zu Comirnaty, Vaxzevria, Nuvaxovid und Spikevax – neue Updates zu Spikevax und Vaxzevria," tkp.at, July 7, 2024, https://tkp.at/2024/07/07/psur-datenarchiv-zu-comirnaty-vaxzevria-nuvaxovid-und-spikevax-neue-updates-zu-spikevax-und-vaxzevria/.

730 Sonia Elijah, "The Tragedy of the Child Deaths: EU's 3rd Damning Vaccine Safety Report, Part 2," Children's Health Defense Europe, June 29, 2023, https://childrenshealthdefense.eu/children-health/the-tragedy-of-the-child-deaths-eus-3rd-damning-vaccine-safety-report-part-2/.

731 Sonia Elijah, "161 CHILDREN DIED following Pfizer/BioNTech 'Vaccination' in Just 12 Months," Substack, June 30, 2023, https://www.soniaelijah.com/p/161-children-died-following-pfizerbiontech.

732 "Graphs and Maps: Pooled by Age Group," EuroMOMO, https://euromomo.eu/graphs-and-maps#pooled-by-age-group.

733 Peter A. McCullough (@P_McCulloughMD), X post, June 12, 2023, https://x.com/P_McCulloughMD/status/1668239438768381952.

734 "FDA Head Dr. Marty Makary Reacts to RFK Jr.'s Contentious Hearing," The Lead with Jake Tapper, CNN, video, September 4, 2025, https://edition.cnn.com/2025/09/04/health/video/the-lead-marty-makary-health-rfk-jr-hhs-congress-hearing-jake-tapper.

735 Vinay Prasad, "Deaths in Children Due to COVID-19 Vaccines and CBER's Path Forward," internal memorandum, Center for Biologics Evaluation and Research, U.S. Food and Drug Administration, November 28, 2025, https://www.washingtonpost.com/documents/3042d15c-676b-48ac-8148-1a2204ef420e.pdf.

736 Dan Diamond and Rachel Roubein, "Blaming Some Child Deaths on Covid Shots, FDA Vows Stricter Vaccine Rules," Washington Post, November 29, 2025, https://www.washingtonpost.com/health/2025/11/29/fda-vaccine-approval-child-covid-deaths/.

737 "Vaccines and Related Biological Products Advisory Committee October 26, 2021 Meeting Announcement," U.S. Food and Drug Administration, https://www.fda.gov/advisory-committees/advisory-committee-calendar/vaccines-and-related-biological-products-advisory-committee-october-26-2021-meeting-announcement.

738 Sonia Elijah, “True Horrors of Covid Vaccine Harm Data NOW Exposed!,” Substack, May 1, 2024, https://www.soniaelijah.com/p/true-horrors-of-covid-vaccine-harm.

739 Wouter Aukema, “Vizzes,” Tableau Public profile, https://public.tableau.com/app/profile/aukema/vizzes.

740 “Keytruda (pembrolizumab),” European Medicines Agency (EMA), https://www.ema.europa.eu/en/medicines/human/EPAR/keytruda.

741 “Inflectra (infliximab),” European Medicines Agency (EMA), https://www.ema.europa.eu/en/medicines/human/EPAR/inflectra.

742 Julie Margetta Morgan and Devin Duffy, “The Cost of Capture: How the Pharmaceutical Industry Has Corrupted Policymakers and Harmed Patients,” Roosevelt Institute, May 22, 2019, https://rooseveltinstitute.org/publications/cost-of-capture-pharmaceutical-industry-corrupted-policymakers-harm-patients.

743 Jen Christensen, “Johnson & Johnson Covid-19 Vaccine Is Safe and Effective, FDA Analysis Finds,” CNN, February 24, 2021, https://edition.cnn.com/2021/02/24/health/johnson-vaccine-fda-analysis.

744 Dr Robert Malone, Inventor of mRNA Technology Interviewed by Sonia Elijah,” YouTube video, uploaded by Sonia Elijah investigates, https://www.youtube.com/watch?v=gHny5-c_Heo.

745 “#1757 - Dr. Robert Malone, MD,” The Joe Rogan Experience, episode 1757, hosted by Joe Rogan, December 31, 2021, https://open.spotify.com/episode/3SCsueX2bZdbEzRtKOCEyT.

746 Alicia Ault, “Baylor Gets Restraining Order Against COVID Vaccine Skeptic Doc,” Medscape, September 16, 2021, https://www.medscape.com/viewarticle/958916.

747 “#1747 - Dr. Peter A. McCullough,” The Joe Rogan Experience, episode 1747, hosted by Joe Rogan, December 13, 2021, https://open.spotify.com/episode/0aZte37vtFTkYT7b0b04Qz.

748 Michael Shellenberger, “Under White House Pressure, Facebook Censored Accurate Covid Vaccine Information,” Public, January 12, 2023, https://www.public.news/p/under-white-house-pressure-facebook.

749 Martin Kulldorff, “Harvard Tramples the Truth,” City Journal, March 11, 2024, https://www.city-journal.org/article/harvard-tramples-the-truth.

750 Sunetra Gupta, “Witness Statement No. 1,” UK COVID-19 Inquiry, INQ000252725, 25 August 2023, https://covid19.public-inquiry.uk/wp-content/uploads/2023/12/18143349/INQ000252725.pdf.

751 “The Advocate, the Mother and the Doctor Raise Concerns Regarding the mRNA Shots | Video,” TrialSite News, December 19, 2022, https://www.trialsitenews.com/a/the-advocate-the-mother-and-the-doctor-raise-concerns-regarding-the-mrna-shots-video-229e1714.

752 “Help Us Push For Life-Saving Help Now! - In Defense of the Vaccine Injured - Cody's Law,” Cody's Law, https://codyslaw.org/help-us-push-for-life-saving-help-now-intl/.

753 Heather Hudson (@Amothersanthem), X post, January 7, 2025, https://x.com/Amothersanthem/status/1876777929688089037.

754 “‘Look me in the EYE!’ - Rishi Sunak HOUNDED by FURIOUS audience member 'left to ROT',” YouTube video, uploaded by GB News, February 12, 2024, https://www.youtube.com/watch?v=nWJyEB7MkkY.

755 “Safe and Effective: A Second Opinion (2022) Oracle Films | News Uncut,” Rumble video, uploaded circa September 2022, https://rumble.com/v1lwbgs-safe-and-effective-a-second-opinion-2022-oracle-films-news-uncut.html.

756 Zoe Kleinman, “Anti-vax Groups Use Carrot Emojis to Hide Facebook Posts,” BBC News, September 16, 2022, https://www.bbc.co.uk/news/technology-62877597.

757 Saskia Mostert et al., "Excess Mortality across Countries in the Western World since the COVID-19 Pandemic: ‘Our World in Data’ Estimates of January 2020 to December 2022," BMJ Public Health 2, no. 1 (2024): e000282, https://doi.org/10.1136/bmjph-2023-000282.

758 Sarah Knapton, "Covid Vaccines May Have Helped Fuel Rise in Excess Deaths," The Telegraph, June 4, 2024, https://www.telegraph.co.uk/news/2024/06/04/covid-vaccines-may-have-helped-fuel-rise-in-excess-deaths/.

759 Short-Term Mortality Fluctuations data series (STMF), Human Mortality Database, Max Planck Institute for Demographic Research (Germany), University of California, Berkeley (USA), and French Institute for Demographic Studies (France), https://www.mortality.org/Data/STMF.

760 "COVID-19 Vaccines Have Saved 20 Million Lives So Far, Study Estimates," Gavi, the Vaccine Alliance, June 27, 2022, https://www.gavi.org/vaccineswork/covid-19-vaccines-have-saved-20-million-lives-so-far-study-estimates.

761 Joseph Fraiman et al., "Serious Adverse Events of Special Interest Following mRNA COVID-19 Vaccination in Randomized Trials in Adults," Vaccine 40, no. 40 (September 22, 2022): 5798–5805, https://doi.org/10.1016/j.vaccine.2022.08.036.

762 Mostert et al., "Excess Mortality," e000282.

763 "The Princess Máxima Center Distances Itself from Publication 'Excess Mortality during COVID-19 Pandemic,'" Princess Máxima Center for Pediatric Oncology, June 11, 2024, https://www.prinsesmaximacentrum.nl/en/news-events/news/the-princess-maxima-center-distances-itself-from-publication-excess-mortality-during-covid-19-pandemic.

764 "Expression of Concern: Excess Mortality across Countries in the Western World since the COVID-19 Pandemic: 'Our World in Data' Estimates of January 2020 to December 2022," BMJ Public Health 2, no. 1 (2024): e000282eoc, https://doi.org/10.1136/bmjph-2023-000282eoc.

765 Harald Walach, Rainer J. Klement, and Wouter Aukema, "The Safety of COVID-19 Vaccinations—We Should Rethink the Policy," Vaccines 9, no. 7 (June 24, 2021): 693, https://doi.org/10.3390/vaccines9070693. Retracted in Vaccines 9, no. 7 (2021): 729, https://doi.org/10.3390/vaccines9070729.

766 M. Nathaniel Mead et al., "COVID-19 mRNA Vaccines: Lessons Learned from the Registrational Trials and Global Vaccination Campaign," Cureus 16, no. 1 (January 24, 2024): e52876, https://doi.org/10.7759/cureus.52876. Retracted in Cureus 16, no. 2 (February 26, 2024): r137, https://doi.org/10.7759/cureus.r137

767 Jessica Rose, "A Report on Myocarditis Adverse Events in the U.S. Vaccine Adverse Events Reporting System (VAERS) in Association with COVID-19 Injectable Biological Products," Current Problems in Cardiology (2021). https://pmc.ncbi.nlm.nih.gov/articles/PMC8483988/. Withdrawn by the author(s) and/or editor.

768 "Are the Scientific Journals Censoring the Science? Part 1: Removal of Myocarditis Report in VAERS," Rumble video, uploaded by [channel/uploader name if specified; often independent or associated with Jessica Rose/Peter McCullough networks], [approximate upload date: November 2021], https://rumble.com/von23w-are-the-scientific-journals-censoring-the-science-part-1-removal-of-myocard.html.

769 Nicolas Hulscher et al., "A Systematic Review of Autopsy Findings in Deaths after COVID-19 Vaccination," Forensic Science International (2024): 112115, https://doi.org/10.1016/j.forsciint.2024.112115.
Withdrawn at the request of the Editors-in-Chief.

770 Rebekah Barnett, "EXCLUSIVE REPORT: Forced Retraction of Covid Vaccine Cancer-Risk Study, Scientist Alleges," Dystopian Down Under (Substack), June 2, 2024, https://news.rebekahbarnett.com.au/p/exclusive-report-forced-retraction.

771 Sonia Elijah, "Exclusive Interview: DNA Contamination in COVID Shots Amidst Retraction Wars and Cyber Censorship," Sonia Elijah Investigates (Substack), January 13, 2026, https://www.soniaelijah.com/p/exclusive-interview-dna-contamination.

772 David J. Speicher, Jessica Rose, and Kevin McKernan, "Quantification of Residual Plasmid DNA and SV40 Promoter-Enhancer Sequences in Pfizer/BioNTech and Moderna modRNA COVID-19 Vaccines from Ontario, Canada," Autoimmunity 58, no. 1 (2025): 2551517, https://doi.org/10.1080/08916934.2025.2551517.
(Under investigation by the publisher.)

773 Brigitte König and Jürgen O. Kirchner, "Methodological Considerations Regarding the Quantification of DNA Impurities in the COVID-19 mRNA Vaccine Comirnaty®," Methods

and Protocols 7, no. 3 (May 8, 2024): 41, https://doi.org/10.3390/mps7030041. (Expression of Concern issued June 25, 2025.)

774 "Shocking Study Linking Covid Jabs and Cancer 'Censored' by Mysterious Cyberattack," Daily Mail, January 9, 2026, https://www.dailymail.co.uk/sciencetech/article-15440249/cancer-Covid-vaccination-journal-cyberattack.html.

775 Wafik S. El-Deiry (@weldeiry), "Freedom of the Press is protected under the First Amendment of the US Constitution. But: Censorship is alive and well in the US and has come into medicine in a big awful way," X (thread), January 3, 2026, https://x.com/weldeiry/status/2007465043437170746.

776 Michael Nevradakis, "'Profound Breach of Trust': Pfizer Omitted Trial Data Showing Higher Mortality, Kidney Failure in Seniors Given mRNA Flu Shot," Children's Health Defense Defender, December 1, 2025, https://childrenshealthdefense.org/defender/pfizer-omitted-trial-data-showing-higher-mortality-kidney-failure-seniors-mrna-flu-shot/.

777 Sonia Elijah, "Piercing the Veil of Silence over Excess Deaths," Sonia Elijah Investigates (Substack), October 22, 2023 (updated October 28, 2023), https://www.soniaelijah.com/p/piercing-the-veil-of-silence-over.

778 "Trends in Excess Deaths," House of Commons Debates, vol. 738, October 20, 2023, cols. 560–567, https://hansard.parliament.uk/commons/2023-10-20/debates/69C5A514-9A04-4ED7-B56B-61A3D40E3226/TrendsInExcessDeaths.

779 Robin Monotti (@robinmonotti), "That the BBC puts slogans which contradict what an MP is saying in Parliament as he is saying it is in my view acting in contempt of the democratic process and should be condemned in the strongest terms by everyone as interference in democracy," X (thread), October 21, 2023, https://x.com/robinmonotti/status/1715628733665554782.

780 "Corrections and Clarifications - Archive 2023," BBC, last updated 2023, https://www.bbc.co.uk/helpandfeedback/corrections_clarifications/archive-2023.

781 "Did UK Office of National Statistics Manipulate Data on Covid Deaths by Vaccination Status?," Rumble video, uploaded by Sonia Elijah (or associated channel), circa December 2021, https://rumble.com/vu3pug-did-uk-office-of-national-statistics-manipulate-data-on-covid-deaths-by-vac.html.

782 Martin Neil et al., "Official Mortality Data for England Suggest Systematic Miscategorisation of Vaccine Status and Uncertain Effectiveness of Covid-19 Vaccination," preprint, ResearchGate, January 12, 2022, https://www.researchgate.net/publication/357778435_Official_mortality_data_for_England_suggest_systematic_miscategorisation_of_vaccine_status_and_uncertain_effectiveness_of_Covid-19_vaccination.

783 Office for National Statistics, "Deaths Involving COVID-19 by Vaccination Status, England: Deaths Occurring between 2 January and 24 September 2021," November 1, 2021, https://www.ons.gov.uk/peoplepopulationandcommunity/birthsdeathsandmarriages/deaths/bulletins/deathsinvolvingcovid19byvaccinationstatusengland/deathsoccurringbetween2januaryand24september2021.

784 Sonia Elijah, "Debate in Parliament Ignites over Excess Deaths and Vaccine Safety Concerns," Sonia Elijah Investigates (Substack), April 19, 2024, https://www.soniaelijah.com/p/debate-in-parliament-ignites-over.

785 Office for National Statistics, "Deaths Involving COVID-19 by Vaccination Status, England: Deaths Occurring between 1 April 2021 and 31 May 2023," August 25, 2023, https://www.ons.gov.uk/peoplepopulationandcommunity/birthsdeathsandmarriages/deaths/bulletins/deathsinvolvingcovid19byvaccinationstatusengland/deathsoccurringbetween1april2021and31may2023.

786 Camilla Turner, "Government 'Withholding Data That May Link Covid Jab to Excess Deaths'," The Telegraph, November 15, 2025, https://www.telegraph.co.uk/politics/2025/11/15/government-withholding-data-covid-jab-link-excess-deaths/.

787 Camilla Turner, "ONS Accused of Overestimating Excess Deaths in First Year

of Pandemic," The Telegraph, February 22, 2024, https://www.telegraph.co.uk/news/2024/02/22/ons-accused-of-overestimating-covid-deaths-in-2020/.

788 Gareth Eve (@garetheve), "As someone who lost his amazing wife to a Covid jab As a Dad of a little boy who lost his Mammy at the age of 6 I can assure you, my heart and my mental health is already very much broken," X (thread), November 16, 2025, https://x.com/garetheve/status/1990179760945971451.

789 "Search for Suspected Adverse Drug Reaction Reports by Active Substance," European Database of Suspected Adverse Drug Reaction Reports (ADR Reports), European Medicines Agency (EMA), accessed via https://www.adrreports.eu/en/search_subst.html.

790 Aukema, "Vizzes," Tableau Public.

791 Sonia Elijah, "Data Crimes: Deleting Covid Vaccine Deaths," Sonia Elijah Investigates (Substack), November 5, 2024, https://www.soniaelijah.com/p/data-crimes-deleting-covid-vaccine.

792 Sonia Elijah, "BREAKING: Data Analyst Faces EMA's Demand to Delete Pharmacovigilance Data!," Sonia Elijah Investigates (Substack), October 25, 2025, https://www.soniaelijah.com/p/breaking-data-analyst-faces-emas.

793 "Back to the Future: Restoring Hippocrates, Trust, and Sovereignty in Modern Medicine," Artsen Collectief (Netherlands Doctors' Collective), October 25–26, 2025, Driebergen, Netherlands, https://backtothefuture.nu/.

794 "Hoe het Lareb cruciale COVID-19-vaccinatiedata liet vertroebelen," blckbx (YouTube channel), October 24, 2024, https://www.youtube.com/watch?v=YYAhKITFiTc.

795 "Bill Maher Drops Stunning Monologue on the COVID Experts Who Got It Wrong," Rumble video, uploaded by Vigilant Fox, March 2024 https://rumble.com/v4me0ne-bill-maher-drops-stunning-monologue-on-the-covid-experts-who-got-it-wrong.html.

796 Johns Hopkins Center for Health Security, World Economic Forum, and Bill & Melinda Gates Foundation, Public-Private Cooperation for Pandemic Preparedness and Response: A Call to Action, January 17, 2020, https://centerforhealthsecurity.org/sites/default/files/2022-12/200117-publicprivatepandemiccalltoaction.pdf.

797 Sonia Elijah, "Mpox, Project Bioshield, Everyone's Dark Winter?," Sonia Elijah Investigates (Substack), September 19, 2024, https://www.soniaelijah.com/p/mpox-project-bioshield-everyones.

798 Sonia Elijah, "Cashing in on a Very 'Dark Winter'," Sonia Elijah Investigates (Substack), September 25, 2024, https://www.soniaelijah.com/p/cashing-in-on-a-very-dark-winter.

799 "FBI Amerithrax or Anthrax Investigation," Federal Bureau of Investigation, accessed via https://www.fbi.gov/history/famous-cases/amerithrax-or-anthrax-investigation.

800 U.S. Department of Justice, Office of Public Affairs, "Justice Department and FBI Announce Closure of Amerithrax Case," press release, August 1, 2008, https://www.justice.gov/archive/opa/pr/2008/August/08-opa-697.html.

801 "Bruce Edwards Ivins," Wikipedia, https://en.wikipedia.org/wiki/Bruce_Edwards_Ivins.

802 Stephen Engelberg, "New Evidence Adds Doubt to FBI's Case Against Anthrax Suspect," ProPublica, October 10, 2011, https://www.propublica.org/article/new-evidence-disputes-case-against-bruce-e-ivins.

803 Prof. Francis Boyle on the 2001 Anthrax Attacks," Qlipoth (blog), July 2007, https://qlipoth.blogspot.com/2007/07/prof-francis-boyle-2001-anthrax-attacks.html.

804 Jack Dolan and Dave Altimari, "Anthrax Missing From Army Lab," Hartford Courant, January 20, 2002, archived at https://web.archive.org/web/20020409022746/http://www.ctnow.com/news/specials/hc-detrick0120.artjan20.story?coll=hc-h.

805 Denise Grady, "Deadly Germ Research Is Shut Down at Army Lab Over Safety Concerns," New York Times, August 5, 2019, https://www.nytimes.com/2019/08/05/health/germs-fort-detrick-biohazard.html.

806 Wuhan University School of Basic Medical Sciences, "Institute of Medical Virology," accessed February 20, 2026, https://wbm.whu.edu.cn/English/Departments/Departments/Institute_of_Medical_Virology.htm.

807 Mackinac Center for Public Policy, "What about Bioport?," January 11, 2002, https://www.mackinac.org/3966.

808 U.S. Congress, House, Committee on Government Reform, The Department of Defense Anthrax Vaccine Immunization Program: Unproven Force Protection, 106th Cong., 2d sess., H. Rept. 106-556, April 3, 2000, https://www.congress.gov/committee-report/106th-congress/house-report/556/1.

809 Project BioShield Act of 2004, Pub. L. No. 108-276, 118 Stat. 835 (July 21, 2004), https://www.govinfo.gov/content/pkg/PLAW-108publ276/pdf/PLAW-108publ276.pdf.

810 "Fauci Addresses Bioterrorism Threats," The Hoya, October 17, 2002, https://thehoya.com/uncategorized/fauci-addresses-bioterrorism-threats/.

811 Robert Kadlec, "Testimony of Robert Kadlec, M.D., Assistant Secretary for Preparedness and Response, U.S. Department of Health and Human Services," submitted to the U.S. House of Representatives, Committee on Energy and Commerce, Subcommittee on Oversight and Investigations, December 4, 2019, https://congress.gov/116/meeting/house/110278/witnesses/HHRG-116-IF02-Bio-KadlecMDMTMHMSR-20191204.pdf.

812 Johns Hopkins Center for Health Security, "Dark Winter: A Training Tabletop Exercise," https://centerforhealthsecurity.org/our-work/tabletop-exercises/dark-winter-a-training-tabletop-exercise.

813 Media Monarchy, "'operation dark winter' 2," YouTube video, https://www.youtube.com/watch?v=VMd4z19IJU0.

814 U.S. Department of Health and Human Services, Office of the Assistant Secretary for Preparedness and Response, Crimson Contagion 2019 Functional Exercise After-Action Report, January 2020, https://www.governmentattic.org/38docs/HHSaarCrimsonContAAR_2020.pdf.

815 Michael D. Shear, Noah Weiland, Eric Lipton, Maggie Haberman, and David E. Sanger, "Before Virus Outbreak, a Cascade of Warnings Went Unheeded," New York Times, March 19, 2020, https://www.nytimes.com/2020/03/19/us/politics/trump-coronavirus-outbreak.html.

816 Bipartisan Commission on Biodefense, "A Manhattan Project for Biodefense: Taking Biological Threats Off the Table," agenda for panel meeting, July 11, 2019, https://biodefensecommission.org/wp-content/uploads/2019/07/LiteratureRetrieve.pdf.

817 U.S. Department of Energy, Office of Classification, Office of History and Heritage Resources, and Office of Scientific and Technical Information, "Manhattan District History," https://www.osti.gov/opennet/manhattan_district.

818 Kim Riley, "Experts Support a Future Manhattan Project for Biodefense to Thwart New Threats," Homeland Preparedness News, July 12, 2019, https://homelandprepnews.com/countermeasures/34774-experts-support-a-future-manhattan-project-for-biodefense-to-thwart-new-threats/.

819 Johns Hopkins Center for Health Security, World Economic Forum, and Bill & Melinda Gates Foundation, "Public-Private Cooperation for Pandemic Preparedness and Response: A Call to Action," January 17, 2020, https://centerforhealthsecurity.org/sites/default/files/2022-12/200117-publicprivatepandemiccalltoaction.pdf.

820 Kadlec, "Biographical Statement."

821 Jon Swaine, Robert O'Harrow Jr., and Aaron C. Davis, "Before Pandemic, Trump's Stockpile Chief Put Focus on Biodefense. An Old Client Benefited," Washington Post, May 4, 2020, https://www.washingtonpost.com/investigations/before-pandemic-trumps-stockpile-chief-put-focus-on-biodefense-an-old-client-benefited/2020/05/04/d3c2b010-84dd-11ea-878a-86477a724bdb_story.html.

822 U.S. Food and Drug Administration, Center for Biologics Evaluation and Research, "Supplement Approval (STN: BL 125158/297)," August 29, 2024, https://www.fda.gov/media/181430/download?attachment.

823 Lisa M. James, Apostolos P. Georgopoulos, Brian E. Engdahl, and Arthur Leuthold, "Anthrax Vaccination, Gulf War Illness, and Human Leukocyte Antigen (HLA)," Vaccines 12, no. 6 (June 4, 2024): 613, https://doi.org/10.3390/vaccines12060613.

824 Meryl Nass, "Testimony on H.98," written comments submitted to Vermont Senate Health and Welfare Committee, April 22, 2015, https://legislature.vermont.gov/Documents/2016/WorkGroups/Senate%20Health%20and%20Welfare/Bills/H.98/Witness%20Testimony/H.98~Dr.%20Meryl%20Nass~Written%20Comments~4-22-2015.pdf.
825 Emergent BioSolutions Inc., ACAM2000 [Smallpox and Mpox (Vaccinia) Vaccine, Live] Package Insert, revised October 2024, https://www.fda.gov/media/75792/download.
826 U.S. Congress, House, Select Subcommittee on the Coronavirus Crisis of the Committee on Oversight and Reform, Examining Emergent BioSolutions' Failure to Protect Public Health and Public Funds, 117th Cong., 1st sess., hearing transcript, May 19, 2021, https://docs.house.gov/meetings/VC/VC00/20210519/112641/HHRG-117-VC00-Transcript-20210519.pdf.
827 Jon Swaine, Robert O'Harrow Jr., and Aaron C. Davis, "Before Pandemic, Trump's Stockpile Chief Put Focus on Biodefense. An Old Client Benefited," Washington Post, May 4, 2020, https://www.washingtonpost.com/investigations/before-pandemic-trumps-stockpile-chief-put-focus-on-biodefense-an-old-client-benefited/2020/05/04/d3c2b010-84dd-11ea-878a-86477a724bdb_story.html.
828 U.S. Department of Health and Human Services, Biomedical Advanced Research and Development Authority, "Newsroom Archive: 2020," archived April 14, 2025, https://us.pagefreezer.com/en-US/wa/browse/9081576a-8b48-4971-8e08-dac55433b3e3?url=https:%2F%2Fwww.medicalcountermeasures.gov%2Fnewsroom%2F2020&timestamp=2025-04-14T18:32:12Z.
829 U.S. Congress, House, Committee on Oversight and Reform, The Coronavirus Vaccine Manufacturing Failures of Emergent BioSolutions, staff report, May 2022, https://coronavirus-democrats-oversight.house.gov/sites/evo-subsites/coronavirus-democrats-oversight.house.gov/files/Coronavirus%20Vaccine%20Manufacturing%20Failures%20of%20Emergent%20BioSolutions.pdf.
830 BBC, "Trusted News Initiative Announces Plans to Tackle Harmful Coronavirus Disinformation," BBC Media Centre, March 27, 2020, https://www.bbc.com/mediacentre/latestnews/2020/coronavirus-trusted-news.
831 U.S. Congress, House, Committee on the Judiciary, Select Subcommittee on the Weaponization of the Federal Government, "Hearing on the Weaponization of the Federal Government," July 20, 2023, https://judiciary.house.gov/committee-activity/hearings/hearing-weaponization-federal-government-3.
832 Dave Rubin, "Exposing the Real Reason Legacy Media Fears Me | Robert F. Kennedy Jr. | POLITICS | Rubin Report," YouTube video, 1:09:09, July 16, 2023, https://www.youtube.com/watch?v=7_gHzPvOpIo.
833 Children's Health Defense et al. v. WP Company, LLC d/b/a The Washington Post et al., Complaint, Civil Action No. 3:23-cv-00720 (W.D. La. filed May 31, 2023), https://childrenshealthdefense.org/wp-content/uploads/Trusted-News-Initiative-Louisiana-Complaint-Dkt-1-05-31-2023.pdf.
834 Sonia Elijah, "TrialSite News Founder Speaks Candidly on the Importance of Transparent Clinical Research Information, Unprecedented Censorship & More," TrialSite News, September 9, 2022, https://www.trialsitenews.com/a/founder-of-trial-site-news-speaks-candidly-about-the-need-for-transparent-clinical-research-information-the-rise-of-unprecedented-censorship-how-tr-a9b984d0.
835 U.S. Department of Justice, Office of Public Affairs, "Justice Department Files Statement of Interest on Suppression of Competition in the Marketplace of Ideas Through Deplatforming of Rival Viewpoints," July 11, 2025, https://www.justice.gov/opa/pr/justice-department-files-statement-interest-suppression-competition-marketplace-ideas.
836 Wikipedia contributors, "Twitter Files," Wikipedia, The Free Encyclopedia, https://en.wikipedia.org/wiki/Twitter_Files.
837 Wikipedia contributors, "Murthy v. Missouri," Wikipedia, The Free Encyclopedia, https://en.wikipedia.org/wiki/Murthy_v._Missouri.
838 "FB Portal," Exhibit 71-9 to Declaration of [Plaintiff/Defendant], Missouri

v. Biden, No. 3:22-cv-01213-TAD-KDM (W.D. La. filed Aug. 31, 2022), https://www.documentcloud.org/documents/23129270-fb-portal.
839 Jenin Younes and Aaron Kheriaty, "The White House Covid Censorship Machine," Wall Street Journal, January 8, 2023. https://www.wsj.com/articles/white-house-covid-censorship-machine-social-media-facebook-meta-executive-rob-flaherty-free-speech-google-11673203704.
840 Emails from Rob Flaherty and Andy Slavitt Regarding COVID-19 Content Moderation, exhibit/document, Wall Street Journal, accessed via https://www.wsj.com/public/resources/documents/17623-0314.pdf.
841 Zolan Kanno-Youngs and Cecilia Kang, "'They're Killing People': Biden Denounces Social Media for Virus Disinformation," New York Times, July 16, 2021. https://www.nytimes.com/2021/07/16/us/politics/biden-facebook-social-media-covid.html.
842 "White House Reviewing Section 230 amid Efforts to Push Social Media Giants to Crack Down on Misinformation," CNN, July 2021, PDF exhibit cited in Murthy v. Missouri, No. 23-411, U.S. Supreme Court. https://www.supremecourt.gov/opinions/URLs_Cited/OT2023/23-411/23-411-20.pdf.
843 Sonia Elijah, "Big Tech Censorship by Order of the White House," Sonia Elijah Investigates (Substack), September 19, 2022. https://www.soniaelijah.com/p/big-tech-censorship-by-order-of-the?utm_source=publication-search.
844 U.S. House Committee on the Judiciary, Select Subcommittee on the Weaponization of the Federal Government, "Hearing on the Weaponization of the Federal Government on the Twitter Files," March 9, 2023. https://judiciary.house.gov/committee-activity/hearings/hearing-weaponization-federal-government-twitter-files.
845 Matt Taibbi, Written Statement for "Hearing on the Weaponization of the Federal Government on the Twitter Files," Select Subcommittee on the Weaponization of the Federal Government, Committee on the Judiciary, U.S. House of Representatives, March 9, 2023. https://judiciary.house.gov/sites/evo-subsites/republicans-judiciary.house.gov/files/evo-media-document/taibbi-testimony.pdf.
846 Michael Shellenberger, "The Censorship Industrial Complex: U.S. Government Support For Domestic Censorship And Disinformation Campaigns, 2016 - 2022," Written Testimony, Select Subcommittee on the Weaponization of the Federal Government, Committee on the Judiciary, U.S. House of Representatives, March 9, 2023. https://judiciary.house.gov/sites/evo-subsites/republicans-judiciary.house.gov/files/evo-media-document/shellenberger-testimony.pdf.
847 Committee on the Judiciary and Select Subcommittee on the Weaponization of the Federal Government, U.S. House of Representatives, The Censorship-Industrial Complex: How Top Biden White House Officials Coerced Big Tech to Censor Americans, True Information, and Critics of the Biden Administration, Interim Staff Report, May 1, 2024. https://judiciary.house.gov/sites/evo-subsites/republicans-judiciary.house.gov/files/evo-media-document/Biden-WH-Censorship-Report-final.pdf.
848 Terry A. Doughty, Memorandum Ruling on Request for Preliminary Injunction, Missouri v. Biden, No. 3:22-cv-01213-TAD-KDM (W.D. La. July 4, 2023). https://ago.mo.gov/wp-content/uploads/missouri-v-biden-ruling.pdf.
849 Amy Coney Barrett, Opinion of the Court, Murthy v. Missouri, No. 23-411 (U.S. June 26, 2024). https://www.supremecourt.gov/opinions/23pdf/23-411_3dq3.pdf.
850 Big Brother Watch, Ministry of Truth: The Secretive Government Units Spying on Your Speech (London: Big Brother Watch, January 2023). https://bigbrotherwatch.org.uk/wp-content/uploads/2023/01/Ministry-of-Truth-Big-Brother-Watch-290123.pdf.
851 Carl Heneghan, "Boris Johnson Needs to Bin the Rule of Six," Spectator, September 13, 2020. https://spectator.com/article/boris-johnson-needs-to-bin-the-rule-of-six/.
852 Center for Countering Digital Hate, "Impact," accessed February 20, 2026. https://counterhate.com/impact/.
853 Center for Countering Digital Hate, The Disinformation Dozen: Why Platforms Must

Act on Twelve Leading Online Anti-Vaxxers (London/Washington, D.C.: CCDH, March 24, 2021). https://counterhate.com/research/the-disinformation-dozen.
854 U.S. House Select Subcommittee on the Weaponization of the Federal Government, Committee on the Judiciary, Hearing on the Weaponization of the Federal Government, 118th Cong., 1st sess., July 20, 2023. https://www.govinfo.gov/content/pkg/CHRG-118hhrg53145/html/CHRG-118hhrg53145.htm.
855 Sonia Elijah, "'Disinformation Dozen' Survivor—Sayer Ji Speaks Out," Sonia Elijah Investigates (Substack), November 25, 2025. https://www.soniaelijah.com/p/disinformation-dozen-survivor-sayer.
856 Biden Rows Back on Facebook 'Killing People' Comment," BBC News, July 20, 2021. https://www.bbc.co.uk/news/technology-57901710.
857 Center for Countering Digital Hate, Building a Safe and Accountable Internet: CCDH's Refreshed STAR Framework (London/Washington, D.C.: CCDH, September 19, 2024). https://counterhate.com/research/star-framework-to-build-a-safe-and-accountable-internet/.
858 Center for Countering Digital Hate, "Our Campaigning Resulted in the Online Safety Act in the UK," CCDH Blog, January 30, 2024. https://counterhate.com/blog/our-campaigning-resulted-in-the-online-safety-act-in-the-uk/.
859 Joint Committee on the Draft Online Safety Bill, Corrected Oral Evidence: Draft Online Safety Bill, Evidence Session No. 1, 9 September 2021. https://committees.parliament.uk/oralevidence/2694/pdf.
860 Paul D. Thacker and Matt Taibbi, "Election Exclusive: British Advisors to Kamala Harris Hope to 'Kill Musk's Twitter,'" The DisInformation Chronicle (Substack), October 22, 2024. https://disinformationchronicle.substack.com/p/election-exclusive-british-advisors.
861 "'The Only Honourable Course': Morgan McSweeney's Resignation Statement in Full," The Guardian, February 8, 2026. https://www.theguardian.com/politics/2026/feb/08/morgan-mcsweeney-resignation-speech.
862 Marco Rubio, "Announcement of Actions to Combat the Global Censorship-Industrial Complex," Press Statement, U.S. Department of State, December 23, 2025. https://www.state.gov/releases/office-of-the-spokesperson/2025/12/announcement-of-actions-to-combat-the-global-censorship-industrial-complex/.
863 International Fact-Checking Network, "International Fact-Checking Network," Poynter Institute, accessed February 20, 2026. https://www.poynter.org/ifcn/.
864 PolitiFact, https://www.politifact.com/.
865 The Poynter Institute, https://www.poynter.org/.
866 International Fact-Checking Network, "International Fact-Checking Network Transparency Statement," Poynter Institute, https://www.poynter.org/international-fact-checking-network-transparency-statement/.
867 Andy Nguyen, "Blog Post Ignores Important Context about COVID-19 Immunity Study," PolitiFact, January 26, 2022. https://www.politifact.com/factchecks/2022/jan/26/blog-posting/blog-post-ignores-important-context-about-covid-19/.
868 Kiannah Sepeda-Miller, "No, the Novel Coronavirus Was Not 'Man-Made,'" PolitiFact, May 21, 2020. https://www.politifact.com/factchecks/2020/may/21/kimberly-lightford/no-novel-coronavirus-was-not-man-made/.
869 Gabrielle Settles, "There's No Basis to Claim Thousands Have Died from COVID-19 Vaccines," PolitiFact, December 10, 2021. https://www.politifact.com/factchecks/2021/dec/10/instagram-posts/theres-no-basis-claim-thousands-have-died-covid-19/.
870 Can We Believe the Lockdown Sceptics?," Full Fact, first published December 18, 2020, updated December 21, 2020. https://fullfact.org/health/can-we-believe-lockdown-sceptics/.
871 Full Fact, Search Results for "vaccine safety" (page 5), https://fullfact.org/search/#gsc.tab=0&gsc.q=vaccine%20safety&gsc.sort=&gsc.page=5.
872 "Andrew Bridgen's Covid-19 Claims Debunked as He Returns to Parliament," Leicester Mercury (Leicestershire Live), January 18, 2023. https://www.leicestermercury.co.uk/news/local-news/andrew-bridgens-covid-19-claims-8044205.

873 "Full Fact Campaign Wins Improved Media Literacy in the Online Safety Bill," Full Fact, July 28, 2023. https://fullfact.org/blog/2023/jul/full-fact-campaign-wins-improved-media-literacy-in-the-online-safety-bill/.

874 Nadine Dorries, "Online Safety Update," Written Ministerial Statement HCWS194, UK Parliament, July 7, 2022. https://questions-statements.parliament.uk/written-statements/detail/2022-07-07/hcws194.

875 Lee Fang, "British AI Firm Helped Censor Activists and Journalists, Poised to Shape 2024 U.S. Elections," Lee Fang (Substack), January 26, 2024. https://www.leefang.com/p/british-ai-firm-helped-censor-activists.

876 Josh Christenson, "Pentagon, Other Agencies Funded Censorship Firm That Blacklisted The Post, House Committee Reveals," New York Post, October 25, 2024. https://nypost.com/2024/10/25/us-news/pentagon-other-agencies-funded-censorship-firm-that-blacklisted-the-post-house-committee-reveals/.

877 "NewsGuard, Publicis Groupe Press Release," Publicis Health Media Perspectives, May 25, 2021. https://www.publicishealthmedia.com/perspective/newsguard-publicis-groupe-press-release/.

878 Sonia Elijah, "NATO's Mind 'Games'—Inoculating Dissent?," Sonia Elijah Investigates (Substack), September 30, 2025. https://www.soniaelijah.com/p/natos-mind-gamesinoculating-dissent.

879 Inoculation Theory and Misinformation (Riga: NATO Strategic Communications Centre of Excellence, October 29, 2021). https://stratcomcoe.org/publications/inoculation-theory-and-misinformation/217.

880 "Cambridge Social Decision-Making Lab | Department of Psychology." University of Cambridge. https://www.sdmlab.psychol.cam.ac.uk/.

881 "GO VIRAL!" Tilt. https://www.tiltstudio.co/solutions/cases/goviral/.

882 Central Intelligence Agency, "Project Mockingbird," Memorandum/Report, Office of Security, declassified January 14, 2020 (document reference C02353962). https://www.cia.gov/readingroom/docs/PROJECT%20MOCKINGBIRD%5b15770719%5d.pdf.

883 "NATO Centres of Excellence – NATO Strategic Communications Centre of Excellence," NATO Allied Command Transformation, https://www.act.nato.int/article/nato-stratcom-coe/.

884 Compton, Josh, Ben Jackson, and James A. Dimmock. "Persuading Others to Avoid Persuasion: Inoculation Theory and Resistant Health Attitudes." Frontiers in Psychology 7 (February 2016): 122. https://pmc.ncbi.nlm.nih.gov/articles/PMC4746429/.

885 "IRIS Academic Research Group." IRIS Academic Research Group. https://www.irisacademic.org/.

886 "Google's Think Tank Is Transforming into a Tech Lab Called Jigsaw." The Verge, February 16, 2016. https://www.theverge.com/2016/2/16/11027444/alphabet-google-ideas-jigsaw-global-policy-think-tank.

887 "JITSUVAX." University of Bristol. https://jitsuvax.info/.

888 Sonia Elijah, "UK Government Admits NATO's Hidden Hand in COVID Censorship But Refuses to Release Files." November 1, 2025. https://www.soniaelijah.com/p/uk-government-admits-natos-hidden.

889 Sonia Elijah, "How the UK and Canada Are Leading the West's Descent into Digital Authoritarianism," Sonia Elijah Investigates (Substack), October 17, 2025. https://www.soniaelijah.com/p/how-the-uk-and-canada-are-leading.

890 United Nations, "Transforming Our World: The 2030 Agenda for Sustainable Development," A/RES/70/1, September 25, 2015. https://sdgs.un.org/2030agenda.

891 "Tempora," Wikipedia, https://en.wikipedia.org/wiki/Tempora.

892 Ewen MacAskill, Julian Borger, Nick Hopkins, Nick Davies, and James Ball, "GCHQ Taps Fibre-Optic Cables for Secret Access to World's Communications," The Guardian, June 21, 2013. https://www.theguardian.com/uk/2013/jun/21/gchq-cables-secret-world-communications-nsa.

893 Investigatory Powers Act 2016, c. 25 (UK). https://www.legislation.gov.uk/ukpga/2016/25/contents.
894 "Five Things You Need to Know About the Online Safety Bill," Big Brother Watch, September 13, 2021. https://bigbrotherwatch.org.uk/blog/five-things-you-need-to-know-about-the-online-safety-bill/.
895 Liv McMahon, "Imgur Blocks Access to UK Users after Proposed Regulatory Fine," BBC News, September 30, 2025, https://www.bbc.co.uk/news/articles/c4gzxv5gy3qo.
896 BitChute, "UK Regulation," May 7, 2025, https://www.bitchute.com/ukregulation.
897 UK Government, Department for Science, Innovation and Technology, "UK Children and Adults to Be Safer Online as World-Leading Bill Becomes Law," news release, October 26, 2023, https://www.gov.uk/government/news/uk-children-and-adults-to-be-safer-online-as-world-leading-bill-becomes-law.
898 UK Government, Department for Science, Innovation and Technology, "Data (Use and Access) Act 2025: Data Protection and Privacy Changes," guidance, June 27, 2025, https://www.gov.uk/guidance/data-use-and-access-act-2025-data-protection-and-privacy-changes.
899 UK Government, Department for Science, Innovation and Technology, "Cyber Security and Resilience Bill," collection, last updated November 18, 2025, https://www.gov.uk/government/collections/cyber-security-and-resilience-bill.
900 Sky News, "Police to Get 40 New Live Facial Recognition Vans and AI Help in Sweeping Reforms," January 26, 2026, https://news.sky.com/story/facial-recognition-technology-to-be-rolled-out-nationally-and-police-to-also-get-ai-support-13499172.
901 Adam Satariano and Lizzie Dearden, "Has Britain Gone Too Far With Its Digital Controls?," New York Times, September 17, 2025, https://www.nytimes.com/2025/09/17/technology/britain-facial-recognition-digital-controls.html.
902 Charlie Parker, Yennah Smart, and George Willoughby, "Police Make 30 Arrests a Day for Offensive Online Messages," The Times, April 4, 2025, https://www.thetimes.com/uk/crime/article/police-make-30-arrests-a-day-for-offensive-online-messages-zbv886tqf.
903 Tony Blair Institute for Global Change, "Time for Digital ID: A New Consensus for a State That Works," paper, September 24, 2025, https://institute.global/insights/politics-and-governance/time-for-digital-id-a-new-consensus-for-a-state-that-works.
904 UK Parliament. House of Commons. "Digital ID." Hansard Parliamentary Debates, vol. 773, cols. October 13, 2025. https://hansard.parliament.uk/commons/2025-10-13/debates/37D3137B-302E-4E1B-A6E4-0676456F26D0/DigitalID.
905 James Melville (@JamesMelville), "Nearly 40 MPs from multiple parties have now signed a letter opposing Keir Starmer's proposed mandatory digital ID. No one voted for this. Massive authoritarian overreach by the Labour government. We must not become 'show us your government digital papers' society.," X, October 10, 2025, https://x.com/JamesMelville/status/1976597279374037072.
906 Rory Tingle, Arthur Parashar, and Greg Heffer, "EVERY Adult in Britain Will Need a Government-Issued ID Card despite Backlash at Starmer's Plan for a 'Dystopian Nightmare'," Daily Mail, September 25, 2025, https://www.dailymail.co.uk/news/article-15133629/Every-adult-Britain-need-new-Government-issued-digital-ID-card-new-Keir-Starmer-plan.html.
907 UK Parliament. "Do Not Introduce Digital ID Cards," e-petition 730194, closed January 9, 2026, https://petition.parliament.uk/petitions/730194.
908 UK Parliament. House of Commons. "Digital ID." Hansard Parliamentary Debates, vol. 777, December 8, 2025. https://hansard.parliament.uk/Commons/2025-12-08/debates/9E01F17C-557A-4D02-8A93-B573721B8B20/a.
909 Chris Mason, "Digital IDs: Starmer's Change of Heart Another 'Almighty Backtracking'," BBC News, January 14, 2026, https://www.bbc.co.uk/news/articles/c14regjvk6no.
910 Government Digital Service, "About GOV.UK One Login," n.d., https://www.sign-in.service.gov.uk/about.
911 Department of Justice Canada, "Bill C-2: An Act Respecting Certain Measures Relating to the Security of the Border between Canada and the United States and

Respecting Other Related Security Measures," Charter Statement, tabled June 19, 2025, https://www.justice.gc.ca/eng/csj-sjc/pl/charter-charte/c2_2.html.
912 Canada. Parliament. House of Commons. Bill C-8: An Act Respecting Cyber Security, Amending the Telecommunications Act and Making Consequential Amendments to Other Acts. First reading, June 18, 2025. https://www.parl.ca/DocumentViewer/en/45-1/bill/C-8/first-reading.
913 Department of Justice Canada, "Bill C-63: An Act to Enact the Online Harms Act, to Amend the Criminal Code, the Canadian Human Rights Act and An Act Respecting the Mandatory Reporting of Internet Child Pornography by Persons Who Provide an Internet Service and to Make Consequential and Related Amendments to Other Acts," Charter Statement, tabled May 30, 2024, https://www.justice.gc.ca/eng/csj-sjc/pl/charter-charte/c63.html.
914 Swikar Oli, "Canada's Public Health Agency Admits It Tracked 33 Million Mobile Devices during Lockdown," National Post, December 24, 2021, https://nationalpost.com/news/canada/canadas-public-health-agency-admits-it-tracked-33-million-mobile-devices-during-lockdown.
915 Canada. Parliament. House of Commons. Bill C-59: An Act to Implement Certain Provisions of the Fall Economic Statement Tabled in Parliament on November 21, 2023 and Certain Provisions of the Budget Tabled in Parliament on March 28, 2023. First reading, November 30, 2023. https://www.parl.ca/documentviewer/en/44-1/bill/C-59/first-reading.
916 Greg McMullen, "Pulling Back the Curtain on Canada's Mass Surveillance Programs – Part Two: The CSE Secret Spying Archive," British Columbia Civil Liberties Association (blog), March 16, 2023, https://bccla.org/2023/03/pulling-back-the-curtain-on-canadas-mass-surveillance-programs-part-two-the-cse-secret-spying-archive/.
917 Government of Canada. Canadian Digital Service. "Trusted Access to Digital Services," last modified December 2, 2024, https://www.canada.ca/en/government/system/digital-government/digital-government-innovations/digital-credentials.html.
918 European Commission, "The Digital Services Act," n.d., https://digital-strategy.ec.europa.eu/en/policies/digital-services-act.
919 David Ingram, "E.U. Hits Musk's X with $140 Million Fine, Says It Broke Hate Speech and Misinformation Rules," NBC News, December 5, 2025, https://www.nbcnews.com/world/europe/elon-musk-x-european-union-fine-content-regulations-misinformation-rcna247498.
920 European Commission, "Digital Markets Act," n.d., https://digital-markets-act.ec.europa.eu/index_en.
921 European Commission. "EU Digital Identity Wallet Home," last modified January 21, 2026, https://ec.europa.eu/digital-building-blocks/sites/spaces/EUDIGITALIDENTITYWALLET/pages/694487738/EU+Digital+Identity+Wallet+Home.
922 European Commission, "EU Digital COVID Certificate," n.d., https://commission.europa.eu/strategy-and-policy/coronavirus-response/safe-covid-19-vaccines-europeans/eu-digital-covid-certificate_en.
923 NHS, "Check Your COVID-19 Vaccine Record," n.d., https://www.nhs.uk/nhs-services/online-services/vaccine-record/.
924 Canada Border Services Agency, "ArriveCAN," last modified July 11, 2025, https://www.canada.ca/en/mobile/arrivecan.html.
925 Centers for Disease Control and Prevention. National Center for Immunization and Respiratory Diseases (U.S.). "Your CDC COVID-19 Vaccination Record and Vaccination Card," updated February 7, 2022, https://stacks.cdc.gov/view/cdc/114211.
926 New York State, "Excelsior Pass," March 2021, PDF brochure, https://www.nysca.org/downloads/files/Excelsior_Pass_V3.pdf.
927 Laurie Baratti, "California Launches Digital COVID-19 Vaccine Verification Tool," TravelPulse, June 18, 2021, https://www.travelpulse.com/news/technology/california-launches-digital-covid-19-vaccine-verification-tool.
928 Sonia Elijah, "Living under Medical Apartheid in Austria," YouTube video, 0:00, November 18, 2021, https://www.youtube.com/watch?v=ikZ6eQ6ALTA.

929 Rachel Gilmore, "'Fringe Minority' in Truck Convoy with 'Unacceptable Views' Don't Represent Canadians: Trudeau," Global News, January 26, 2022, https://globalnews.ca/news/8539610/trucker-convoy-covid-vaccine-mandates-ottawa/.

930 Canadian Anti-Hate Network, "The 'Freedom Convoy' Is Nothing But A Vehicle For The Far Right," January 27, 2022, https://www.antihate.ca/the_freedom_convoy_is_nothing_but_a_vehicle_for_the_far_right.

931 Sonia Elijah, "Canadian Truckers Are Driving Freedom Home," The Conservative Woman, January 30, 2022, https://www.conservativewoman.co.uk/canadian-truckers-are-driving-freedom-home.

932 Sonia Elijah, "Canadian Truckers Make a Stand for Freedom," Sonia Elijah investigates (Substack), February 3, 2022, https://www.soniaelijah.com/p/canadian-truckers-make-a-stand-for.

933 Catharine Tunney, "Federal Government Invokes Emergencies Act for First Time Ever in Response to Protests, Blockades," CBC News, February 14, 2022, https://www.cbc.ca/news/politics/trudeau-premiers-cabinet-1.6350734.

934 BBC News, "Trudeau Vows to Freeze Anti-Mandate Protesters' Bank Accounts," February 15, 2022, https://www.bbc.co.uk/news/world-us-canada-60383385.

935 Canada. Federal Court. Canadian Frontline Nurses v. Canada (Attorney General), 2024 FC 42, January 23, 2024, https://www.fct-cf.ca/Content/assets/pdf/base/2024.01.23-306-22-T-316-22-T-347-22-T-382-22.pdf.

936 World Health Organization, "Global Digital Health Certification Network," n.d., https://www.who.int/initiatives/global-digital-health-certification-network.

937 World Health Organization, International Health Regulations (2005), A77/A/CONF./14, adopted June 1, 2024, https://apps.who.int/gb/ebwha/pdf_files/WHA77/A77_ACONF14-en.pdf.

938 Sonia Elijah, "Censorship & Control, Under the Guise of Promoting Public Health? A Breakdown of the WHO's New Pandemic Treaty & IHR Amendments with Attorney, Philipp Kruse," Sonia Elijah investigates (Substack), February 16, 2024, https://www.soniaelijah.com/p/attorney-philipp-kruse-breaks-down.

939 U.S. Department of Health and Human Services and U.S. Department of State, "Joint Statement by Secretary of State Rubio and Secretary of Health and Human Services Kennedy on the Termination of U.S. Membership in the World Health Organization (WHO)," news release, January 20, 2025, https://www.hhs.gov/press-room/joint-statement-by-secretary-of-state-rubio-and-secretary-of-health-and-human-services-kennedy-on-the-termination-of-us-membership-in-the-world-health-organization-who.html.

940 Klaus Schwab (@ProfKlausSchwab), "Our societies face a decline of truth and trust. Without truth, we lose a shared reality; without trust, we lose our capacity to act together.," X, January 17, 2026, https://x.com/ProfKlausSchwab/status/2012446440404951521.

941 Jenny Strasburg and Shalini Ramachandran, "Probe of Davos Founder Finds Unauthorized Spending, Inappropriate Behavior," Wall Street Journal, July 23, 2025. https://www.wsj.com/business/world-economic-forum-probe-of-klaus-schwab-finds-unauthorized-spending-and-inappropriate-behavior-bec3dc4f.

# INDEX

# B

## C

## D

# E

# F

## G

# H

# I

## J



## K

## L

## M

## N

# O

# P

# Q



# R

## S

# T

## V

# X



# Y



# Z

Made in United States
Troutdale, OR
04/19/2026

48629565R00266

# *References*


Abend, S., Porder, M., & Willick, M. (1983), *Borderline Patients: Psychoanalytic Perspectives*. New York: International Universities Press.

Adler, G. (1985), *Borderline Psychopathology and Its Treatment*. New York: Jason Aronson.

Bak, R. (1946), Masochism in paranoia. *Psychoanal. Quart.*, 15:285–301.

Bettelheim, B. (1950), *Love Is Not Enough*. Glencoe: Free Press.

——— (1976), *The Uses of Enchantment: The Meaning and Importance of Fairy Tales*. New York: Knopf.

Bibring, E. (1954), Psychoanalysis and the dynamic psychotherapies. *J. Amer. Psychoanal. Assn.*, 3:745–770.

Bion, W. R. (1957), Differentiation of the psychotic from non-psychotic personalities. *Internat. J. Psycho-Anal.*, 38:266–275.

Bleuler, E. (1911), *Dementia Praecox or the Group of Schizophrenias*. New York: International Universities Press, 1950.

Bonaparte, M., Freud, A., and Kris, E. (1954), *The Origins of Psychoanalysis: Letters to Wilhelm Fliess, Drafts and Notes, 1887–1902 by Sigmund Freud*. London: Image Publishing Company, Ltd.

Bornstein, B. (1935), Phobia in a two-and-a-half year old child. *Psychoanal. Quart.*, 4:93–119.

Brenner, C. (1982), *The Mind in Conflict*. New York: International Universities Press.

Breuer, J., & Freud, S. (1893–1895), Studies on Hysteria. *Standard Edition*, 2:1–305. London: Hogarth Press, 1955.

Deutsch, H. (1965), *Neuroses and Character Types*. New York: International Universities Press.

Dostoyevsky, F. (1916), *Crime and Punishment*. New York: Macmillan.

Dowling, S. (1977), Seven infants with esophageal atresia: A developmental study. *The Psychoanalytic Study of the Child*, 32:215–256. New Haven, CT: Yale University Press.

——— (ed.) (1991), *Conflict and Compromise: Therapeutic Implications*. Madison, CT: International Universities Press.

Fairbairn, W. R. D. (1952), *Psychoanalytic Studies of the Personality*. London & Boston: Routledge & Kegan Paul.

Fraiberg, S. (1959), *The Magic Years*. New York: Charles Scribner's Sons.

——— (1977), *Insights from the Blind*. New York: Basic Books.

Freud, A. (1928), *Introduction to the Technique of Child Analysis*. New York & Washington, DC: Nervous & Mental Disease Publishing Company.

——— (1936), *The Ego and the Mechanisms of Defense*. New York: International Universities Press, 1966.

——— (1941), Infants without families. Reports of the Hampstead Nurseries, 1939–1945. In: *The Writings of Anna Freud*, Vol. 3. New York: International Universities Press, 1966.

——— (1963a), Assessment of childhood disturbances. *The Psychoanalytic Study of the Child*, 17:149–158. New York: International Universities Press.

——— (1963b), The concept of developmental lines. *The Psychoanalytic Study of the Child*, 18:245–265. New York: International Universities Press.

Freud, S. (1895), Project for a scientific psychology. In: *The Origins of Psycho-Analysis: Letters to Wilhelm Fliess, Drafts and Notes: 1887–1902*, ed. M. Bonaparte, A. Freud, & E. Kris. New York: Basic Books, 1954, pp. 355–445.

——— (1900), The Interpretation of Dreams. *Standard Edition*, 5. London: Hogarth Press, 1953.

——— (1905), Three essays on the theory of sexuality. *Standard Edition*, 7:135–245. London: Hogarth Press, 1953.

——— (1909), Analysis of a phobia in a five-year-old boy. *Standard Edition*, 10:155–318. London: Hogarth Press, 1955.

——— (1914), On narcissism: An introduction. *Standard Edition*, 14:69–102. London: Hogarth Press, 1957.

——— (1923), The ego and the id. *Standard Edition*, 19: 12–66. London: Hogarth Press, 1961.

——— (1924), The dissolution of the Oedipus complex. *Standard Edition*, 19:173–179. London: Hogarth Press, 1961.

——— (1925), An autobiographical study. *Standard Edition*, 22:7–74. London: Hogarth Press, 1959.

——— (1926), Inhibitions, symptoms and anxiety. *Standard Edition*, 20:87–156. London: Hogarth Press, 1964.

Furman, R., & Katan, A. (1969), *The Therapeutic Nursery School*. New York: International Universities Press.

Gay, P. (1988), *Freud: A Life for Our Time*. New York: W. W. Norton.

Goldstein, J., Freud, A., & Solnit, A. (1973), *Beyond the Best Interests of the Child*. New York: Free Press.

Greenacre, P. (1952), *Trauma, Growth, and Personality*. New York: International Universities Press.

Hartmann, H. (1939), *Ego Psychology and the Problem of Adaptation*. New York: International Universities Press.

Jacobson, E. (1964), *The Self and the Object World*. New York: International Universities Press.

Kempe, C. H., & Helfer, R. E. (1980), *The Battered Child*. Chicago: University of Chicago Press.

Kernberg, O. (1975), *Borderline Conditions and Pathologic Narcissism*. New York: Jason Aronson.

Klein, M. (1923), *The Psycho-Analysis of Children*. London: Hogarth Press.

——— (1975), *Envy and Gratitude and Other Works*. New York: Delacorte Press, 1975.

Kohut, H. (1977), *The Restoration of the Self*. New York: International Universities Press.

Kraepelin, E. (1913), *General Paresis*. New York: J. of Nervous & Mental Disease Publishing Co.

Lowenstein, R. M. (1957), A contribution to the psychoanalytic theory of masochism. *J. Amer. Psychoanal. Assn.*, 5:197–234.

Mahler, M., Pine, F., & Bergman, A. (1975), *The Psychological Birth of the Human Infant*. New York: Basic Books.

McDonald, M. (1970), *Not by the Color of Their Skin*. New York: International Universities Press.

Modell, A. (1976), 'The holding environment' and the therapeutic action of psychoanalysis. *J. Amer. Psychoanal. Assn.*, 24:285–307.

Money, J., & Ehrhardt, A. (1972), *Man and Woman, Boy and Girl: The Differentiation and Dimorphism of Gender Identity from Conception to Maturity*. Baltimore: Johns Hopkins University Press.

Piaget, J. (1951), *Play, Dreams, and Imitation in Childhood*. New York: W. W. Norton.

Plank, E. (1962), *Working with Children in Hospitals*. Cleveland: Western Reserve University Press.

Porder, M. S. (1987), Projective identification: An alternative hypothesis. *Psychoanal. Quart.*, 56:431–451.

——— (1990), On beginning with borderline patients. In: *On Beginning an Analysis*, ed. T. J. Jacobs & A. Rothstein. Madison, CT: International Universities Press, pp. 163–178.

Rado, S. (1933), Fear of castration in women. *Psychoanal. Quart.*, 2:425–475.

Robbins, M. (1983), Toward a new model of the mind for primitive personalities. *Internat. J. Psycho-Anal.*, 64: 457–473.

Robertson, J. (1952), *A Two-Year-Old Goes to Hospital* (Film: 16mm, b & w, Sound, 45 & 30 minute versions; English/French; Guide booklet). New York: New York University Film Library.

——— (1958), *Young Children in Hospitals*. New York: Basic Books.

——— (1968), *Jane, 17 Months: In Foster Care for 10 Days* (Film No. 2, 16mm, b & w, Sound, 37 minutes; Guide booklet). New York: New York University Film Library.

——— (1969), *John, 17 Months: For 9 Days in a Residential Nursery* (Film No. 3: 16mm, b & w, Sound, 45 minutes; Guide booklet). New York: New York University Film Library.

——— (1971), *Thomas, 2 Years 4 Months: In Foster Care for 10 Days* (Film No. 4: 16mm, b & w, Sound, 38 minutes; Guide booklet). New York: New York University Film Library.

——— Robertson, J. (1967), *Young Children in Brief Separation. Kate, 2 Years 5 Months: In Foster Care for 27 Days* (Film No. 1: 16mm, b & w, Sound, 33 minutes; Guide booklet). New York: New York University Film Library.

——— ——— (1971), Young children in brief separation: A fresh look. *The Psychoanalytic Study of the Child*, 26:264–315. New York: Quadrangle.

Rothstein, A. (1980), *The Narcissistic Pursuit of Perfection.* New York: International Universities Press.

——— (1984), The fear of humiliation. *J. Amer. Psychoanal. Assn.*, 32:99–116.

——— (1991a), Sadomasochism in the neuroses conceived of as a pathologic compromise formation. *J. Amer. Psychoanal. Assn.*, 39:2:363–375.

——— (1991b), On some relationships between fantasies of perfection and the calamities of childhood. *Internat. J. Psycho-Anal.*, 72:313–323.

Searles, H. F. (1965), *Collected Papers on Schizophrenia and Related Subjects.* New York: International Universities Press.

Seminov, P. V. (1986), *The Emotional Brain.* New York: Plenum Press.

Solnit, A. (1987), Book review of D. N. Stern: *The Interpersonal World of the Infant: A View from Psychoanalytic and Developmental Psychology. Amer. J. Psychiat.*, 144: 1508–1509.

Spitz, R. (1945), Hospitalism: An inquiry into the genesis of psychiatric conditions in early childhood. *The Psychoanalytic Study of the Child*, 1:53–74. New York: International Universities Press.

Steele, B. F. (1982), Effects of abuse and neglect on psychological development. In: *Frontiers of Infant Psychiatry*, ed. J. Call, E. Galensen, & C. R. Tyson. New York: Basic Books, pp. 235–244.

Stern, D. (1985), *The Interpersonal World of the Infant: A View from Psychoanalysis and Developmental Psychology.* New York: Basic Books.

Tyson, P. (1982), A developmental line of gender identity, gender role, and choice of love object. *J. Amer. Psychoanal. Assn.*, 30:61–86.

Willick, M. S. (1983), On the concept of primitive defenses. *J. Amer. Psychoanal. Assn.*, 31:175–200.

——— (1990), Psychoanalytic concepts of the etiology of severe mental illness. *J. Amer. Psychoanal. Assn.*, 38: 1049–1081.

——— (1991), Working with conflict and deficit in borderline and narcissistic patients. In: *Conflict and Compromise: Therapeutic Implications*. Madison, CT: International Universities Press, pp. 77–94.

Winnicott, D. W. (1958), *Through Pediatrics to Psychoanalysis*. New York: Basic Books.

# Name Index

# Subject Index